MAN, HEALTH, AND NURSING:

Basic Concepts and Theories

MAN, HEALTH, AND NURSING:

Basic Concepts and Theories

Irene Makar Joos, RN, BSN, MN, PhD
Ramona Nelson, RN, BSN, MN, PhD
Ann Lyness, RN, BSN, MPH, PhD

School of Nursing
University of Pittsburgh

RESTON PUBLISHING COMPANY, INC.
A Prentice-Hall Company
Reston, Virginia

Library of Congress Cataloging in Publication Data

Joos, Irene Makar.
   Man, health, and nursing.

    1. Nursing.   2. Nursing—History.   3. Nursing—
Philosophy.   I. Nelson, Ramona.   II. Lyness, Ann.
[DNLM: 1. Education, Nursing.   2. History of Nursing.
3. Nursing   4. Philosophy, Nursing. WY   16 J81m]
RT41.J66   1985   610.73   84-18256
ISBN 0-8359-4177-9

*Design and editorial/production supervision
by Norma Miller Karlin*

© 1985 by
Reston Publishing Company, Inc.
A Prentice-Hall Company
Reston, Virginia 22090

All rights reserved. No part
of this book may be reproduced in
any way, or by any means, without
permission in writing from the publisher.

10 9 8 7 6 5 4 3 2 1

PRINTED IN THE UNITED STATES OF AMERICA

Dedicated to
Brian and Brian Michael Joos
Glenn, Kurt, Dorianne, and Leslie-Ann Nelson
and the memory of
Jonathan Lyness

Contents

Preface xi

Acknowledgments xiii

UNIT I   **CONCEPT OF NURSING**   1

Chapter 1   **Introduction to Nursing**   3
Definitions of Nursing, 5
Purpose and Goal of Nursing, 11
Components of Nursing, 12

Chapter 2   **Development of Nursing: Religious, Military, and Secular Forces**   21
Religious Forces, 22
Military Forces, 29
Secular Forces, 35

Chapter 3   **Development of Nursing's Early Leaders and Studies**   47
Nursing Leaders, 48
Educational Studies, 54

Chapter 4   **Development of Nursing Education**   65
The English Influence, 65
Early American Schools, 66
University Education, 69
Mid Century, 70
Conceptual Framework, 72

viii   Contents

UNIT II   SELECTED THEORIES UTILIZED IN NURSING   77

Chapter 5   **Systems Theory**   79

Definition of Terms, 79
System Defined, 81
Structure in an Open System, 83
Function in an Open System, 86
Change in an Open System, 89
Purpose of an Open System, 91

Chapter 6   **Stress-Adaptation Theory**   95

Definition of Terms, 95
Stress Defined, 96
Factors Influencing Stress, 97
Classification of Stressors, 98
Stress Response, 100
Stress Adaptation and Systems Theory, 108

Chapter 7   **Learning Theory**   119

Definition of Terms, 119
Behavioral Approach, 121
Information Processing Approach, 124
Developmental Approach, 131
Application to Nursing Practice, 135

Chapter 8   **Communication Theory**   147

Definition of Terms, 147
Defining Communication, 149
Reason for Communicating, 150
Components of a Communication Model, 151
Levels of Communication, 154
Influences on Communication, 158
Facilitators and Inhibitors to Communicating, 160

Chapter 9   **Change Theory**   173

Definition of Terms, 173
Change Defined, 174
Change Models, 177
Assessment of the Need to Change, 178
Identification of Change Reactions, 181
Change Principles, 184
Strategies for Implementing Change, 185

Chapter 10	**Role Theory** 189
	Definition of Terms, 189
	Role Defined, 190
	Role Theory Defined, 192
	Role Structure, 193
	Role Socialization, 194
	Role Stress, 198

UNIT III	**SELECTED CONCEPTS UTILIZED IN NURSING** 203

Chapter 11	**Man as a System** 205
	Man Defined, 205
	The Structure of Man as an Open System, 209
	The Function of Man as an Open System, 213
	Change and the System of Man, 217
	Purpose of Man, 220

Chapter 12	**Health** 225
	Definitions, 226
	Assessing Health, 230
	Factors Influencing Health Behaviors, 235
	Nursing Role, 240

Chapter 13	**The American Health Care System** 245
	Purpose, 246
	Structure, 247
	Function of the Health Care System, 261

Chapter 14	**Nursing's Future** 269
	Societal Trends, 270
	Economic Pressures, 273
	Educational Trends, 274
	Technological Advances, 276
	The Profession Moves Forward, 281
	Making Predictions, 284
	Index 289

Preface

As nurses have moved from being the physicians' handmaidens into their own delineated field of practice, they have been increasingly concerned with developing and understanding the theories and concepts which guide the practice of nursing. This book focuses on three concepts and six theories that underlie the practice of nursing in all settings. These three concepts—man, health, and nursing—are the main concepts identified in almost all nursing programs. Although nurses use many theories in their practice, the six theories selected—systems, stress, learning, communciation, change, and role—are the theories that frequently provide a framework for us in our practice.

While much has been written on these concepts and theories, this book utilizes an introductory approach. This means that the information is presented in clear, understandable terms for those students of nursing who have had limited opportunity to study or utilize these concepts and theories.

Unit I introduces the concept of nursing through an analysis of nursing history. The emphasis is on understanding how nursing's history influenced current practice and education rather than a chronological accounting of historical events. Unit II presents each of the six theories. Although each theory is presented in a separate chapter, where appropriate, the interrelatedness that exists between and among the theories is discussed. These theories are then utilized in Unit III to present the concepts of man and health. Unit III concludes with an overview of the health care system in which nursing functions and a analysis of forces influencing nursing's future.

You, as professional nursing students, will be involved in and affected by nursing's future. Knowledge gained about basic concepts and theories will serve you well as you enter the world of professional nursing and continue your development as a professional nurse.

Acknowledgments

This textbook, a synthesis of the efforts of three colleagues, was made possible only with the help of a number of people and we are grateful to them. First, we would like to thank Sandra Johnson for her consistent help in typing the manuscript. She took pages, often a little rough around the edges, and turned them into sheets of neatness and readability. We would like to thank our reviewers who made many relevant suggestions. In addition to making enlightening comments, the reviewers shared citations, which permitted us to develop certain sections more completely. One reviewer in particular was exemplary in providing revised sentences and excellent examples. We are deeply appreciative for the time taken to do this. We would like to thank our students whose diverse questions and comments over the years have impressed on us the need for an organized body of material addressing basic concepts and theories used in nursing. We also wish to express sincere thanks for the administrative support given by the school of nursing. Their encouragement toward creative endeavors helped to inspire us in the beginning and gave us the steadfastness needed to complete the work. Finally, we would like to thank Stuart Horton, our editor, whose patience and intelligent communciations assisted the entire process.

MAN, HEALTH, AND NURSING:

Basic Concepts and Theories

UNIT I
CONCEPT OF NURSING

Ideas and events occurring over time make up the study of history. The events can be pictured as a concrete structure. They occur in a time and place; they are observable and recordable. But it is the intangible—the ideas—that give meaning to the events. The ideas which surround the events in history are like the family which makes a house a home. The purpose of this unit is to assist the student in developing an appreciation of what nursing is as well as the events and ideas that have brought us to this place in history.

Chapter 1 introduces the unit by defining and briefly describing the components of nursing as they currently exist. While there are many myths and beliefs about nursing, the chapter clarifies the modern concept of professional nursing. With this as a background, Chapter 2 describes three major forces that brought nursing to its current state. Chapter 3 continues by introducing the reader to selected early nursing leaders who led nursing in its march through history. In many cases the direction chosen by nursing leaders was based on research they had both supported and attempted to follow. Chapter 3 includes many of the studies conducted on the state of nursing practice and education. Chapter 4 traces the educational development that has produced the practitioner of nursing. This chapter focuses on the development of programs and the organization of knowledge as taught in the nursing programs. This chapter concludes by defining and explaining conceptual frameworks, the current organizational themes in nursing curricula.

1

Introduction to nursing

Most of us entered nursing with a preconceived idea or perception of what nursing is. These ideas and perceptions developed over time and were influenced by many people and events. Most people who enter nursing have had some direct contact with nurses. Frequently, this contact is with employed nurses in schools, doctors' offices, and clinics. Many times the contact is more personal when family members or friends are nurses. Each direct contact with nurses influenced your perceptions and ideas of nursing. You have also been influenced by a variety of books, television programs, and movies.

These interactions allowed you to add, to rearrange, to think, and to change your perceptions and ideas about nursing. Many of you talked to career counselors, attended career days, or joined a future nurses club to broaden your understanding of nursing and its requirements. Some of you worked in hospitals or health care centers. From each experience your ideas and perceptions grew, expanded, and changed. Finally, you liked what you believed about nurses and nursing well enough to give it a try.

When you made the decision to be a nurse, your friends and family probably responded in one of two ways. They either congratulated you saying that nursing is a fine profession, "I'm proud of you. You will find many excellent opportunities in nursing." Or they frowned saying, "You can do better than that. Nursing is a low, menial occupation requiring a lot of hard work with few rewards. Why don't you become a doctor?" These two tracks present two polar views about nursing. Movies, television programs, and books rarely characterize the nurse as an intelligent, independent person who influences health care, who makes decisions, and who is responsible and accountable for more than pleasing the physician. Nurses traditionally are characterized as either sexy, dumb handmaidens who rarely provide nursing care, who always flirt with the doctors, and who spend their time answering phones, holding charts, and taking coffee breaks, or as old-maid, battle-ax nurses who demean and demoralize subordinates, who spend time making sure units run like tight ships, and who are concerned about nursing care only as it reflects managerial abilities (Muff, 1982).

Considering the many and varied perceptions about nursing, why do people become nurses? In many beginning nursing courses students are asked why they entered nursing, what they believe nursing is, and what characteristics they believe make a good nurse. Take a few minutes now to reflect on these three questions. Why did you decide to study nursing? How would you define nursing and how would you describe a nurse?

When answering the question why am I studying nursing, many students reply, "I want to help people." Some students elaborate on some personal experience or some nurse they know and admire. Others state that they believe nursing offers job security and mobility; that they want to be able to find employment after their formal education. Still others reply that they were undecided about what they wanted to do and family and friends influenced them to try nursing. Some students tried other things and then decided on nursing. Some of you are currently registered nurses back in school for additional education for the purpose of improving your skills and job opportunities. All of these responses are typical of why people study nursing.

Many students have a difficult time responding to the definition question. Defining nursing is not an easy task. Nursing leaders continue to define and redefine nursing. While defining nursing is not easy, all nursing students have some ideas or beliefs about nursing which can serve as a base or beginning for developing a definition. Many students' ideas or beliefs about nursing are similar to those listed below. Nursing is

1. Giving nursing care.
2. Carrying out doctors' orders.
3. Meeting the needs of the patients in hospitals.
4. Managing the patients' environment.
5. Teaching people how to take care of themselves.

Many of these ideas or beliefs are task statements—things the students believe the nurse does. As you learn more about nursing, you will expand, delete, and rearrange your ideas and beliefs about nursing.

In regard to describing a nurse, how many of you used such words as caring, concerned, kind, dedicated, pleasant, devoted, ethical, honest, stable, or compassionate? Did you also include words reflective of appearance, such as neat, dignified, well groomed, or clean? Or words of action—competent, calm, hardworking, organized, or punctual?

In this discussion on your beliefs about nursing and the nurse, we alluded to the idea that nurses provide services to people in the area of health. The recipient of these services is frequently referred to as the patient or client. Some people use the term *patient* to refer to an individual(s) who is ill and experiencing a significant degree of dependence on the nurse. The term *client* is used to refer to a healthy individual(s) who exercises a significant degree of independence in how the services of the nurse are utilized. Other people use these two terms interchangeably. When using the terms interchangeably, the definition encompasses an individual(s), either ill or well, who needs the services of the nurse. In this book we tend to use the term *client* for people who are mostly healthy and *patient* for those who are mostly ill. However, in those situations when we are talking about groups of people who may be placed anywhere on the health continuum, the term *client* is used.

Since there are many and varied perceptions of nursing and nurses, the purpose of this chapter is to explore the concept of nursing. At the completion of this chapter the reader will be able to

1. Recognize various definitions of nursing.
2. Develop a personal definition of nursing.
3. Identify the goals of nursing.
4. Identify and discuss the components of the concept *nursing:* nurse, client, interaction, and environment.

DEFINITIONS OF NURSING

What is nursing? While this question appears simple, you have already discovered in the introduction to this chapter that it is not. Nurses have been struggling for a long time to answer it. Definitions of nursing have been analyzed, reworked, and are still not without controversy. Why? First, it is difficult to develop one definition of nursing acceptable to all because the purpose or reason for the definition varies. For example, defining nursing for the purpose of communicating what nursing is to other professionals or prospective students requires a different emphasis and terminology from defining nursing for the purpose of identifying the legal scope of practice. Second, personal beliefs about nursing vary from individual to individual. Although commonalities can be found in personal definitions, the terminology and focus of nursing actions vary. Third, nursing is changing. Newer definitions are attempting to reflect the changing practice of nursing.

When examining various definitions of nursing, remember that the intent of writing any definition is to make the phenomenon being described clear and to identify the essential nature of that phenomenon. When comparing one definition with another, two questions to ask yourself are

1. What is the purpose of this definition?
2. Does the definition achieve the purpose by describing the phenomenon clearly?

This section of the chapter focuses on definitions of nursing from three perspectives: legal, professional, and personal.

Legal

Nursing had no legal definition until the 1930s. The early laws (1903-1923) did not define nursing, nor describe the scope of nursing practice; instead, they described the nurse. The nurse was of good character, graduated from an approved nursing school, and passed an examination given by the State Board of Nursing (Bullough & Bullough, 1977).

In the 1930s, the revised professional nursing laws or nurse practice acts began defining nursing by focusing on the scope of nursing practice. Since nursing is legally defined at the state level, states differ in these definitions and scopes of practice. Because of these differences, nurses must familiarize themselves with the definition of the state in which they practice. What may be permitted or required in one state may be prohibited in another. For instance, in most states nurses make a nursing diagnosis; in a few states, they do not.

In an attempt to minimize difficulties and provide some national standards, the American Nurses' Association (ANA) in 1955 adopted a model legal definition of nursing practice:

> The practice of professional nursing means the performance for compensation of any act in the observation, care and counsel of the ill, injured, or infirm, or the maintenance of health or prevention of illness of others, or in supervision and teaching of other personnel, or the administration of medications and treatments as prescribed by a licensed physician or dentist; requiring substantial specialized judgment and skill and based on knowledge and application of the principles of biological, physical, and social science. The foregoing shall not be deemed to include acts of diagnosis or prescription of therapeutic or corrective measures. (ANA, 1955, p. 1474)

Since the purpose of this definition is to define the scope of practice, the definition described functions or tasks of the nurse, i.e., observation, care of ill, maintenance of health, teaching and supervision of other personnel, and administering medications and treatments. Not only did this model act include what nurses can do but it also included a disclaimer—what nurses cannot do. In this model practice act, nurses cannot make a diagnosis or prescribe therapeutic or corrective measures.

In 1976 and 1979, ANA revised the model practice act to reflect the changing role of the nurse (see Table 1-1). The 1976 model definition was similar to the 1955 one except that it accommodated for the expanding role of the nurse by providing for the addition of functions as recognized by the nursing profession. The 1979 definition adds or recognizes the importance of the nursing process in the practice of nursing, including making a nursing diagnosis, spelling out additional roles of the nurse, and recognizing the nurses' accountability and responsibility to the consumer. Most states used some of

TABLE 1-1
ANA model practice acts

1976
PRACTICE OF NURSING BY A REGISTERED NURSE The practice of nursing as performed by a registered nurse is a process in which substantial specialized knowledge derived from the biological, physical, and behavioral sciences is applied to the care, treatment, counsel, and health teaching of persons who are experiencing changes in the normal health processes; or who require assistance in the maintenance of health or the management of illness, injury, or infirmity or in the achievement of a dignified death; and such additional acts as are recognized by the nursing process as proper to be performed by a registered nurse

From: Suggestions for Major Provisions to be Included in a Nursing Practice Act. Kansas City: American Nurses' Association, 1976, p. 1. Used with permission.

1980
The practice of nursing means the performance for compensation of professional services requiring substantial specialized knowledge of the biological, physical, behavioral, psychological, and sociological sciences and of nursing theory as the basis for assessment, diagnosis, planning, intervention, and evaluation in the promotion and maintenance of health; the casefinding and management of illness, injury, or infirmity; the restoration of optimum function; or the achievement of a dignified death. Nursing practice includes but is not limited to administration, teaching, counseling, supervision, delegation, and evaluation of practice and execution of the medical regimen, including the administration of medications and treatments prescribed by any person authorized by state law to prescribe. Each registered nurse is directly accountable and responsible to the consumer for the quality of nursing care rendered

From: The Nursing Practice Act: Suggested State Legislation. Kansas City: American Nurses' Association, 1980, p. 6. Used with permission.

the language contained in these model acts, but variations from state to state exist.

As a student you will be presented with the legal definition of nursing from your state. Remember that legal definitions focus on nursing practice, i.e., what the nurse does in the exercise of the profession. One state practice act definition of nursing is presented here as an example. In New York, nursing practice is defined as

> ... Diagnosing and treating human responses to acute or potential health problems through such services as casefinding, health teaching, health counseling, and provision of care supportive to or restorative of life and well-being, and executing medical regimens as prescribed by a licensed physician or otherwise legally authorized physician or dentist. A nursing regimen shall be consistent with and shall not vary any existing medical regimen. (New York State Nurse Practice Act 1972 Section 6902)

This definition reflects a movement of nursing from a dependent profession to one of growing independence. This definition also expands the scope of nursing practice to include healthy people, with real or potential problems. Of interest is also the inclusion of diagnosis and treatment. In other words, a nurse in New York is required by law to make a nursing diagnosis and to prescribe nursing treatments.

If you examine the practice act from your state, you will be able to find statements that describe functions and roles of the nurse. You will also be able to find a reference concerning to whom the nurse is accountable. You may find statements that deal with the expanding scope of practice and responsibility to consumers.

Professional

While nursing is legally defined at the state level, professional nursing associations, through work being done in many subcommittees, are also involved in defining nursing. In 1973, the American Nurses Association defined nursing in *Standards of Nursing Practice.* Nursing was defined as a "... direct service, goal directed and adaptable to the needs of the individual, family and community during health and illness" (ANA, 1973, p. 1). Some students entered nursing thinking that nursing care was only provided to individuals; they did not think in terms of families or communities. Another important point in this description of nursing is that nursing care is provided to healthy and ill people. Many students think of nursing in terms of acute care patients, critical care units, trauma care, transplant patients—not as also providing for the needs of the healthy population.

In 1980, ANA in *Nursing: A Social Policy Statement* defined nursing as the "... diagnosis and treatment of human responses to actual or potential health problems" (ANA, 1980, p. 9). Once again, you see that nursing included providing care to ill and healthy people who are experiencing real or potential problems. A new point made in this statement is the inclusion of a nursing diagnosis.

To more fully describe the scope of nursing responsibilities, the ANA has also published a code for professional nurses (see Table 1-2). This code reflects nursing's responsibility to the client's uniqueness, values, and rights. While the Code does not address the definition of nursing nor the specific functions of the nurse, it addresses the relationship of nurses to their clients and thereby explains the responsibilities of nurses with regard to their ethical obligations and quality care obligations.

The ANA's definition of nursing and the Code for Nurses guide the education and practice of nurses. Although no legal basis or support exists for these statements, they are many times used in court testimonies regarding the professional organizations' stand on nursing. These statements also serve to guide the direction of nursing. They are not considered minimal standards but reflect the ideal.

TABLE 1-2
AMERICAN NURSES' ASSOCIATION CODE FOR NURSES

Preamble

The Code for Nurses is based on belief about the nature of individuals, nursing, health, and society. Recipients and providers of nursing services are viewed as individuals and groups who possess basic rights and responsibilities, and whose values and circumstances command respect at all times. Nursing encompasses the promotion and restoration of health, the prevention of illness, and the alleviation of suffering. The statements of the Code and their interpretation provide guidance for conduct and relationships in carrying out nursing responsibilities consistent with the ethical obligations of the profession and quality in nursing care.

1. The nurse provides services with respect for human dignity and the uniqueness of the client unrestricted by consideration of social or economic status, personal attributes, or the nature of health problems.
2. The nurse safeguards the client's right to privacy by judiciously protecting information of a confidential nature.
3. The nurse acts to safeguard the client and the public when health care and safety are affected by the incompetent, unethical, or illegal practice of any person.
4. The nurse assumes responsibility and accountability for individual nursing judgments and actions.
5. The nurse maintains competence in nursing.
6. The nurse exercises informed judgment and uses individual competence and qualifications as criteria in seeking consultation, accepting responsibilities, and delegating nursing activities to others.
7. The nurse participates in activities that contribute to the ongoing development of the profession's body of knowledge.
8. The nurse participates in the profession's efforts to implement and improve standards of nursing.
9. The nurse participates in the profession's efforts to establish and maintain conditions of employment conducive to high quality nursing care.
10. The nurse participates in the profession's effort to protect the public from misinformation and misrepresentation and to maintain the integrity of nursing.
11. The nurse collaborates with members of the health professions and other citizens in promoting community and national efforts to meet the health needs of the public.

From: Code for Nurses with Interpretive Statements. Kansas City: American Nurses' Association, 1976. Used with permission.

Personal

Each practicing nurse and nursing student must define what nursing is to them. This personal definition more closely reflects the nurse's practice. While legal and professional definitions will help guide you in developing your own definition, no discussion of the definition of nursing would be complete without examining some of the personal definitions espoused by nursing leaders (see Table 1-3).

Early definitions of nursing took a circuitous route in defining nursing (Nightingale, 1946; Henderson, 1966). These early definitions did not state

TABLE 1-3
Selected nursing leaders' definitions of nursing

Nursing Leader	Definition of Nursing
Florence Nightingale (1946, p. 6)	...providing an environment that allowed nature to act on behalf of the patient
Hildegard Peplau (1952, pp. 4-6)	...human relationship between an individual who is sick or in need of health services, and a nurse especially educated to recognize and to respond to the need for help
Virginia Henderson (1966, p. 415)	...assisting the individual, sick or well, in the performance of those activities contributing to health or its recovery (or to peaceful death) that he could perform unaided if he had the necessary strength, will or knowledge
Martha Rogers (1970, pp. 84-85)	...humanistic and humanitarian science directed toward describing and explaining the human being in synergistic wholeness and in developing the hypothetical generalizations and predictive principles basic to knowledgeable practice
Imogene King (1971, p. 25)	...process of action, reaction, interaction and transaction whereby nurses assist individuals of any age and socioeconomic group to meet their basic needs in performing activities of daily living and to cope with health and illness at some particular point in the life cycle
Dorothea Orem (1971, pp. 1-2)	...way of overcoming human limitations...its special concern...man's need for self care action and the provision and management of it on a continuous basis in order to sustain life and health, recover from disease or injury, and cope with their effects
Sister Callista Roy (1976, p. 4)	...theoretical system of knowledge which prescribes a process of analysis and action related to the care of the ill or potentially ill person
Betty Neuman (1982, p. 14)	...a unique profession...concerned with all of the variables affecting an individual's response to stressors.

what nursing was but instead described the nurse and the functions of the nurse. They also focused on the ill client and care and comfort functions of the nurse. The major differences were in the complexity of the definitions and the perceptions of the client, i.e., passive recipient of care or promotion of independence.

Later definitions of nursing were not circuitous (Roy, 1976; King, 1971; Orem, 1971). These definitions began with "Nursing is..." and then went on to describe nursing. They did not describe nurses. In addition, several definitions also acknowledged that nursing practice has a theory or knowledge base (Roy, 1976; Rogers, 1970). Most of these definitions then went on to describe the goal of nursing and the functions of nurses. Commonalities in these definitions include that nursing is a process-oriented, goal-directed service and has as its clients individuals along the total health continuum. Differences in the definitions reflect philosophical beliefs about man, health, and society. Goals of nursing tend to be similar—achievement of optimal health for all clients.

As you progress through your program you will be exposed to many more definitions of nursing than were presented here. Your faculty have their own definitions that guide them in their practice and in developing your educational program. As you grow professionally, you too will develop a definition of nursing which you will continuously modify to reflect your current beliefs, values, and practices.

PURPOSE AND GOAL OF NURSING

Most definitions of nursing also included statements of goals or directions to nursing. Throughout our history one basic element that has remained constant is the goal of nursing. Regardless of the changes occurring in nursing, the goal of nursing remains fairly constant. Few people would disagree that the goal of nursing is to promote health, to optimize the level of functioning of the client, to prevent disability, and, when necessary, to contribute to a peaceful death. One could argue that this is the goal of most health professionals. How does this make nursing different? Unique? How one achieves this goal will differ from profession to profession and even within professions.

Let's go back to the nursing leaders presented earlier. Table 1-4 lists the goal of nursing as identified by these leaders. Take a few minutes now and read them. What would the nurse do for each of these goals? What responsibilities would the nurse have in moving the client toward these goals? What would be the focus of nursing care?

Goals give direction and focus to nursing care. They determine the roles and functions of the nurse. They help identify responsibilities. Take Orem's goal (see Table 1-4) as an example. The focus of nursing care is promoting client's self-care. The functions of the nurse would emphasize education of the client, option presenting, assisting with client decision making, and so on. Although giving total nursing care when the client is unable is not ignored, the nurse spends energy on moving the client to self-care.

Contrast Orem's goals with those of Nightingale (Table 1-4). The focus of nursing care under the Nightingale model is environmental manipulation. The nurse's role is to provide a safe, healthy environment through proper hygiene, sanitation, ventilation, and such, so that nature can take its course. The client in this model is a passive recipient of care.

These two examples demonstrate extreme differences in goals. What is apparent is that goals help determine the focus of care, the functions and roles of the nurse, and the nurse's responsibilities. Each of you will be oriented to the goal of nursing as identified by your educational program. This goal helps the faculty identify your plan of study, your clients and the settings for your

TABLE 1-4
Selected nursing leaders' goals for nursing

Nursing Leader	Goal
Florence Nightingale (1946, p. 6)	...to put the individual in the best possible condition for nature to act upon him... aim at prevention of unnecessary suffering
Hildegard Peplau (1952, p. 12)	...forward movement of the personality and other ongoing human process in the direction of creative, constructive, productive, personal, and community life
Virginia Henderson (1969, p. 8)	...to substitute for what the patient lacks in physical strength, will, or knowledge to make him a complete whole
Martha Rogers (1970, p. 86)	...to promote harmony between man and his environment for the ultimate goal of reaching the highest state of health possible
Imogene King (1971, p. 67)	...goal of nursing is health, it is recognized that the roles and responsibilities of the nurse include giving assistance to individuals and families during illness, crisis, and in death
Dorothea Orem (1971, p. 48)	...health and well being of the individual, the focus of nursing is helping the individual to achieve health results ...move the individual toward responsible actions in matters of self-care
Sister Callista Roy (1976, p. 18)	...to promote adaptation in the four adaptive modes: physiological needs, self-concept, role function, and interdependence
Betty Neuman (1982, pp. 4-5)	...retention and/or attainment of client system stability.

clinical experience, and the skills necessary to guide you in assessing your clients and planning their nursing care.

COMPONENTS OF NURSING

While goals help provide direction to nursing, analysis of the component parts of nursing helps identify the specifics of nursing care. The four components of nursing are: clients, nurse, interaction, and environment (see Figure 1-1). Each of these components will be discussed here.

Clients

Man (*man* as used in this book refers to a generic term to mean human beings as individuals or groups) is the first component of nursing. In other words nursing exists to help people, human beings. Two key questions which will be addressed here are what is a person and what makes a person a client?

A person consists of a set of attributes that are uniquely human. Human beings are differentiated from animal life by two basic attributes—the capac-

Introduction to Nursing 13

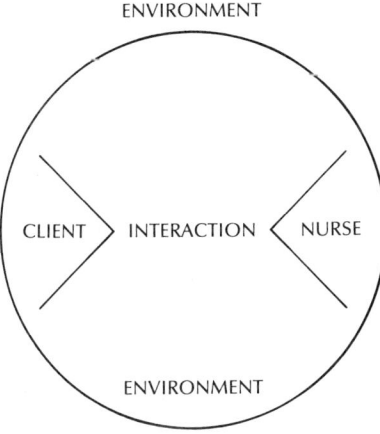

Figure 1-1 Components of Nursing.

ity to think (abstract reasoning) and the use of language (Anderson & Carter, 1974). Man has two attributes in common with animals—forming families and staking out their own territory. A man shares with all other persons a biological structure. With some other persons are shared a sociocultural and ethnic heritage. Man is unique and thus is like no other man in relation to his internal environment, thoughts, values, beliefs, and emotions (Kluckholn, 1953). These ideas related to man will be more fully addressed in Chapter 11, "Man as a System."

What makes a person a client? Historically, patients were persons who for whatever reasons were not able to meet their basic needs or whose family members were unable to meet these needs. Ill persons have always received some form of nursing care. Who provided the care has varied over time.

Today, clients are any persons or groups of persons who need assistance in meeting their health needs. Health needs include the total health continuum from maintenance of optimal wellness to peaceful death. While there are many kinds of needs, when these health needs are for nursing care, the health provider is the nurse.

Nurse

Who is the nurse? While this question was at one point relatively easy to answer, today it is much more difficult. Nurses are no longer a homogeneous group. Probably, the best data collected to answer this question was done by the American Nurses' Association (*Facts About Nursing*, 1981). Most of the data here reflect this study.

The majority of nurses (98 percent) are female and married (66 percent). This is not surprising as nursing has for a long time been considered a female profession and considered by many as a "nice" preparation for marriage. The current trend seems to be that more men are entering nursing and more nurses see nursing as a lifelong commitment, not just a stepping stone to marriage.

Ninety-two percent of nurses are white. Of the 8 percent who are not, 40 percent are black, 33 percent Asiatic, 22.2 percent Hispanic, 3.8 percent American Indian, and 1 percent other. Many schools of nursing now have active recruitment programs to increase the admission and retention of minorities in nursing.

The majority of nurses are graduates of hospital schools of nursing (60 percent). This is also not surprising as this was the major method of educating nurses since the founding of education for nurses. With the cost containment push and the drive for the BSN as the entry degree, many hospital schools of nursing are closing. Other schools are merging with degree granting institutions. More nurses are seeking baccalaureate degrees and pursuing graduate education.

As far as work goes, the majority of nurses work full-time (58 percent) in hospital settings (65 percent). The majority of the nurses who work part-time are married. More nurses work in medical-surgical nursing (40 percent) than in any other specialty.

Identification of personality characteristics is difficult and often confusing and misleading. Many studies that have attempted to describe nurses' personalities are difficult to evaluate because of many limitations—sample size, methodology used, or instrument used. However, many stereotypes exist about the personality makeup of nurses.

In 1700, an English physician described the ideal nurse

1. Of middle age, fit and able to go through with the necessary Fatigue of her Undertaking.
2. Healthy, especially free from Vapours, and Cough.
3. A good Watcher, that can hold sitting up the whole Course of the Sickness.
4. Quick in Hearing, and always ready at the first Call.
5. Quiet and Still, so as to talk low, and but little, and tread softly.
6. Of good Sight, to observe the Pocks, their Colour, Manner and Growth, and all Alterations that may happen.
7. Handy to do every Thing the best way, without Blundering and Noise.
8. Nimble and Quick a going, coming, and doing every Thing.
9. Cleanly, to make all she dresseth acceptable.
10. Well-tempered, to humour, and please the Sick as much as she can.
11. Cheerful and Pleasant; to make the best of Every Thing, without being at any time Cross, Melancholy, or Timorous.
12. Constantly careful, and diligent by Night and by Day.
13. Sober and Temperate; not given to Gluttony, Drinking, or Smoking.
14. Observant to follow the Physician's Orders duly; and not be so conceited of her own Skill, as to give her own medicines privately.

15. To have no Children, or other to come much after her.
(Bullough & Bullough, 1969, p. 67).

Some of these characteristics still abound today. Many people today believe that nurses should be competent, caring, conscientious, kind, dependable, and compassionate. If you recall, earlier in this chapter you probably used these same adjectives. However, in the final analysis, answering the question of who is the nurse is not best done through demographic data or personal characteristics. Rather this question might best be answered by analysis of the roles of the nurse.

The majority of nurses function in the role of care-giver. In this role of care-giver, nurses assess their clients (collect information to help determine their needs, problems, or stressors), analyze this information to formulate a nursing diagnosis, plan the appropriate nursing care needed, carry out the plan, and evaluate the impact of the care given (commonly referred to as the nursing process). Examples of specific functions carried out in the care-giver role include interviewing, supporting clients, setting mutual goals, carrying out procedures, monitoring clients' progress, and supervising others.

Increasing numbers of nurses are assuming more responsibility for teaching, research, and leadership roles. The teaching role means enhancing the clients' health by expanding their knowledge base of health-promotion activities, diseases, and specific treatments. Teaching implies assessing educational needs, developing teaching plans, doing the teaching, and evaluating the results. Teaching occurs with both individuals and groups and formally and informally.

In the area of research, nurses are becoming more concerned with expanding nursing's knowledge base through research. Although many undergraduate programs do not prepare the graduate to be a researcher, they do prepare a research consumer. A research consumer evaluates research studies and interprets the implications of these results to specific practice settings. A research consumer also has an appreciation for research. As a graduate you may be involved in identification of clinical problems and participation in research studies. If your agency has an active nursing research department, you may become further involved in the research process.

In the area of leadership, the nurse is expected to demonstrate skills related to management, change process, advocacy, and collaboration. Management skills are needed to ensure proper functioning and coordination of all the activities occurring in the nursing-care areas. As a change agent the nurse is involved in identifying areas in need of change, planning the change, and implementing it. Change process is used for both individuals and institutions. The advocacy function means doing what the client would do to protect his rights if he were able. As a collaborator, the nurse facilitates health professionals in working together toward achievement of specific clients' goals.

As you continue your studies, these various roles presented will be elaborated on as appropriate to your clinical experiences and theories being introduced. In addition, the skills necessary for effectively using this interactive process will be introduced, refined, and perfected in your clinical nursing courses.

Interaction

Between the nurse and the client exists a reciprocal role relationship. Just as there is no such thing as mother without child, there is no such thing as nurse without client. The one role is reciprocal of the other. The relationship that exists between these roles is termed interaction. Historically, the relationship consisted of the nurse providing services to a passive recipient, the patient. Today, the interaction is more reciprocal.

Many factors have influenced the change to the type of relationship that exists between the client and the nurse today. One of the major factors has been the development of the nursing process (a systematic way of providing nursing care). As this process evolved, nurses became increasingly aware of the need for clients' involvement in defining their needs, planning goals, and identifying ways of achieving them. At the same time, changes in the concept of consumer rights have stimulated clients' interests in having a more active role in managing their health care.

Although all clients have a more active role in their care, the actual degree of client or nurse involvement in solving health problems varies with the situation. A patient who is critically ill may of necessity delegate almost all decisions. A client with a new health problem may depend on the nurse for information on which to base his decisions. For example, a newly diagnosed diabetic may have many questions that need answering before he is ready to plan his own meals.

Since the relationship in all situations is at all times reciprocal, the effectiveness of the care is dependent upon the quality of the communication between the client and the nurse. This is the reason such strong emphasis is placed on communication within all nursing programs.

Environment

The last component of nursing is the environment. The environment refers to the setting for nursing practice. Historically, nurses practiced nursing in the homes of their clients. Hospitals were seen as places to go to die or if your family was unable to care for you. In the homes, nursing care was given by one nurse. This private duty nurse was responsible for the nursing care of the client seven days a week, twenty-four hours a day. Many of these private duty nurses lived in the clients' homes and provided services from cooking to washing the laundry to cleaning the house. In addition, this private duty nurse observed the client, provided for the physical care, instructed the family, and carried out the physician's orders.

As medical care became more organized and institutionalized, nurses moved into these settings—the hospitals. Hospitals are the single largest employer of nurses. Approximately 65 percent of nurses are employed in hospitals (*Nurses Today—A Statistical Portrait*, 1982). In this setting, the nurse works with the other health care providers in providing health care in all phases of client care. The practice of nursing in hospitals is influenced by a variety of factors. Some of these influential factors are the philosophy of the institution, organization and control, physical facility, and personnel and administrative practices. These factors will be discussed in Chapter 13, "The American Health Care System." Generally the nursing staff is under the control of the director of nursing or associate administrator for nursing. Within the nursing department a variety of nurses are employed. Included in most hospitals are nurses in the positions of staff nurses, team leaders, head nurses, supervisors or managers, clinical specialists, and assistants to the director.

The methods used for assignment of nurses to client care varies among hospitals. The three most common methods of assignment are functional, team, and primary. The functional method of assignment emphasizes tasks to be done in providing the nursing care to the clients. Therefore, the nursing staff is organized around the tasks to be completed. As a nurse you would be assigned as the charge nurse responsible for the management tasks for the day; treatment nurse responsible for all the treatments, such as dressing changes, baths, temperatures, etc.; or medicine nurse responsible for administering all the medications ordered. Although this method of assignment tends to facilitate the completion of tasks, it falls short on providing continuity of care and comprehensive care.

Team nursing, another method of assignment, organizes health care providers into teams. Each team, consisting of registered nurses, licensed practical nurses, and aides and/or orderlies, is responsible for providing the care to a group of clients. Each team is headed by a team leader who is generally a registered nurse. The team nursing method of assignment is an attempt at providing continuity and comprehensive nursing care.

The last and most recent popular method of assignment is primary nursing. Primary nursing is the method of assignment where the total care for a client is the responsibility of one nurse. Each client entering the hospital system is assigned a primary nurse. This primary nurse is responsible for the development of the nursing care plan, providing the nursing care when on duty, monitoring the care provided when off duty, and evaluating the client's progress. Some nurses believe this is the old case method of assignment except that the nurse is responsible for multiple clients.

Although the majority of nurses work in hospitals, dissatisfaction with this environment exists. Many nurses are concerned about the increasing emphasis on cost containment at the expense of quality care. Decisions are being made regarding what is necessary care and what is optional, sometimes without concern for individualized, comprehensive care. Additional concerns include the lack of status nursing has in many hospital organizations, the lack of control over nursing care the nurse has, and the lack of involvement in direct client care the nurse experiences as she progresses in this organizational structure.

The second largest practice setting for nurses is the nursing home. Approximately 8 percent of registered nurses work in nursing homes or extended care facilities (*Nurses Today—A Statistical Portrait*, 1982). Nursing homes are health facilities that provide long-term nursing care to clients predominantly over sixty-five. The practice of nursing in these facilities varies greatly depending upon their philosophy, finances, and administrative practices. The nursing staff is generally under the control of a nurse and includes nursing positions similarly to those found in hospitals. Many nurses see the advantage of working in a nursing home as the opportunity to work with the same clients on a long-term basis. With the increasing interest in gerontological nursing and the numbers of elderly and chronically ill clients, more nurses are seeing this environment as a challenging alternative to traditional nursing in a hospital setting.

Public health or community health nursing is the third largest practice setting for nurses. Approximately 6.5 percent of nurses are employed in this setting (*Nurses Today—A Statistical Portrait*, 1982). Nurses employed in these agencies generally work in teams consisting of the nurse, social workers, nutritionists, dentists, physical therapists, speech therapists, physicians, and others. Programs offered in this setting include maternal-child care, communicable disease control and monitoring, family planning, drug and alcohol abuse, mental illness care, diagnostic and prevention care, and home health

TABLE 1-5
Practice settings for nurses

Practice Setting	Approximate Percent
Hospital	65.6
Nursing home/extended care facility	8.0
Public/community health	6.5
Physician's or dentist's office	5.7
Student health service	3.5
Nursing education	3.6
Occupational health	2.3
Private duty	1.6
Self-employed	.9
Other—health planning agencies, state boards, etc.	2.3

From: "Nurses Today—A Statistical Portrait." *American Journal of Nursing* 82 (1982):448–451.

nursing care. The responsibility and influence of the nurse in this setting is considerable. Many of these agencies require a minimum of a baccalaureate degree (BSN) for employment.

Although many other practice settings exist, these three represent the top employment settings. Table 1-5 presents a summary of where nurses practice. The current trend is a movement from the traditional settings (hospital) to nursing homes, community agencies, and independent practice. This movement is not surprising. With the increased emphasis on health and maintaining health, community agencies and independent practice provide opportunities to implement care aimed at health maintenance. In addition, these three growing practice settings facilitate nurses' independence in practicing nursing and assuming responsibility for this nursing care.

SUMMARY

This chapter presented an introduction to nursing through the presentation of definitions of nursing, various goals of nursing, and the components of nursing. The definitions of nursing presented included those from three perspectives: legal, professional, and personal. The goal of nursing was presented by briefly describing the purpose of goals and comparing two goal statements. The components of nursing presented included: client, nurse, interaction, and environment. Each of these components was discussed as it relates to nursing.

Some key points to remember about nursing are

1. There is no one accepted legal, professional, and personal definition of nursing.
2. Although there is no one accepted definition, commonalities do exist: nursing is service-oriented, nursing is goal-directed, clients include individuals and groups, and nursing deals with health and illness.
3. Each nurse develops a personal definition that influences nursing practice.
4. The goal of nursing determines the focus of nursing care, functions and roles of the nurse, and nursing responsibilities.
5. The components of nursing provide a basis for beginning to understand the complexity of nursing practice.

REFERENCES

American Nurses' Association. *Nursing: A Social Policy Statement*. Kansas City: American Nurses' Association, 1980.

American Nurses' Association. *The Nursing Practice Act: Suggested State Legislation*. Kansas City: American Nurses' Association, 1980.

American Nurses' Association. *Code for Nurses with Interpretive Statements.* Kansas City: American Nurses' Association, 1976.

American Nurses' Association. *Suggestions for Major Provisions to be Included in a Nursing Practice Act.* Kansas City: American Nurses' Association, 1976.

American Nurses' Association. *Standards of Nursing Practice.* Kansas City: American Nurses' Association, 1973.

American Nurses' Association. "A.N.A. Board Approves a Definition of Nursing Practice." *American Journal of Nursing* 55 (1955):1474.

Anderson, R., and Carter, I. *Human Behavior in the Social Environment.* Chicago: Aldine Publications, 1974.

Bullough, B., and Bullough, V., eds. *Expanding Horizons for Nurses.* New York: Springer Publishing Co., 1977.

Bullough, B., and Bullough, V. *The Emergence of Modern Nursing.* London: The Macmillan Co., 1969.

Facts about Nursing 1980–1981. New York: American Journal of Nursing Co., 1981.

Henderson, V. *The Nature of Nursing.* New York: The Macmillan Co., 1966.

King, I. *Toward a Theory for Nursing.* New York: John Wiley and Sons, 1971.

Kluckholn, C. *Personality in Nature, Society and Culture.* New York: Alfred Knopf, 1953.

Muff, J., ed. *Socialization, Sexism, and Stereotyping.* St. Louis: The C. V. Mosby Co., 1982.

Neuman, B. *The Neuman System Model.* Application to Nursing Education & Practice. Norwalk, CT: Appleton-Century-Croft, 1982.

New York State Nurse Practice Act. Article 139, Section 6902, 1972.

Nightingale, F. *Notes on Nursing: What It Is and What It Is Not.* Philadelphia: Stern Co., 1946.

Nurses Today—A Statistical Portrait. *American Journal of Nursing* 82 (1982): 448–451.

Orem, D. *Nursing: Concepts of Practice.* New York: McGraw-Hill Co., 1971.

Peplau, H. *Interpersonal Relations in Nursing.* New York: G. P. Putnam and Sons, 1952.

Rogers, M. *An Introduction to the Theoretical Basis of Nursing.* Philadelphia: F. A. Davis Co., 1970.

Roy, C. *Introduction to Nursing: An Adaptation Model.* Englewood Cliffs: Prentice-Hall, Inc., 1976.

2

Development of nursing: religious, military, and secular forces

Historical remains and written records of man go back thousands of years. A wealth of information about man has accumulated and been analyzed. For many students this wealth of information has been both overwhelming and boring. The idea of studying nursing's past does not usually generate great excitement. Many students of nursing as well as graduate nurses believe there are too many other, more important things to be learning. They demand to know how studying nursing's past could in any way make them a better nurse.

The major reason this information is valuable is that the present state of nursing is incomprehensible without understanding the past. If any profession does not know from whence it came, it cannot identify where it is or the forces which are influencing tomorrow's directions. For example, people who meet you today, and know you only in this setting and this time do not really begin to know you. They do not know your values, your beliefs, your dreams, your fears. Sometimes we will say they do not really know where you are coming from. The same is true for nursing as a profession. As a professional nurse, you need to know how the past is influencing what you are. You need to know where you as a nurse are coming from. You need this information so that you can understand your power to influence the future of nursing.

Through the years many forces have influenced nursing; and many ways exist for examining these forces. Since the purpose is to examine the past so that you might understand the present, this chapter will focus on selected religious, military, and secular forces which have influenced the development of nursing. Although a general description of the time will be given where appropriate, the major focus is the impact on nursing. For a more detailed description of events, the reader is referred to history of nursing textbooks.

At the completion of this chapter, the reader will be able to

1. Explain the value of studying nursing history.
2. Recognize the impact of selected religious forces on the development of nursing.
3. Identify the impact of military forces on the development of nursing.
4. Recognize and discuss the impact of secular forces on the development of nursing.

RELIGIOUS FORCES

Pre-Christian Era

Since the beginning, man has devised ways to live, assimilate problems, and work on improvements. This has meant actively expending energy and fighting for life. The biggest threats to life have been labeled by historians as disease, famine, and war (Cartwright & Biddiss, 1972). Materials have been uncovered as far back as the Stone Age which have helped to show how these threats were managed.

Health care practices have been identified or inferred from these earliest records. When trying to understand how nursing and nursing care practices developed, no clear picture emerges. Several reasons may explain this. First, some ancient materials such as fossilized remains give up their information reluctantly, and incompletely. Many times artifacts create more questions than answers to the questions. A second possible reason why nursing's beginnings are unclear is that care providers of ancient times may have had such a different scope of function that their activities do not easily fit any one, current-day role or position. The same person could have served as helper, healer, protector, and counselor. That one person may have been nurse, doctor, pharmacist, and spiritual advisor. A third reason why early nursing is unclear may have to do with past historical searchers tending to focus on health care by females thereby missing male participation. A fourth reason is that care giving prior to Christianity may not have been considered noteworthy for documentation.

During the Stone and Bronze Ages, corrective interventions involving the skull took place. Women surgeons of Sumeria, Egypt, and Greece had developed knowledge to the degree of using flint chisels and stick drills on the head in an effort to relieve disorders (Marks & Beatty, 1972). If these procedures were being done, who then assisted the patient to recovery? Someone had to monitor and assist this individual back to self-care and health.

Ancient Egyptians of about 2700 BC left records of both men and women healers who used techniques to improve health (Marks & Beatty, 1972; Dolan, Fitzpatrick, and Herrmann, 1983). Egypt has recorded evidence of being one of the healthiest of ancient civilizations. Egyptians developed hygienic and sanitation measures. Who then instructed the population on proper hygiene and sanitation? Did these healers perform both medical and nursing functions? Again, the answer to these questions is unclear. Someone was involved in this teaching and healing. Herbal remedies in pill and suppository form were also dispensed (Dietz, 1967). The Papyrus Ebers of 2500 BC contained 700 prescriptions for different diseases (Dolan, et al., 1983). Someone must have been involved in dispensing these and monitoring the patients.

During the same period, health interests have been recorded for other parts of the world. The Mayan Indians left evidence of advanced civilized life. The Mayans are thought to have used sweat baths for health purposes (Dolan, et al., 1983). Ancient Aztecs, other American Indians, and inhabitants of the Pacific and Africa employed women in the healing arts and left artifacts revealing their skills (Marks & Beatty, 1972).

In the Eastern part of the world, *The Great Herbal*, the earliest known medical textbook, dates back to 3000 BC (Cartwright & Biddiss, 1972). This document represents an effort to capture and control losses of health knowledge in the Eastern hemisphere. A few hundred years later, Emperor Huang-Ti wrote four steps for examining the sick: look, listen, ask, and feel. This interactive method resembles assessment techniques used today. Chinese health care flourished early and then regressed for a period (Dietz, 1967).

The Hindus of India brought together people with diverse needs, experiences, and knowledge. They used the team concept as far back as 1200 BC. The team included the doctor, the male nurse, patient, and drugs. The suitable nurse was described as having knowledge, cleverness, devotion, and purity (Dietz, 1967). No evidence currently exists that describes how these male nurses achieved this knowledge. The Hindus' health team was a form of organized care. The members interacted in applying their combined knowledge.

The ancient Hebrews used substantial knowledge to combat disease. Isolation techniques against diseases thought to be communicable were used. The Hebrews were aware of prevention of illness and instructed their people in hygiene and sanitary measures (Dolan, et al., 1983). They helped to control losses of knowledge from the culture by emphasizing teaching and learning. Again, little is known about the people who cared for the isolated patients or who instructed the population on hygiene and sanitation.

Greek health records date back to about 2000 BC and contain a mixture of myths with real events that cannot always be differentiated. The ancient Greeks believed in a number of gods with specialized attributes, some relating to health. There was Apollo, the god of health; Asklepios, the god of medicine; Hygeia, the goddess of health; and Panacea, the goddess of medications. The Greeks were known for a spirit of inquiry and later sparked the scientific approach to thinking (Dolan, et al., 1983).

At this time Greek scientific thought grew and progressed. Progress was rapid for about 600 years, or until the first century AD (Baly, 1973). One sees male scholars coming to the forefront. Pythagoras (580–496 BC) advanced mathematics and medicine. Hippocrates (460–355 BC) began a period of rational medical care.

Hippocrates promoted making clinical observations with inferences and described how this was to be done. He spoke against magic in treating the sick. A school of his followers developed later to continue his ideas about the scientific laws governing health and illness (Cartwright & Biddiss, 1972; Dietz, 1967; King, 1963).

Ancient Rome gave considerable attention to health and health care. The Romans enlisted the assistance of both men and women healers and tapped into health knowledge from other cultures. Greek medical terms were translated into Latin, and this translation is still in use today (Dietz, 1967). The early Romans developed engineering skills which assisted the health of the population. They maintained cleanliness by a generous water supply provided through aqueducts (Cartwright & Biddiss, 1972).

Records from these earliest civilizations indicate that medicine tended to be (1) primitive, (2) tied to beliefs about the supernatural, and (3) practiced by healers who also had other roles. In many of these earliest civilizations health was an important value, and achieving health depended on the belief systems in existence in that civilization. Also valued in many of these civilizations were education, culture, medicine, and sanitation.

Care of the sick at this time is inferred. There are no written records of organized nursing from this time; however, there are indications that individuals within the household performed nursing functions. What were those nursing functions and who performed them? Nursing tasks probably included administering treatments, such as hot or cold packs, massage, purifying baths, medications; teaching about hygiene and sanitation; fostering tender, loving care; conserving the patient's energy; and observing the patient (Fitzpatrick, 1983). The treatment followed beliefs in the evil spirits and how to drive out these spirits.

Who performed these tasks? The word nurse in Latin (*nutrix*) means to nourish and is associated with nourishing functions of caring, cherishing, and fostering (Fitzpatrick, 1983). The nurse then was probably the individual(s) who was/were responsible for nurturant functions. Most probably they were females, but they may have also been males, especially in civilizations where nursing was integrated with other roles of healers and priests.

The primary influence from this period of our history was the belief that nursing was intuitive and equated with mothering and nurturing; a formal education was not needed to practice nursing. Education was available only to the elite. Most likely nursing practice was communicated among families and from one generation to another by word of mouth and observation. If you look at some of the current nurse practice acts, you will see indications of this influence. For example, the Pennsylvania Nurse Practice Act, Section 4 states

> This act confers no authority to practice dentistry . . . nor does it prohibit home care of the sick by friends, domestic servants, nursemaids, companions, or household aids of any type, so long as such persons do not represent or hold themselves out to licensed nurses . . . or use in connection with their names, any designation tending to imply that they are licensed to practice under the provisions of this act. . . . (*Professional Nursing Law*, 1974, p. 2)

What this means is that nursing care can be provided by family members in the home as long as they do not call themselves nurses. Does this imply then that anyone can perform some aspects of nursing without being a nurse? Can you see the same type of provision applied to law, dentistry, or medicine?

Early Christian Era (AD 1-500)

From the time of the first century BC and into the succeeding several centuries, Rome experienced serious disease (Cartwright & Biddiss, 1972). A potent form of malaria disabled the population, and it has been thought by historians that Rome's decline may have been greatly influenced by this epidemic. Not only did Romans suffer from malaria, but by the second century AD they also had sweeping encounters with plague, probably contacted first by their armies on the march. In addition, Rome was ruled by a series of powerful and ruthless rulers: The common man was unmercifully exploited. Christianity began spreading and taking hold among greater numbers of people. New hope spawned and provided a new sense of direction to a people weakened by disease. The sick, distressed, and disabled were highlighted through Christian teachings and writings, e.g., "I was sick and ye visited me" (Matthew 25:36). Records from this time period exist that seem to be in contradiction. On the one hand, women were thought to decline in status as the early church rose to power. At one point women were not considered reasoning individuals by church fathers (Marks & Beatty, 1972). Men were seen at the helm of church organization and control. On the other hand, reference has been made to women of status, particularly in Rome, who initiated high level help to the sick. They exerted influence and in addition to visiting the sick in their homes, a forerunner to public health, they founded hospitals.

These early church laymen were called deaconesses. The deaconesses, women of good social standing, were appointed by bishops. Phoebe (AD 55) of Rome became well known as a helping Christian and has been called the first deaconess and first nurse (Dietz, 1967). In using "first nurse," Phoebe's activities must have been viewed as more similar to nursing as it is known today—using a judgment factor and working within a recognized structure of care capable of promoting positive health changes. The prime goal of these deaconesses was to provide care for the sick in their homes and to care for the needy. They functioned as visiting nurses and social workers. In this capacity, these women provided care that probably included attending to the hygiene, sanitation, nourishment, and spiritual needs of the patient.

In addition to the deaconesses, a group of wealthy Roman women and some war widows established hospitals. The purpose of these hospitals was to provide a place for the sick and needy to receive proper care and spiritual guidance. At times, some of these women provided care for the needy in their own homes. Some of the more noted of these Roman women were St. Helena, St. Marcella, and St. Fabiola. As Christianity spread, more and more settings for the sick were established in various places by individuals or church groups. For example, a well-known hospice, the Hospice of Turmanin, was established in Syria in AD 475 as a Christian monastery and refuge for the sick (Thompson & Cantile, 1975). Deaconesses were known to work in Syria, Asia Minor, Italy, Spain, Gaul, and Ireland (Marks & Beatty, 1972).

What was the impact of this early Christian Era on nursing? This early Christian Era was the beginning of organized nursing. In addition, these early nurses believed in the sanctity of life, charity, and visiting the sick. The deaconesses, women of high social status, viewed nursing as a proper activity for women of status. However, nursing was also connected with free service. Nursing was seen as work of mercy. Probably the major influence from this era was that nursing became associated with religious motives for selflessness and backbreaking servile labor. Note the following from the current Pennsylvania Nurse Practice Act which is a continuation of the previously quoted section

> This act confers no authority to practice dentistry . . . nor does it prohibit . . . (2) Care of the sick, with or without compensation or personal profit, when done solely in connection with the practice of the religious tenets of any church by adherents thereof. (*Professional Nursing Law*, 1974, p. 2)

Does part of our past surface when we are told nurses work for the love of humanity, because they want to help those in need? Is this what others mean when they say nursing should not be concerned with benefits and salary?

Religious Orders (AD 500-1500)

Rome fell in AD 476. It was a time of confusion for the people; neighboring tribes invaded and captured Roman territories. This confusion created unsettling movements of people. A large number of way stations were built to accommodate the travelers on their treks. Traveling could not have been an easy matter with rough roads, exposure to climate factors, and marginal supplies. More people gravitated into closer communities. Cities began to develop a whole way of life distinct from the rural ways previously known. Disease, famine, economic insecurity, and lack of personal freedoms created an undercurrent of violence in all segments of society (Hale, 1977).

During the medieval period individuals clung to old traditional beliefs. Philosophers slanted ideas based on the views of their ancestors rather than from their own observations (Brody, 1974). This slanting of ideas applied to illness as well as to other facets of life. The church was attributed with being both help and hindrance. The church gave unceasing care to the sick but also held back advances through dogmatism (Ehrenreich & English, 1973; Marks & Beatty, 1972; Cartwright & Biddiss, 1972).

Monasteries developed. They offered men and women an opportunity to live a better, safer, Christian life than existed in the general society (Notter & Spalding, 1976). One of the most famous monasteries established was the order of Benedictines.

These monasteries were strongly fortified and almost inaccessible because of the terrain surrounding them. Most of them were self-sufficient; providing for their own survival needs. Order and authority prevailed, and everyone worked long, hard days at the tasks assigned to them. Manual labor was encouraged, no work was beneath them. The need for sacrifice, work, and discipline was stressed. Although everyone worked, attention was also paid to preserving the culture.

Since these monasteries attempted to meet all the needs of the inhabitants, health care was also provided. Not only did the monasteries provide for the care of their own, but many also provided care for large numbers of sick people who lived outside their walls. The task of giving care to large numbers required a system of organization and education, so an apprentice learning system was developed. In it, students served under a master and did not ask questions. Nursing care included anything required to keep the hospital or infirmary running well—from nursing care, to cooking, washing, and cleaning.

During the late Middle Ages, the population was increasingly active as they made pilgrimages to Jerusalem to rescue the holy land. The movement of large numbers of people accelerated the growth of cities and commercial enterprises. Supplies were needed, and someone was needed to deliver them. However, travelers were exposed not only to new articles and food, but also to disease and pestilence. Leprosy was rampant, and epidemics were common. In addition, wounded crusaders needed help. Therefore, hospitals grew at a rapid rate. Religious orders of the mendicant type developed—orders of Friars Minor, Poor Clares, Augustine Sisters, and Dominicans. The members of these mendicant orders took vows of poverty, donating their earthly goods to the needy. These men and women did not live in monasteries secluded from the real world; much of their time was spent caring for the ill in hospitals and their homes. These religious orders contributed much to the care of the sick during the epidemics and furthered the knowledge of communicable disease care. They were the forerunners of community health care.

What impact did these religious orders have on nursing? Nursing was seen as a righteous, proper sacrifice; a calling; a service to God. Obedience and devotion were maintained through rigid discipline and a hierarchy of authority. Until the 1950s, nursing students were taught to stand when the doctor entered the room, to not question those in authority, and to anticipate the needs of the doctor. Failure to obey rules could result in dismissal from some schools of nursing.

Nursing tasks included anything that needed to be done. Nursing care today many times includes activities not directly related to nursing care. For example, in some hospitals nurses are expected to perform housekeeping tasks—cleaning the linen closets, supply closets, wheelchairs, and so on.

Lastly, these religious orders instituted the apprentice form of learning. While this was an improvement over no education, it is far from ideal. Today some people believe that nursing can only be learned in the clinical setting by watching other nurses perform the tasks.

Renaissance (1436–1600)

The Renaissance is known for the birth of the scientific method of inquiry. This was a time of quest for new knowledge and beauty. While the Renaissance saw the development of libraries, universities, medical schools, and the printing press, there was little change in the state of health (Dolan, et al., 1983). Poverty, unsanitary living conditions, and plagues continued to spread throughout Europe. Nursing was basically in a holding pattern. Nurses were uneducated and continued to provide custodial care under the authority of the church.

During the sixteenth century, a major religious upheaval occurred called the Reformation (1500–1650). This movement began as a religious reform but progressed to a major political revolt. Numerous hospitals and community settings served by nursing sisters of the Roman Catholic church closed. Care givers with religious ties fled. In the midst of the confusion illness continued to occur, but few places existed to provide the care needed. It was a dire scene and has been called the "dark age in nursing" (Dietz, 1967). The main influences from the Reformation on nursing were that (1) nursing became predominantly a female profession, (2) nursing became associated with domestic service, and (3) nurses were drunk, heartless, or immoral women. How many of you have seen movies, get well cards, or read books that depict nurses as less than professional?

These influences from the reformation continued without interruption until the 1800s. This was a time when no respectable woman worked outside the home. For the very poor women who did work the only jobs available were in domestic service. Nursing was one type of domestic service with even less status than some of the other domestic jobs. To deal with the shortage of nurses women were frequently assigned to nursing duties in lieu of serving jail sentences. Sairey Gamp and Betsy Prig in *Martin Chuzzlewit* by Charles

Dickens are excellent examples of the type of crude and ignorant women who provided care in the Protestant countries. Despite the hardships of the period, there were many who lived exemplary lives in the care of the sick and needy: St. Vincent de Paul and the Sisters of Charity of France; St. John of God in Spain; St. Camillus DeLellis of Italy; Marie Herbert Hubon in Nova Scotia; Augustinian Sisters in Quebec; and Jeanne Mance in Montreal, to name a few.

Revival of Religious Influences (1836-present)

Pastor Theodor Fliedner, a Lutheran pastor, and his wife, Friederike, opened Kaiserswerth Institute in Germany in 1836. During Pastor Fliedner's travels abroad and at home, he noted the lack of good nurses. He and his wife believed revival of the deaconesses would be a good solution to providing quality nursing care. With little money and much hard work the Kaiserswerth Institute opened to provide patient care and clinical experiences for the deaconesses. Later, many schools patterned themselves after Kaiserswerth. This model school included a three-year course of instruction, minimum age eighteen, letters of reference for entrance, probationary period, pocket money, theory classes, rotation through several clinical departments, classification of students by years, and uniform dress (Notter & Spalding, 1976). The impact of this revival movement on nursing included increasing respect for nurses, providing a model for a system of educating nurses, and providing Florence Nightingale with formal training.

Many of the current nursing history references provide little information concerning religious influences on nursing after the emergence of Florence Nightingale. Since many hospitals and schools of nursing developed in this country with religious affiliations, many of the nurses were educated in religious-related schools. What specific influence this had on the profession of nursing has not been identified. This may be the subject of future nursing historical research.

MILITARY FORCES

Crusades (1095-1270)

For almost 200 years, a series of Crusades were carried out to recapture Jerusalem for the Christians. With the long trip to the holy land came sickness and disease. Nutrition and sanitary conditions were poor. Thousands of Crusaders died before reaching the holy land. Many Crusaders who made it to Jerusalem were injured during the fighting. Who was to provide assistance to these people? In addition to the religious orders mentioned earlier, military nursing orders were established.

Three of the better known military orders established were the Knights

Hospitallers, Teutonic Knights, and Knights of St. Lazarus. Members of these orders were knights and monks who served mainly as nurses but when needed also performed as soldiers. On the battlefields these men were distinguished by their Maltese Cross. All of the military orders established a standard uniform.

These nurses established hospitals in strategic locations en route to Jerusalem as well as in Jerusalem. These military orders are well known for the excellent nursing care they provided to all in need. Strict sanitation measures were enforced to control communicable disease. Proper nutrition and hygiene were encouraged.

What impact did these military nursing orders have on nursing? First, they brought recognition to nursing by elevating the status of being a nurse. This also was a time when many men practiced nursing. Second, they brought organization to the practice of nursing. Hospitals utilized their good administrative practices in bringing order to providing care. Lastly, they instituted uniforms and the symbol of the cross. Many nurses today continue to wear uniforms. How many of you have seen the cross on nursing pins worn by nurses?

Crimean War (1854-1856)

In 1854, England, France, and Turkey declared war on Russia. Newspapers were filled with reports of the neglect of the English soldiers wounded in battle. Soldiers suffering from cholera, pain from wounds, and infections after amputations lay on the floors in bug and lice-infested coverings. Sanitation conditions were deplorable and rats and mice were everywhere. Ventilation was inadequate and the food was of such poor quality no one could eat it. The death rate was 42 percent (Marks & Beatty, 1972). The English were appalled at this treatment. Questions were asked regarding why England had no Sisters of Charity or Sisters of Mercy to provide care for the soldiers as the French and Russians had.

Florence Nightingale, who is discussed in more detail in Chapter 3, was sent to the Crimean War to see what could be done to improve these conditions. When Nightingale and thirty-eight sisters of religious orders and lay nurses arrived at Scutari, they were met with hostility from the medical personnel who believed women did not belong there. There were no hospital facilities at Scutari. The wounded were housed in converted artillery barracks. Conditions were worse than anticipated. Supplies—blankets, beds, utensils, food, soap, towels, etc.—were nonexistent. Through much hard work and persistence, these nurses set about cleaning the hospital, setting up a diet kitchen and laundry and obtaining the supplies necessary to care for the sick. Within a few months, conditions in the hospital improved tremendously. The death rate was cut to 2 percent.

The major impact of the Crimean War on nursing was to elevate the standards acceptable for good nursing care as well as for the conduct of the nurses. Concern for proper nutrition and sanitation was stressed. Today, as a student in nursing, you will take courses in nutrition, microbiology or epidemiology, public health principles, and hygiene measures. In addition, the Crimean War provided Florence Nightingale with the opportunity to demonstrate what good nursing care could do. It laid the groundwork for the establishment of the Florence Nightingale system of education to be discussed later.

Civil War (1861-1865)

When the Civil War broke out in the United States in 1861, the only nurses with any training were Catholic and Protestant sisters. While these nurses provided competent care, they could not begin to meet the needs of the soldiers. Besides battle casualties, illnesses consisting largely of dysentery, infections, and deficiency diseases existed. Men wounded in battle lay in the fields receiving practically no care.

In 1861, Dorothea Dix, known for her fight for insane asylum reform, accepted an appointment as Superintendent of Women Nurses for the Union Army. She was charged with recruiting nurses for the Army. Some of the standards she set for these nurses included: 35-50 years old, plain dress, and plain appearance. Women across the country volunteered to assist in these efforts. Some of the more noted ladies included Clara Barton, Mary Livermore, Mother Mary-Ann Bickerdyke, Woolsey sisters, Louisa Alcott, Mary Breckinridge, and Sojourner Truth. These untrained ladies assisted in distributing clothing and comforts, attending to families of servicemen, and giving care to the sick in the hospitals.

The major impact on nursing from the Civil War was the impetus it gave to the development of schools of nursing. While the intent of the army nurses was honorable, their lack of education in nursing highlighted a critical need in nursing. Three schools of nursing, patterned after the Nightingale School, opened in the United States in 1873. The first was connected with Bellevue Hospital in New York City. Another was founded in Boston at Massachusetts General Hospital and the third, called the Connecticut Training School, was established in New Haven, Connecticut (Anderson, 1981). By the end of the century, nursing schools were growing rapidly. Hospital training programs were opened one after the other. In the United States by 1890 there were 15 schools and by 1900, there were 432.

After the Civil War, there was a surge of interest to improve the health of the black population and to increase the education of black nurses. Spellman Seminary in Atlanta, Georgia, opened in 1886. The School of Nursing at Hampton Institute, Virginia, was founded in 1891. In the same year the school at Providence Hospital in Chicago, Illinois, began. Finally, Tuskegee Institute, Alabama, opened a school of nursing in 1892. Financial needs were met partly by well-to-do benevolent individuals and also the local black communities. These trained nurses provided health care to the poor sick. There were over 250 graduates from the programs by 1906 (Sloan, 1978).

Spanish-American War (1898)

Once again at the inception of a war, no organized army nurse corps existed nor was there a system by which nurses could be recruited. Dr. Anita McGee was appointed to head this recruitment effort through her association with the Daughters of the American Revolution. Criteria established for recruitment of nurses included being a graduate nurse and having recommendations attesting to character. Initially, the army surgeons did not support these nurses.

Because of the excellent care and devotion given by these nurses, they won recognition and support of all in the service. The nursing care included nonwar injuries such as typhoid and yellow fever. At the end of the war and with the urging of several organizations and nursing leaders, federal legislation was passed to establish a permanent corps of nurses ready to provide care in time of war. In 1901, the Army Nurse Corps was established and in 1908, the Navy Nurse Corps was begun.

World War I (1914-1918)

Unlike the situation in all the other wars to date, the nurses of this country were prepared for the United States' entry into World War I in 1917. Through the American Red Cross Nursing Service and Jane Delano, its chairman, 8,000 nurses were available for service. In addition, existing schools of nursing stepped up their enrollment and graduation to provide additional graduate nurses.

Nursing care problems in this war were related to the type of warfare used. Large numbers of patients were seen with tetanus, respiratory diseases (related to gas warfare), parasites, and typhoid fever. The type of injury received necessitated advances in plastic surgery.

In civilian hospitals, serious problems occurred with the enlistment of many doctors and nurses in the armed services. In addition, the great influenza epidemic of 1918 was claiming many lives. Those nurses remaining in the civilian hospitals were taking on more and more responsibilities, responsibilities once thought the domain of medicine.

Although these nurses performed admirably, they received less recognition than those nurses serving in previous wars. The major impact on nursing from World War I was that nurses could competently assume tasks once reserved for doctors and that knowledgeable nurses are a must in providing quality nursing care. In an attempt to supply nurses over a long term, the Army School of Nursing and the Vassar Training Camp were opened in 1918. Both of these programs produced some of nursing's greatest leaders. In 1920, for the first time nurses were granted relative rank in the armed services. Lastly, the government continued employment of nurses. After the war, nursing services were established in the U.S. Public Health Service in 1919, in the Veterans Bureau in 1919, and in the Indian Bureau in 1924.

World War II (1941-1945)

World War II was a time of great patriotism. Men enlisted in the service. Civilians worked long, hard hours in factories, on farms, and as volunteers in civilian hospitals. Nurses too arose to the occasion. The National Nursing Council for War Service established plans to develop a national inventory of nurses, expand existing nursing schools, and provide alternative nursing services to civilian hospitals and agencies.

Although the federal government had financially supported private nursing education previous to World War II, the War served as a stimulus for major funding of nursing education. In 1941, the federal government appropriated $1,800,000 for nursing education. The goal of this appropriation was to ensure an adequate supply of well-trained nurses (Kalisch & Kalisch, 1978). This initial appropriation was followed by additional funds until 1943 when Congress passed the Bolton Act establishing the Cadet Nursing Corps. Students who enrolled in the Corps had their education subsidized in return for agreeing to engage in essential military or civilian service for the duration of the war. Between July 1943 and October 1945, almost 170,000 cadets entered 1,125 participating schools, making the U.S. Cadet Nursing Corps the largest uniformed women's services in the United States (Bullough & Bullough, 1978).

Nurses provided care to the soldiers wherever military operations existed. Nurses assisted in field hospitals, underground operating rooms, hospital ships, tropical jungles, and airlift operations. Some were taken prisoner and some died in the line of duty.

Communicable diseases such as malaria and typhoid took their toll. Anxiety neuroses and emotional instability accompanied mass evacuations and intolerable field conditions. Many medical advances were made, such as in the treatment of shock (giving of blood plasma in the field), treatment of infection (use of penicillin and sulfonamides), and the use of quinine for malaria and vaccines for tetanus and yellow fever.

Along with the nurses in the armed services, nurses in industry were contributing to the war effort. Industrial nurses were providing safety education and accident prevention programs to the workers in an effort to keep them productive. Civilian hospitals found themselves in dire need of people to provide nursing care. Many people offered their services as aides, gray ladies, and orderlies.

What impact did World War II have on nursing? World War II encouraged the first direct financing of nursing education by the federal government. The U.S. Cadet Nurse Corps was established. The government's financing of nursing education continued indirectly after the war through the GI Bill, which applied to nurses who had served their country. Many nurses took advantage of it. This was the first time there developed a significant group of nurses with higher education. The nursing curricula expanded to include content on rehabilitation and psychiatric concepts in an effort to provide care to the returning veterans.

World War II is frequently considered the beginning of contemporary nursing practice. Certainly, many changes which began then are still with us today. Although physicians were already well specialized, the post-war period was a time of increasing nursing specialization. As the nurse's role grew, delegation of tasks occurred. The use of auxiliary personnel became well established in World War II. In order to deal with the various levels of health care providers, team nursing was developed; it continues to be one of the main methods of delivering nursing care.

Korean (1950) and Vietnam (1968) Wars

Having learned from the other wars, when the Korean War broke out, immediate care for the wounded soldiers was available through the United Nations. The U.S. Army supplied nurses through the Army Corps as well as from the reserves. The United States supplied MASH (Mobile Army Surgical Hospital) units for front-line duty. These MASH units included physicians, nurses, and corpsmen. They were responsible for setting up the mobile units as close to the battlefield as possible. Care centered around stabilization of the injured and included shock treatment and surgery. Once stabilized the injured soldiers were evacuated to army hospitals where additional care was provided. Those soldiers requiring extensive rehabilitation were sent back to the United States; those able to return to active duty did so.

With the involvement of the United States in Vietnam in 1968, these mobile units (now called Medical Unit, Self-contained, Transportable or MUST units) continued providing trauma care. More and more corpsmen were trained to care for these injured soldiers. An amazing number of lives were saved through the use of blood or plasma, antibiotics, and immediate surgery for severe injuries to the chest, abdomen, and extremities.

What impact did these two wars have on nursing? When these nurses returned to the United States they were increasingly discontented with their working situation and the lack of independent decision making. At the same time, coronary care units and trauma units were being developed. Many of these nurses saw these units as an opportunity to specialize, to take on the additional responsibility that had provided them with much satisfaction in the service. Today these nurses with advanced clinical education and preparation are called clinical specialists and nurse practitioners.

In addition to the returning nurses, we also had returning corpsmen.

These corpsmen had received extensive training in providing trauma care. Where did they fit into the civilian health care scene? At the same time these corpsmen were returning, a critical shortage of doctors and nurses existed. Emerging from all of this was the development of physicians' assistants (PA's).

SECULAR FORCES

Industrialization (Philanthropy Movement)

The beginning of the twentieth century was a time when this country was interested in reform, especially in finding new and better ways of meeting the needs of individuals in the new industrial order. The interdependence resulting from industrialization challenged the values and beliefs of a country that emphasized individual independence. The issue to be dealt with was the protection of the individual, in many cases the helpless individual, as he dealt with "great aggregations of capital in enormous industrial establishments" (Morrison, 1965, p. 811). Wages were low and housing and working conditions horrendous.

Changes occurred at all levels of government. On the federal level these changes were reflected in the political slogans and new laws enacted. Theodore Roosevelt called his policies the "Square Deal," and Woodrow Wilson called his the "New Freedom." These slogans reflected a belief in the need for government intervention to provide protection for the individual in dealing with business, transportation, and finance. In 1906, the Pure Food and Drug Act provided federal regulation of food and drugs; the Meat Inspection Act provided federal regulation of the interstate meat packing industry. The variety of new laws directed at protecting the individual also occurred at the state level. For example, in 1911, the first state welfare law for mothers with dependent children was adopted in Illinois. A year later the first state minimum wage law was adopted by Massachusetts.

Although much of the government control and intervention which is so questioned today can be traced to the early 1900s, this country maintained a strong belief in the need to limit or control the effect of government on the individual. Many people believed that the private sector should deal with society's problems. Many of the wealthy industrialist wives were looking for a cause, something to occupy their time. Many of the private foundations (e.g., Carnegie Foundation in 1910) and social service organizations (e.g., Boy Scouts of America in 1910), were established to help meet the needs of the common worker and the millions of immigrants who migrated to this country.

What impact did this philanthropy movement have on nursing? The major impact of this movement was the impetus given to the development of public health nursing. Sporadically throughout the late 1800s, various professionals and lay volunteers were concerned with the health and poor quality of life of the immigrants. Included in those concerned for the immigrants were many nurses. Two of the most famous were Lillian Wald and Mary Brewster. These two nurses set up the famed Henry Street Settlement and offered nursing care to the immigrants (more details about Lillian Wald and the Henry Street Settlement will be discussed in Chapter 3). Maternal child programs were set up, and the public health nurse became the backbone for implementing these programs. These nurses carried case loads and functioned as independent practitioners concerned with the welfare of the community.

In order to function effectively these nurses were encouraged to seek additional education in universities. Courses were developed to assist these nurses to provide quality care and to fill the gap in their education. Many articles in the *American Journal of Nursing* (AJN) and the *Visiting Nurse Quarterly* were directed to these public health nurses. The National Organization for Public Health Nursing (NOPHN) was formed in 1912 and served as a major force in determining the practice and education of public health nurses for the next four decades. Today, public health and community health nurses continue to provide nursing care aimed at families and community groups.

Women's Movement (1800-present)

Education for females emerged sluggishly and usually concentrated on preparing women to be wives and mothers. Advanced education was not thought to be relevant for women, who were viewed as domestically based. Any instruction beyond that environment was held to be artificial, unnecessary, and remote (Watson, 1977). Against this background, it is not surprising that information for nurses often focused on domestics.

By the mid-nineteenth century, women's groups, both here and abroad, formed to improve conditions in hospitals and almshouses. They aroused public reaction, and subsequent investigations began bringing about improvements (Bingham, 1979). This was the beginning of a demand for emancipation and enfranchisement of women. In 1848, a women's rights convention was held in New York. The purpose of this convention was to fight for the rights of women to be treated as human beings, to have access to higher education, and to have an opportunity for careers in professions other than teaching and nursing (Dolan, et al., 1983). The significance of this convention and movement it represented was that it would provide support for the concept of an educated nurse.

Suffrage, however, was not an easy route. Much opposition was experienced. Newspapers portrayed women suffrage leaders as old maids, childless women, and unsexed persons. This was a time of much exploitation of women and children. Since nursing was a predominantly female profession, it was only natural that the American Nurses' Association and the National League for Nursing would be asked to take a stand. What is surprising is the stand taken—refusal to support the movement. The women's movement was seen as a controversial issue that nurses should avoid. Some nursing leaders, however, were actively involved in the movement.

The nineteenth amendment finally passed in 1920 giving women the right to vote. The law, however, did nothing to stop discrimination against women. For the next few years, things seemed to be quiet as everyone was caught up in the depression and wars.

In 1966, the National Organization for Women (NOW) was founded. The purpose of this organization was to assist in the consciousness raising of people to the fact that women did not have full equality. What the organization did for nursing was to make many nurses aware of their status. It was through the efforts of nurses in NOW that assertiveness skills were developed. This organization also provided a stimulus for nurses to become more politically involved.

State and Federal Legislation

Through the years many pieces of legislation have influenced the practice of nursing. A few of them will be presented here. The licensing laws are state laws, but all the remaining laws are federal ones.

In 1901, at the International Council of Nurses Meeting a resolution was passed calling for nursing professions in all countries to work for enactment of laws to regulate nursing education and for laws to protect the public from incompetent nurses. Prior to 1903, anyone could practice as a nurse. Nursing leaders worked long and hard to fight the opposition–doctors and hospital administrators who did not want these laws. Considering the lack of women's rights, what was accomplished was a credit to our leaders. In 1903, the first nurse practice act was passed. By 1923, all states had some form of licensing laws.

What impact did nurse practice acts have on nursing? These practice acts gave recognition to nursing as an organized service requiring some standards—nursing practice was restricted to qualified practitioners. Support for the acts led to the formation of state associations that lobbied for the passage of these state laws. Starting in about 1938, the revised laws set higher standards for nursing and eventually led to legal definitions of nursing.

As discussed earlier under World War II, the Bolton Act was passed in 1943. This piece of legislation was the federal government's first involvement in financing nursing education. Criteria were established for who could qualify for this federal assistance: 17–35 years old, good high school record, and good health status. This law forbade discrimination based on race and marital status, and many nurses received their nursing education through this act.

In 1956, the Health Amendments Act was passed after 14 years of effort by various people interested in health professional education. This act provided money for graduate education and served as the stimulus for development of nursing leaders in administration, teaching, and public health. As more nurses became vocal and politically sophisticated and as the professional organizations grew in strength, nurses were more instrumental in obtaining federal funds.

In 1964, the first nurse training act was passed. This act provided federal funds for construction of collegiate schools of nursing, grants for improving nursing curricula, and educational strategies and capitation grants for every student in the programs. This legislation was an attempt at improving nursing practice by facilitating quality educational programs and increasing the numbers of qualified nurses. This training act contained antidiscrimination provisions and included all types of nursing programs leading to registration as a nurse. The nurse training acts have been extended and altered many times. Each time the act is up for renewal much discussion occurs regarding the need for this financial support to nursing. Several presidents have vetoed the bill extensions. Each time to date Congress successfully overrode the veto through the efforts of active lobbying by our organizations and leaders.

This law provided assistance to many people who otherwise could not afford to become nurses. It also served to improve the educational facilities and upgrade the faculty teaching in them.

Civil Rights Legislation of the 1960s

In the 1960s, a number of civil rights acts were passed in an attempt to end discrimination by sex, race, or color. These laws were especially important to nurses since the profession is predominantly female. The first of these laws was the Equal Pay Act of 1963. The intent of this act was to end wage inequities based on sex. Women were to receive the same financial return as men doing the same things. The major problem with this act was that it excluded hospital employees, who were predominantly female.

In 1964, the Civil Rights Act was passed. This act prohibited job discrimination in the hiring and promotion of women and minorities. This act, unlike the Equal Pay Act, included hospitals and colleges. The act covered all places which accepted federal grants. While the effect of these two acts helped lessen hiring and pay discrimination for women and minorities, it did not eliminate the problem. Many people believe this discrimination still exists as evidenced by the number of suits against employers for violation of the Equal Pay and Civil Rights Acts.

The 1974 amendments to the Taft-Hartley Act had the effect of increasing pay and benefits for hospital employees including nurses. These amendments for the first time gave employees in nonprofit health care facilities the right to unionize.

Today, concern still exists for discrimination of women and minorities. Efforts to ratify an Equal Rights Amendment have failed. Suits continue to be filed regarding sex discrimination. While progress has been made in equalizing the status of women and nurses, much has yet to be done.

Professional Organizations

By the turn of the century two professional nursing groups had been organized. These groups were the first professional groups to be organized and controlled by women in the United States (Bullough & Bullough, 1978). These two organizations developed under the direction of nursing leaders to reform nursing education and practice. Serious conditions existed in the hospitals and nursing schools. Most schools of nursing were dependent on the hospitals for their financial support. These hospitals found a new source of cheap labor which led to exploitation of the students. Service was their primary objective; not the education of the students. Graduate nurses were not employed by the hospitals but sought employment in private duty or public health. There were no standards or control of nursing education or practice. Improvement in the system of educating future nurses was seen as the first in many steps to improving nursing practice.

The American Society of Superintendents of Training Schools of Nursing (changed to the National League of Nursing Education [NLNE] in 1912) was founded in 1893. This organization, which limited membership to superintendents, had three objectives (Flannagan, 1976)

1. To promote fellowship of members
2. To establish and maintain a universal standard of training
3. To further the best interest of the nursing profession.

Three years later, with support from the superintendents, a second organization was formed. Many schools of nursing had alumnae associations. This second organization, the Nurses Associated Alumnae of the United States and Canada, limited membership to alumnae associations of schools connected with general hospitals of not less than 100 beds and giving not less than two full years of training (Flannagan, 1976).

The superintendents focused their reform on the establishment of educational standards. The Associated Alumnae (changed to the American Nurses' Association in 1911) focused their reform on the control of nursing practice. This can be seen in the priorities set at the third annual convention of the Associated Alumnae (Bullough & Bullough, 1978)

1. Growth of the professional organization.
2. Registration for nurses in each of the states.

By 1912, both organizations had clearly directed their areas of interest. The superintendents focused on the education of nurses and the Alumnae focused on nursing practice. Although these organizations existed as distinct ones, they maintained a close relationship. For example, the president of each organization was an ex-officio member of the board of directors of the other (Goostray, 1969).

A number of the reforms which nursing experienced during this time were directly related to the effectiveness of these organizations. No other single force has contributed to the development of professionalism as much as these organizations. Two of these reforms maintain their influences today: the development of an official nursing journal and the licensure of nurses.

The first of these reforms, the development of a magazine which was controlled by the nursing profession and promoted nursing was made possible by the formation of the American Journal of Nursing Company in 1900. Control of their own publication was thought important for two reasons. First, a publication was needed to facilitate communication between members and inform them about issues occurring that would affect nursing. Secondly, a publication was needed to inform nurses about new and better ways for providing nursing care (Fitzpatrick, 1983). This journal has remained to the present day the official publication of the American Nurses' Association.

The second major reform, licensure, also began early in the 1900s. Before 1903, no licensure laws existed; there was no way for the public to distinguish a trained nurse from the untrained attendants. By 1923, all states in the union, the District of Columbia, and Hawaii had licensure laws. However, this success was not without opposition and, in turn, compromise. The opposition came from those who trained and utilized nurses: hospital administrators, physicians, people who ran correspondence schools in nursing, and charitable organizations that sponsored home nursing programs (Bullough & Bullough, 1978). Two compromises resulted. The first was the acceptance of permissive laws. A permissive nurse practice act permits anyone to work as a nurse as long as she does not call herself registered. These laws, therefore, did not define what nursing was, but rather defined who could be registered.

The second compromise involved membership on the state nursing boards. Nurses believed the state boards should be comprised of all nurses. Membership was rarely limited to nurses. In fact, in many cases, physicians were in control of the state boards instead of the nurses being in control.

In 1939, the American Nurses' Association was petitioned by a state association to consider the matter of amalgamation of all existing professional organizations (Goostray, 1969). This was followed in 1944 by a decision of the boards of the ANA, the NLNE, and the National Organization for Public Health Nursing (NOPHN) to undertake a joint survey of their organizational structures. They were joined in this venture by the National Association of Colored Graduate Nurses (NACGN), the Association of Collegiate Schools of Nursing (ACSN), and the American Association of Industrial Nurses (AAIN) (Bullough & Bullough, 1978). The final restructuring decision in 1950 created two organizations, the ANA and the NLN. Included in the NLN were the NLNE, NOPHN, and ACSN. The formation of two organizations was required because there were nonnurse members in the NLNE and NOPHN. This type of membership was unacceptable to the ANA. The goal of reorganization was to reduce the number and increase the strength of nursing organizations.

During the 1960s and into the 1970s, the American Nurses' Association and the National League for Nursing continued as the main nursing organizations. However, the increasing specialization in nursing resulted in a number of new small specialty organizations (e.g., the American Association of Critical Care Nurses founded in 1969, National Intravenous Therapy Association, and the American Urological Association, formed in 1972). These new groups compete with the ANA and the NLN. In 1966, the ANA and NLN issued a joint statement delineating their roles. This was repeated in 1970 and reaffirmed in 1973 (Kelly, 1981).

The developments within the American Nurses' Association demonstrate two trends. The first trend is a formal effort to improve the quality of nursing care by improving the standards of nursing practice and nursing education. The second trend is a formal effort to improve the quality of nursing for nurses by improving their role and rewards in the marketplace. Several events track these trends.

The ANA effort to improve standards was demonstrated in 1965 when the ANA issued a formal position statement on nursing education.

> The education for all those who are licensed to practice nursing should take place in institutions of higher education.
> The minimum preparation for beginning professional nursing practice at the present time should be baccalaureate degree education in nursing. The minimum preparation for beginning technical nursing practice at the present time should be associate degree education in nursing. (American Nurses' Association, 1965)

Although the history of nursing had shown a persistent move toward higher education and the position paper paralleled in many ways the Brown Report from eighteen years earlier, the reaction of nurses indicated many in nursing were not ready for this move. The position paper did not mention diploma education, and many professional nurses saw themselves excluded or as less than professional. The position paper resulted in some closings of diploma schools but also caused much conflict in nursing about the best place to educate nurses.

Though the position paper of 1965 became the best known of the ANA stands, several other statements have been issued since 1965 and demonstrate this same effort at improving quality. One of the most significant of these involves the establishment of standards. This began in 1965 when the ANA issued its *Standards for Organized Nursing Service*. This was followed in 1973 by *Standards for Nursing Service*, and *Standards for Nursing Practice*. This concern with standards considered not only nursing practice but also education. In 1974, the ANA issued *Standards for Nursing Education* which addressed associate degree, diploma, baccalaureate, and continuing education. This was followed in the same year by the ANA's *Statement of Continuing Education* and the *Standards for Continuing Education Guidelines* for State Nurses' Associations. The main significance of these publications on continuing education is that they are related to the beginning move of ANA into accreditation of educational programs for nurses, a role that had traditionally belonged to the NLN.

The ANA's move to improve the quality of nursing involved not only formal positions and standards but also mechanisms for recognition of individuals. Two specific events demonstrate the ANA efforts to provide for recognition. These events were the establishment of the Academy of Nursing and a certification program. Although discussion concerning both the Academy of Nursing and the certificate program date back to the late 1950s, these were not established until 1973. The Academy was created to provide for recognition of professional achievement and excellence in nursing. Fellows in the Academy include researchers, academicians, administrators, and practitioners. Certification, on the other hand, was established to provide recognition for professional achievement and excellence in practice. The process of certification was open to all nurses who met the specific preparation and guidelines as to practice and include a written examination in their area of specialization. Because of the time and money involved in development of the examinations only two areas of specialization, pediatric and geriatric, were included the first year (Kelly, 1981). Each year since this has seen new areas for certification established.

The establishment of positions, standards, and recognition involved the ANA in working for improvement within the profession of nursing. During this same time, the organization also became much more aggressive in working for the improvement of nursing for nurses. One of the more effective efforts in this trend involved collective bargaining. Although the ANA usually did not function as a bargaining unit, it moved to improve the laws related to bargaining and to support the state associations that functioned as bargaining units. In 1962, employees in federal health care institutions gained the right to bargain collectively. This right was extended to profit-making hospitals and nursing homes in 1967, to nonprofit nursing homes in 1970, and to nonprofit hospitals in 1974 (Kalisch & Kalisch, 1978). Although the ANA first called on state associations to represent nurses in collective bargaining in 1946, little action occurred before these changes in the laws. From 1963 to 1973, the number of state associations that had negotiated contracts increased from eight to thirty-two (Schutt, 1973). By 1975, state nursing associations had negotiated 515 bargaining contracts (Kalisch & Kalisch, 1978).

Although the developments within the ANA reflect the more significant trends within the professional nursing organizations during this time period, the number of other groups which have moved into representing nurses reflect a significant trend in itself. The future of this organization and, in turn, nursing will be greatly influenced by how the ANA functions with its competitors, mainly labor unions.

Although the ANA is noted for its contributions to the improvements in nursing practice, the NLN's most important contributions were to the improvement of nursing curricula and the standards set for accrediting the various nursing schools. Several guides were published to provide assistance to nurse educators in development and revision of nursing programs. The NLN has supported all types of preparation for nursing education. Through the years these two organizations have contributed to the development of nursing through the efforts of its leaders, studies, position statements, and political activities.

SUMMARY

This chapter presented an introduction to nursing history by examining three forces which have influenced the development of nursing. The three forces presented were religious, military, and secular. A general description of the situation was given, followed by the involvement of nurses. Each section concluded with a discussion of the specific impact this force had on nursing.

Some key points to remember about the development of nursing are

1. The major impacts on nursing of religious forces were
    a. Nursing is a calling involving a dedication to serving mankind.
    b. Nurses should not be too concerned with money and benefits; more concern should exist for self-sacrifice.
    c. All tasks even menial are appropriate for nurses.
    d. Two views of nurses exist: one, an angel of mercy, and the other, a loose, sexy person.
2. The major impacts of military forces were
    a. Hierarchical organization and obedience to authority figures was emphasized in the education of nurses.
    b. Nurses' responsibilities expanded with the development of specializations.
    c. The Army Nurse Corps became a respectable division of the armed services and established some of the first standards for nursing practices and nurses.
    d. Nurses wore uniforms when providing nursing care.

3. The major impacts on nursing of secular forces were
   a. Nurses became involved in politics.
   b. The U.S. government stimulated improvements in nursing practice and education through financial support.
   c. Nurses gained increased control over their practice through laws.
   d. The general welfare of nurses increased through a series of federal laws.

REFERENCES

"American Nurses' Association, First Position for Nursing Education." *American Journal of Nursing* 65 (1965): 107–108.

Anderson, N. "The Historical Development of American Nursing Education." *Journal of Nursing Education* 20 (1) [1981]: 18–36.

Baly, M. *Nursing and Social Change.* London: William Heinemann Medical Books, 1973.

Bingham, S. *Ministering Angels.* Oradell, N.J.: Medical Economics Co., 1979.

Brody, S. *The Disease of the Soul.* Ithaca, N.Y.: Cornell University Press, 1974.

Bullough, V., and Bullough, B. *The Care of the Sick: The Emergence of Modern Nursing.* New York: Prodist, 1978.

Cartwright, F., and Biddiss, M. *Disease and History.* New York: Thomas Y. Crowell Co., 1972.

Dietz, L. D. *History and Modern Nursing.* Philadelphia: F. A. Davis Co., 1967.

Dolan, J., Fitzpatrick, M., and Herrmann, E. *Nursing in Society: A Historical Perspective.* Philadelphia: W. B. Saunders, 1983.

Ehrenreich, B., and English, D. *Witches, Midwives and Nurses: A History of Women Healers.* Old Westbury, N.J.: The Feminist Press, 1973.

Fitzpatrick, M. *Prologue to Professionalism.* Bowie, MD: Robert J. Brady Co., 1983.

Fitzpatrick, M., ed. *Historical Studies in Nursing.* New York: Teachers College Press, 1978.

Flannagan, L. *One Strong Voice: The Story of the American Nurses' Association.* Kansas City: American Nurses' Association, 1976.

Goostray, S. *Memoirs: Half a Century in Nursing.* Boston: Nursing Archive, Boston University Mugar Memorial Library, 1969.

Hale, J. R. *Renaissance Europe.* Berkeley: University of California Press, 1977.

Kalisch, P., and Kalisch, B. *The Advance of American Nursing.* Boston: Little, Brown and Co., 1978.

Kelly, L. *Dimensions of Professional Nursing.* New York: The Macmillan Co., 1981.

King, L. S. *The Growth of Medical Thought.* Chicago: The University of Chicago Press, 1963.

Marks, G., and Beatty, W. *Women in White.* New York: Charles Scribner's Sons, 1972.

Matthew 25:36, *Holy Bible.*

Morrison, S. *The Oxford History of the American People.* New York: Oxford University Press, 1965.

Notter, L., and Spalding, E. *Professional Nursing: Foundations, Perspectives and Relationships.* Philadelphia: J. B. Lippincott Co., 1976.

Schutt, B. "Collective Action for Professional Security." *American Journal of Nursing* 73 (1973): 1946–1951.

Sloan, P. "Commitment to Equality: A View of Early Black Nursing Schools." In *Historical Studies in Nursing.* Edited by M. L. Fitzpatrick. New York: Teachers College Press, 1978.

The Professional Nursing Law. Act #69 and Amendments. Harrisburg, PA: Pennsylvania Nurses' Association, 1974.

Thompson, J., and Cantile, G. *The Hospital: A Social and Architectural History.* New Haven: Yale University Press, 1975.

Watson, J. "The Evolution of Nursing in the United States: 100 Years of a Profession for Women." *Journal of Nursing Education* 16 (7) [1977]: 31–38.

3

Development of nursing's early leaders and studies

In the development of any profession, there are people who point the way to the future. These people are not always in charge but they are almost always related to the authority figures of the times; to the sources of power. Although leaders demonstrate a wide variety of personality types, they possess some innate, undefined ability to plan for the future, to excite others to follow. However, the development of a profession cannot be explained solely by a study of the prominent people of that profession. Numerous studies and positions impact on the growth of any profession. Nursing is no exception to these influences.

Chapter 2 presented religious, military, and secular influences on nursing. This chapter will focus on selected early leaders as well as on key studies and positions. The purpose of this chapter is to provide a brief introduction, a foundation to the development of the profession as it relates to people and studies. No attempt is made to present an in-depth analysis of these influences but, rather, to focus on their major impact. The leaders are presented in chronological order by date of birth. The studies are presented in chronological order by date of publication.

At the completion of the chapter, the reader will be able to

1. Identify selected early nursing leaders.
2. Relate selected nursing leaders to their major influence on the nursing profession.
3. Recognize selected studies, proposals, and positions which have influenced nursing.
4. Discuss the impact of selected studies, proposals, and positions on the development of nursing.

NURSING LEADERS

In order to appreciate these early leaders and their accomplishments, one needs to consider the era in which they functioned. For our purposes, this era (1800–early 1900s) includes the general state of the times, the status of women, and the state of nursing.

During this time, the industrial revolution was in full force. As a result, the life style of the population was undergoing massive change: cities were growing with inadequate food and housing; and epidemics of infectious diseases were rampant, with a shortage of trained and untrained doctors and nurses. Life was particularly harsh for women and children of the poor. While the industrial revolution produced these horrendous conditions, it also produced the wealth that would lead to improvements for all. Given the state of the times and the status of women, it is amazing these leaders were able to accomplish as much as they did. For example, they started schools of nursing at a time when many people believed that women should not be educated. They obtained licensure legislation in most states when women could not vote. While most of these early leaders had good classical or liberal educations, some had no opportunity to attend schools of nursing. Those who did were among some of the earliest graduates from the newly formed schools of nursing.

Dorothea Dix (1802-1887)

Born in New England to a wealthy family, Dorothea Dix was a school teacher in a New England private school until almost forty years of age. In addition to teaching school, she also taught Sunday School lessons in jails. In these settings Dix was appalled by the conditions and treatment of both the insane and the imprisoned criminal. However, she was not stimulated to change conditions until she herself suffered a major trauma. With the public school movement, Dix lost her job and subsequently suffered a physical breakdown. To recover from her illness, she went abroad. Upon her return to the United States a year later, she started a twenty-year battle that produced markedly improved conditions and nursing care of the mentally ill. From this battle, Dix became a well-known humanitarian.

With the advent of the Civil War, Dix volunteered her services as a nurse. While a volunteer nurse, she was appointed, at age sixty, as the Superintendent of Female Nurses in the U.S. Sanitary Commission. In this position, Dix set the first standards for Army nurses. These standards included thirty years old, plain dress, plain hair, no jewelry, and dark-colored clothing, as well as good morals and common sense.

Florence Nightingale (1820-1910)

Florence Nightingale is considered the founder of modern nursing. She established nursing as a field of study requiring a planned program of preparation. Books have been written on her life and recent articles recount her accomplishments (Woodham-Smith, 1951; Kalisch & Kalisch, 1983; Palmer, 1983).

Born to wealthy parents, Nightingale was directly influenced by her father who provided an education for his two daughters in the classics, mathematics, philosophy, and languages. Given the Victorian era in which she lived, this was a considerable feat. Nightingale was also exposed to intellectual stimulation and varied cultural pursuits through the people visiting at home and travel abroad.

Being from a wealthy family and considering the status of nursing, Nightingale's parents were opposed to her becoming a nurse. Her mother believed she should take her rightful place in society. Nightingale, however, believed that women had an obligation to contribute to the betterment of society. Every opportunity that presented itself was taken to increase and stimulate her pursuit of a nursing career. Her frequent contact with care givers from a variety of countries increased her knowledge and interest in nursing; however, she limited her nursing practice to family members.

Under the guise of going to Germany to assist her sick sister, Nightingale spent three months studying at Kaiserswerth. When she returned to England, she became superintendent of a charity hospital.

Nightingale became involved in military nursing when England, France, and Turkey declared war on Russia. Nightingale went to the Crimea and was dismayed when she observed the conditions. She used all the skills she possessed to effect change. Her accomplishments in the Crimean War established her reputation as an administrator and reformer. In addition, she is also credited with being the first nurse researcher. Upon her return, she used facts, figures, and her observations to support recommendations for improvement of nursing care. It is interesting to note that her total nursing experience was three years. After that her time was spent in organization and administration (Palmer, 1983).

Based on her recommendation, the Nightingale Fund was established to start a training school for nurses. By 1860, the first class began their program. The first fifteen students found themselves in a highly supervised environment. Nightingale believed that the strict discipline was necessary to establish respect for these new nurses. The organization and the curriculum of the school became the model for schools of nursing on several continents.

While Nightingale is noted for her contribution to the concept of an educated nurse, much conflict surrounds why she did some of the things she did. She has been portrayed in a variety of ways in the media and her personality analyzed by many (Kalisch & Kalisch, 1983). What did she do to arouse so many people today? First, she placed nursing directly under the control of medicine and hospital administration. Secondly, she did not emphasize the importance of independent practice. Thirdly, she established nursing as belonging to the servant class by nature of the hours of service and dress; and lastly, she emphasized strict discipline and obedience (Palmer, 1983).

Why then do people so honor Florence Nightingale today? Why does she remain our most famous leader? She overcame social obstacles to elevate the status of nursing from what it was. She made revolutionary changes in the educational system for nurses by her belief in separation of school and hospital, that control over the nursing school rests with the matron, and that nurses needed to be educated. She made contributions to the development of nursing theory through her publications and research. Much can be learned today by analyzing her methods of change and beliefs about nursing.

Clara Barton (1821-1912)

The American Red Cross, which is so well known to the general public for its relief efforts in times of disasters as well as its many public education courses, began in this country through the efforts of Clara Barton. Barton was a former school teacher who volunteered her services as a nurse during the Civil War. As a nurse she directed relief operations and occasionally provided nursing care. The Civil War gave her the opportunity to observe the health problems related to war; however, it was a trip to Europe after the war that gave her the opportunity to observe first hand the advantages of the Red Cross in dealing with these problems.

Convinced that the United States needed a Red Cross, Barton lobbied successfully to persuade Congress to ratify the Treaty of Geneva (1882). She served as a relief worker with the Red Cross during several disasters: the yellow fever epidemic in 1888 and the Johnstown Flood in 1889. In addition to her assistance during disasters, she was also instrumental in establishing a training course for nurses serving with the Red Cross. Her efforts were directed to formation of the Red Cross. She was not actively involved with the nursing leaders' efforts to promote the profession of nursing.

Melinda Ann (Linda) Richards (1841-1930)

Linda Richards, famous for being America's first trained nurse, was born in New York in 1841. As a young girl she was known as a born nurse. Born nurses were women who had a natural instinct for ministering to the sick, making keen observations, and giving sympathy.

Prior to being admitted to the New England Hospital for Women and Children in Roxbury, Massachusetts, she was a nurse at Boston City Hospital. She was greatly disappointed in the role of the nurse—a handmaiden lacking education. She refused a position of head nurse claiming she needed more education. In mid August 1872, she was the first student admitted to the New England Hospital School of Nursing (Dolan, et al., 1983).

The program Linda Richards entered was one year in length and included twelve lectures by doctors. Students spent three months each in medical nursing, surgical nursing, and maternity nursing, two months doing private duty, and one month working nights (Richards, 1915). No other theory was presented and no textbooks existed. Students conducted classes on their own time to share experiences. The days started at 5:30 AM and ended at 9:00 PM. Students slept in little rooms off the wards and many times awoke several times during the night to provide care. In 1873, Richards received the first diploma granted to a nurse in the United States. Upon graduation, she became the night supervisor at Bellevue Hospital. She is credited with starting several training schools in the United States and Japan. She served as the first president of the American Society of Superintendents of Training Schools and worked long and hard to improve the education of nurses.

It is interesting to note that she was called the first trained nurse, not educated. Many people today refer to nursing education as nursing training. What implications can you draw from use of the word training instead of education?

Mary Mahoney (1845-1926)

Mary Mahoney was born in the free state of Massachusetts sixteen years before the Civil War. She became interested in nursing at the age of eighteen; however, the only occupation open to black women at this time was domestic service. After being rejected by several other schools, she was admitted to the New England Hospital for Women and Children (Chayer, 1954). On August 1, 1879, Mahoney, at the age of thirty-four, graduated from nursing school after sixteen months of study. Her course of study was similar to Linda Richards', i.e., rotating through the various services; however, Mahoney spent additional time in private duty nursing in homes around Boston. Thirty-nine other students were admitted with Mahoney. She was considered an excellent student as demonstrated by the fact that she was one of the four applicants who graduated.

Mahoney's professional life was spent as a private duty nurse in the Boston area. Although she served as a model for other black nurses, discrimination among the general public as well as in nursing continued. Many schools of nursing did not accept black nurses. Black nurses especially in the South were forced to go to segregated nursing schools. The quality of these schools ranged from excellent to very poor.

Mahoney served as the chaplain to the National Association of Colored Graduate Nurses, and she spent time furthering the cause of black nurses. As a tribute to Mahoney, the Mary Mahoney Award was established in 1936 by the National Association of Colored Graduates, and she gave the opening address at the first conference of this association. This award is currently given by the ANA.

Mary Adelaide Nutting (1858-1948)

Mary Adelaide Nutting, thought by many to be second only to Florence Nightingale in her influence on nursing, was born in Canada in 1858

(Christy, 1969). Like many of our early leaders, she was born into a prominent family and received her early education in private schools. Nutting was exposed to a liberal education, was schooled in the arts, piano, and voice, and spent her early years traveling.

Her interest in nursing was stimulated by the care she gave her mother during a terminal illness. At the age of thirty-one, she applied and was accepted at Johns Hopkins School of Nursing. Immediately after graduation (1891), she became a head nurse on a medical ward at Johns Hopkins. By 1894, she was superintendent of the school of nursing. While this quick advancement was common in the early 1900s, it is virtually impossible today for a nurse to go from student to director of a nursing program in three years.

Nutting was active in social and professional activities early in her professional career. She served twice as president of the American Society of Superintendents of Training Schools and several times as the secretary. She was also active in the public health movement and establishment of an international council of nurses, but her most noted contribution to nursing is in the area of nursing education.

Nutting was the first professor of nursing at Teachers College, Columbia University (1907), where she remained until 1925. Her goal for nursing education was to establish university education as the base for nursing. Some of her accomplishments towards this goal included expanding the nursing program to three years, establishing a preclinical period where theory was taught, limiting the day to eight hours, introducing social subjects into the curriculum, requiring tuition, setting up scholarships and loans and paying faculty. In working with her peers and students, she encouraged and supported intellectual skills, a broad knowledge base, and a commitment to research and publication.

Acknowledging her contributions to nursing education, especially baccalaureate education, the NLN set up the M. A. Nutting Award for excellence in nursing education. She received the first award. In addition, she was listed by the American Association of University Professors for her contributions to nursing and education. Her honors go on and on. Nutting, indeed, was a nursing leader with much foresight and drive.

Lavinia Dock (1858–1956)

Lavinia Dock, frequently referred to as a feminine activist, was born in Harrisburg, Pennsylvania, in 1858. She was one of six children born into a cultivated, well-to-do family. Her parents were well educated for the times and liberal in their thinking. Lavinia Dock was educated in private schools but was described by her teachers as lacking in ambition and application.

Dock's interest in nursing stems from her experiences in caring for her sick mother and an article about infection written by Isabel Robb, a famous nursing leader. She entered Bellevue Hospital School of Nursing in 1884 at the age of twenty-eight and graduated in 1886. Friends of the family were shocked at this decision because ladies did not work outside the home.

Upon graduation, Dock worked as a night supervisor at Bellevue, typical of graduates at this time. While in that position, she wrote one of the first nursing textbooks, *Materia Medica for Nurses*. She held several other positions during her career, including assistant to Isabel Hampton Robb at Johns Hopkins Training School, Baltimore, Maryland, and was one of the early nurses at the Henry Street Settlement.

Her contributions to nursing include a noted history of nursing book, secretary of the International Council of Nurses, secretary of the American Society of Superintendents, and editor of the foreign department for AJN for twenty years. She also helped improve nursing through assisting in the passage of the suffrage amendment and nurse practice acts. Dock devoted her last twenty years to improvements of the status of women and the poor. She believed in organizational efforts to improve conditions, as evident through her participation in a wide variety of organizations.

While Dock was modest about her accomplishments, she was an excellent role model for exerting change through legislation. The ICN established a Lavinia Dock Fund to help finance exchange of ideas among nurses at the international level.

Isabel Hampton Robb (1860-1910)

Isabel Robb, born in Ontario, was a teacher for three years before becoming a nurse. She entered Bellevue Hospital Training School for Nurses in 1881 at the age of twenty-one, making her younger than most of the other leaders at the time they entered nursing. She, like many other leaders, had traveled abroad.

Professionally, she served as superintendent of the Illinois Training School in Chicago and Johns Hopkins Training School. She introduced new concepts to the educational scene, such as grading the students, affiliations to other institutions for specific clinical experiences, and granting school holidays and vacations.

The professional community mourned the loss of Robb when she married and retired from nursing in 1894. As the custom of the day, Robb was never again employed as a nurse. However, some of her greatest contributions to nursing came after her marriage. She is noted for founding the two professional nursing societies in America, serving as the first president of the forerunner to the ANA. In addition, she authored several textbooks and was involved in teaching the hospital economics course at Teachers College, Columbia University, in New York. Her untimely accidental death was a great loss to the nursing profession.

Lillian Wald (1867-1940)

Lillian Wald, born in Cincinnati, Ohio in 1867, is best noted for her founding of the Henry Street Visiting Nurse Service in New York City. This was the first public health nursing service in the United States.

Professionally, Wald began her education at New York Hospital Training School in 1891 at the age of twenty-four. Her first assignment was as a graduate nurse in a Juvenile Asylum in New York. She was appalled at the conditions and treatment of the immigrants. Wald attended medical school for a while but decided that her love was nursing. In 1893, with the financial help of two wealthy friends, the Henry Street Settlement was opened.

Wald's contributions to nursing include organizing and serving as the first president of the National Organization of Public Health Nursing, serving actively on many committees related to public health nursing and social welfare, serving as a stimulus for the first college course offered in public health nursing at Teachers College, and writing two books on the Henry Street Settlement.

EDUCATIONAL STUDIES

Nursing and Nursing Education in the United States (Goldmark Report 1923)

Nursing leaders in the early 1900s were aware that nursing was facing a variety of problems. Proliferation of nursing schools of questionable quality, poor quality nursing care, and lack of placement for graduate nurses were three of these problems. Since one of the obvious problems facing nursing was the inconsistent quality of education offered, it was believed that if this problem could be documented a solution would be found.

A committee chaired by C. A. Winslow, professor of public health at Yale University, was established with funds from the Rockefeller Foundation. This committee was comprised of six nurses, ten physicians, one public health administrator, and three lay persons. The committee decided the scope of the investigation should include nursing education in general, not just the preparation of the public health nurse, and Josephine Goldmark was employed as the researcher (Goldmark, 1923). This report titled *Nursing and Nursing Education in the United States* (Goldmark Report) is significant in what it did as well as what it did not recommend. Ten recommendations were made.

Although the report did document a number of poor educational practices, no recommendation was made to move schools of nursing out of the hospital setting. A suggestion was given that the schools be separated from hospitals by separate governing boards and that the objective of the schools should be education, not service. However, university education was not recommended except for a small body of nursing leaders.

> It should be made quite clear that the Committee does not recommend that nursing schools in general should work toward the establishment of courses of character that a university would accept for a degree.... The value we see at present in the university schools is that they will furnish a body of leaders who have the fundamental training essential in administrators, teachers, and the like. (Goldmark, 1923, p. 26)

While the Goldmark Report did not recommend university education for most nurses, two university schools were endowed as a direct result of this study. These were the Yale University School of Nursing in 1924 and Vanderbilt University School of Nursing in 1930 (Deloughery, 1977).

A second result of the Goldmark Report was a revision of the National League of Nursing Education curriculum guide. The revised guide, *Curriculum for Schools of Nursing*, was issued in 1927 and tried to include many of the Goldmark Report recommendations. Since this revised guide was seen by many faculty as the bible of nursing education, it did influence the quality of education in many of the schools (Dolan, et al., 1983). Finally, the Goldmark Report influenced the establishment of yet another committee, the Committee on the Grading of Nursing Schools. Many nursing leaders were disappointed that this study did not revolutionize nursing education, like the Flexner Report did for medicine. The Flexner report changed medical education from a diploma mill set-up to a university discipline within a decade.

Nursing Schools, Today and Tomorrow (1934)

The Committee on the Grading of Nursing Schools was formed for the purpose of studying "... ways of insuring an ample supply of adequately trained nursing personnel who could render quality care at a reasonable price" (Flanagan, 1976, p. 83). This purpose defined the three areas that encompassed the scope of the study:

1. The supply and demand for nursing service.
2. A job analysis of nursing practice and nursing education.
3. The grading of schools of nursing. (Goostray, 1969, p. 91)

This committee was composed of two representatives from each of the three nursing organizations—ANA, NLN, and NOPHN; one representative from the American Medical Association (AMA), the American College of Surgeons, the American Hospital Association, the American Public Health Association; four representatives from university education; and three members at large (Committee on the Grading of Nursing Schools, 1934). The committee functioned over the next eight years and issued three reports. The first report dealing with the supply and demand of nurses, *Nurses, Patients and Pocketbooks,* was issued in 1928. The report concluded that although the country was experiencing an over supply of nurses, there was a shortage of adequately prepared nurses. The second report was titled *An Activity Analysis of Nursing* and was published in 1934.

The final report of the Committee's eight-year study, *Nursing Schools Today and Tomorrow,* went into great detail on the problems involved in nursing education. The practical results of this study were a smaller number of better schools and the closing of some of the poorer schools. The schools were further guided towards improvement by the third of the National League of Nursing Education curriculum guides. The guide issued in 1937 and titled *A Curriculum Guide for Schools of Nursing* called for a broader and enriched presentation of scientific and nursing content (Dolan, et al., 1983).

Considering the name of the Committee on Grading of Nursing Schools, it is interesting to note they never graded the schools. However, they did produce much of the ground work for accreditation. Table 3-1 presents a com-

TABLE 3-1
Comparison of selected essentials and criteria for quality nursing programs

Essential for Basic Professional Schools*	NLN Criteria for Accreditation**
FACULTY	
Majority of faculty should have a nursing background	Faculty are academically and professionally qualified: meet the institution's requirements for faculty appointment; they have graduate preparation and experience appropriate to their areas of responsibility; and they continue to improve expertise in areas of responsibility
Graduate of college	
Teaching ability	
Special training in the subject teaching	
Practice experience	
STUDENTS	
Entrance requirements should be those of the college or university	Qualified applicants are admitted
Students have ability to do work	
Students should abide by university policies	The general policies in school of nursing are consistent with those of the university
ORGANIZATION AND ADMINISTRATION	
Program under the control of nursing	The school is administered by a nurse educator
Independently financed	
	The school receives financial support

*Committee on the Grading of Nursing Schools. *Nursing Schools Today and Tomorrow.* New York: National League of Nursing Education, 1934.

**National League for Nursing. *NLN Criteria for the appraisal of baccalaureate and higher degree programs.* New York: National League for Nursing, 1977. Note: These criteria are currently under revision.

parison of some of the essentials of a good nursing school identified in 1934 and NLN criteria for accrediting of nursing programs today.

Nursing for the Future (Brown Report, 1948)

The most important change in nursing education between 1945 and 1960 was in the role of collegiate education. Before 1945, the main purpose of this type of education was the preparation of nursing leaders. By 1960, colleges and universities had started to become the setting for the preparation of the beginning practitioner. The first major study or report to recommend this change was known as the *Brown Report* or *Nursing for the Future*, published in 1948.

After World War II, the nation had neither the quality nor quantity of nurses necessary to meet the needs of society. Application was made to the Carnegie Corporation to finance a study investigating the causes of these problems. Esther Brown, PhD, a social anthropologist at the Russell Sage Foundation, was appointed to conduct this study. The final report contained twenty-eight recommendations covering the areas of nursing service, future role of nurses, education for nonprofessional nurses, education for professional nurses, and resources for the future. Three of these recommendations regarding professional nursing education stand out:

1. Schools of nursing become affiliated with universities.
2. Professional nurses be educated at the baccalaureate level and practical nurses be educated in two-year vocational programs.
3. Schools of nursing be officially examined and accredited. (Brown, 1948)

Many physicians and hospital administrators reacted negatively to these recommendations. They believed the report represented an attempt by nurses to seek economic security (Davis Graham, 1948). However, by 1960, many of these recommendations had started to become reality. Many American college and university schools of nursing had their origins in the 1950s as a result of this report. A committee was formed and charged with developing a plan to propose and implement solutions to the problem areas in nursing.

Nursing Schools at Mid Century (1950)

Instituted by the Joint Committee on Implementing the Brown Report (name changed to National Committee for the Improvement of Nursing Services in 1949), the purpose of this study was to analyze the practices in schools of nursing. Recall the purpose of this committee was to implement the recommendation of the Brown Report, i.e., to improve schools of nursing to meet the needs of society for more and better educated nurses. To accomplish this task, a questionnaire was developed and administered to schools of nursing to determine their current practices. Criteria for analyzing this data were established. Those schools in the top 25 percent were placed in group 1; those in the next 50 percent were placed in group 2; and in the last 25 percent in group 3. However, group 3 schools were not listed. In November 1949, the Interim Classification of Schools of Nursing Offering Basic Programs was published in the *American Journal of Nursing*. This publication resulted in much misunderstanding; many people believed the intent of the report was to close diploma schools and not to stimulate schools to raise their standards.

What impact did this study have on nursing education? This study influenced the accreditation procedures. Early in 1949, the National Nursing Accreditation Service Organization accepted responsibility for the accreditation process. This study provided a base for these procedures.

Collegiate Education for Nurses (1953)

Dr. Margaret Bridgman, a noted educational researcher and academic dean of Skidmore College in New York, was contracted by the Russell Sage Foundation in 1949 to provide a consultation service to college and university faculty and administration interested in improving their nursing programs. In 1952, she worked with the NLN Accrediting Service in conducting an extensive study of collegiate programs in nursing. This study revealed many weaknesses in these educational programs.

To correct the problems, Bridgman identified many responsibilities that colleges and universities should assume if they offer a nursing program. These responsibilities related to space and equipment, faculty, curriculum, financial support, students, and graduates. Many of the school programs offered no or little upper division nursing courses (courses taken in the junior and senior years). Bridgman disagreed with this practice stating:

> The purpose for which higher education is sought is to heighten the qualifications of candidates for professional functions. This purpose is defeated unless policies applied to nursing are consistent with general standards of colleges and universities, nursing students receive the benefits of genuine college education, and nursing degrees are authentically representative of the completion of an upper-division major in the degree-granting institution. (Bridgman, 1953, p. 97)

In this study, Bridgman emphasized the need for upper division courses in nursing. The impact of this study was that it served as an impetus for the improvement of baccalaureate education.

Community College Education for Nursing (1959)

Mildred Montag, EdD, noted for the impetus she gave to the associate degree movement, studied the differences in nursing functions in 1951. These functions ranged on a continuum from assisting to technical to professional. It was the technical functions that interested her the most. How do you prepare the nursing technician? This study resulted in a publication titled *The Education of Nursing Technicians*.

This study was timely in that nursing was experiencing a shortage of qualified nurses to staff the hospitals. Many people believed there was a better and quicker way to educate the nurse who was needed to perform these technical skills. In 1952, an advisory committee established by the American Association of Junior Colleges and the NLN was charged with examining the problems confronting nursing, proposing solutions to these problems, and differentiating the various functions of the nurse. A research study was designed to examine the feasibility of educating this technical nurse in two-year community and junior colleges. The research project ran for five years and involved seven community and junior colleges. In 1958, the results of the five-year study indicated that it indeed was feasible to prepare this technical nurse in two years. This, however, was seen as a terminal degree and did not prepare the nurse to complete two more years and receive a bachelor of science in nursing degree (BSN).

The impact of this study was that it assisted the movement to place nursing education in the mainstream of our educational system. This study created an uproar in the hospital schools of nursing and angered many of the diploma nurses who had graduated from these schools. Many nurses questioned the clinical competence of these nurses, feeling that the diploma nurse was more technically competent than the associate-degree graduate. However, by 1980, there were over 707 associate degree (AD) programs in the United States.

An ANA Position Paper on Education for Nursing (1965 Position Paper)

Although this position paper is not a study, it was the result of many years of self-study and is many times referred to as a landmark position. Since one of the purposes of the ANA is to promote professional and educational advances of nurses, it is only appropriate that the ANA have a position on education.

In 1960, the ANA's Committee on Current and Long-Term Goals recommended that the basic educational level for the professional nurse be a baccalaureate degree (Fitzpatrick, 1983). This goal was adopted for study by the ANA and supported at the 1964 convention. In addition the Committee on Education was formed in 1962 and charged with developing basic educational principles that would result in competent nurses.

The Committee on Education wrote the first position paper in 1965. This position paper was accepted by the ANA Board in September 1965. What was this famous position? Basically, the position was that education for nurses should take place in institutions of learning within the general system of education and that the minimum preparation for the professional nurse should be the BSN; for the technical nurse the AD; and for the assistants, a certificate from a vocational program (ANA, 1965). The paper goes on to present many assumptions explaining the position.

This paper aroused intense controversy within the profession, which continues today. Instead of leading to a plan for implementation, the position paper resulted in widening the gap in nursing education. While many diploma schools closed between 1965 and the present, some nursing educators, hospital administrators, and physicians continue to support diploma school education.

An Abstract for Action; From Abstract into Action; and Action in Affirmation: Toward an Unambiguous Profession (Lysaught Reports, 1970, 1973, and 1981)

In 1961, the Surgeon General of the United States Public Health Service appointed a consultative group on nursing to advise him on nursing needs and the appropriate government role. Their report, *Towards Quality in Nursing: Needs and Goals*, was issued in 1963. One of the recommendations made was for a study of the nursing education system to determine the responsibilities and skills needed to provide quality nursing care. This report served as a stimulus for the establishment of the National Commission for the Study of Nursing and Nursing Education. This commission was an independent agency funded by the American Nurses' Foundation, the Kellogg Foundation, and the Avalon Foundation and an anonymous benefactor. Over the next three years, the commission planned and implemented a study of (1) the supply and demand for nurses, (2) nursing roles and functions, (3) nursing education, and (4) nurses' careers. The results of this study, *An Abstract for Action*, was published in 1970, and contained fifty-eight recommendations addressing four priorities: increased research, improved education, clarification of roles, and increased financial support (Lysaught, 1970, pp. 1-23).

As the mood of the country turned more conservative, a follow-up report was done on the study. This follow-up report, issued in 1973, was called *From Abstract into Action* and described efforts to implement the original study. This implementation phase emphasized three areas: development and expansion of nursing practice, re-patterning of the educational system, and emergence of an unambiguous profession (Lysaught, 1973). As a result of the implementation phase, joint practice commissions between nursing and medicine were established, master planning committees were established in nine target states; and the second report was published.

In 1981, *Action in Affirmation: Toward an Unambiguous Profession of Nursing* was published. This was a follow-up on the recommendations made in the original report. These series of reports received mixed reaction from the nursing profession and other health professionals. Many people felt that nothing new was recommended. This study concluded that slow but steady progress is being made in the nursing profession, but much is yet to be done. Additional recommendations were given regarding research, collegiate education, and certification (Lysaught, 1981).

Nursing Roles—Scope and Preparation
(NLN 1982 Position Statement)

While this position statement is not a study, it is the result of the NLN's commitment to quality nursing and health care. In line with this commitment is the commitment to quality education for professional nurses who provide the nursing care.

This position statement was approved in February 1982. This historic statement was

> ... professional nursing practice requires the minimum of a baccalaureate degree with a major in nursing. Preparation for technical nursing practice requires an associate degree or a diploma in nursing. Preparation for vocational nursing requires a certificate or diploma in vocational/practical nursing. (*NLN Position Statement on Nursing Roles—Scope and Preparation*, 1982, p. 1)

This position brings nursing in line with other professionals on the health team such as dietitians, social workers, and physical therapists, who all begin with the baccalaureate degree as the basic educational preparation. However, this statement caused a fury among the membership. Diploma programs threatened to withdraw their membership while baccalaureate programs were pleased that the NLN had finally taken a stand on education. Finally, at the 1983 biennial convention in Philadelphia, the membership supported this position statement. Although the impact of this support is yet to be seen, it should be noted that this position is for nurses prepared in the future and will not discredit nurses presently licensed as registered nurses.

SUMMARY

This chapter presented the development of nursing by reviewing the impact of early leaders and selected studies on nursing. The focus of this chapter was historical in nature, so no attempt was made to analyze the impact of some of our current nursing leaders. The contributions of each of these early leaders was presented as well as some personal and professional data. When looking at some of these early leaders several points seem to stand out

1. Many of these leaders were from wealthy to upper middle class families with contacts in high places.
2. The education of these leaders included private schools and liberalizing courses, i.e., classics, philosophy, and travel abroad.
3. Several of the leaders became interested in nursing after personal experiences with the health care system.
4. Almost all of these leaders entered nursing at an older age than is common today.
5. All of these leaders were women, all but one remained single.

6. Advancement in nursing was rapid, i.e., from graduation to night supervisor to director of a nursing service or program within 3 to 10 years.
7. Many of these leaders were atypical of women of their time. Although the personalities of these early leaders were different, they all possessed some characteristics that made them leaders.

Although each of these leaders contributed to nursing, so too did a variety of studies.

Each selected study was presented with emphasis on the findings and impact the study had on the development of nursing. When viewing these studies the major point that stands out is that nursing has been studied by a variety of people and through a variety of time periods and, although many recommendations were made, change in nursing was slow to occur. No one study had the impact on nursing as the Flexner Report did on medicine. Some additional points that should be remembered are

1. Many of these studies were conducted by nonnurses. Each of them had nurse members on the committee as well as other health care providers and lay persons.
2. Most of these studies had financial support from private foundations, professional organizations, or the government.
3. All of these studies made multiple recommendations, but only one to three of the recommendations gained national attention.
4. Many of these studies created a controversy both within and outside the nursing profession.

REFERENCES

"American Nurses' Association First Position Paper on Education for Nursing." *American Journal of Nursing* 65 (1965): 106–111.

"ANA's First Position Paper on Education for Nursing." *American Journal of Nursing* 66 (1966): 515–517.

Bridgman, M. *Collegiate Education for Nursing.* New York: Russell Sage Foundation, 1953.

Bridgman, M. "Patterns of Collegiate Nursing Education." *Nursing Outlook* 1 (1953): 525–528.

Brown, E. L. *Nursing for the Future.* New York: Russell Sage Foundation, 1948.

Burgess, A. *Nurses, Patients, and Pocketbooks.* New York: Committee on the Grading of Nursing Schools, 1928.

Chayer, M. "Mary Elizabeth Mahoney." *American Journal of Nursing* 54 (1954): 429–431.

Christy, T. "Portrait of a Leader: Isabel Hampton Robb." *Nursing Outlook* 17 (3) [1969]: 26–29.

Christy, T. "Portrait of a Leader: Lavinia Lloyd Dock." *Nursing Outlook* 17 (6) [1969]: 72–75.

Christy, T. "Portrait of a Leader: M. Adelaide Nutting." *Nursing Outlook* 17 (1) [1969]: 20–24.

Committee on the Grading of Nursing Schools. *Nursing Schools Today and Tomorrow*. New York: National League for Nursing Education, 1934.

"Davis Graham Attacks Brown Report on 'Nursing for the Future,' " *Modern Hospital* 71 (1948): 138.

Deloughery, Grace S. *History and Trends of Professional Nursing*. 8th ed. St. Louis: C. V. Mosby Co., 1977.

Dock, L. "Lavinia L. Dock: Self-Portrait." *Nursing Outlook* 25 (1977): 22–23.

Dolan, J., Fitzpatrick, M., and Herrmann, E. *Nursing in Society: A Historical Perspective*. Philadelphia: W. B. Saunders, 1983.

Elmore, J. "Black Nurses: Their Service and Their Struggle." *American Journal of Nursing* 76 (1976): 435–437.

Fitzpatrick, M. *Prologue to Professionalism*. Bowie, MD: Robert J. Brady Co., 1983.

Flanagan, L. *One Strong Voice: The Story of the American Nurses Association*. Kansas City: American Nurses' Association, 1976.

Goldmark, J. *Nursing and Nursing Education in the United States*. Report of the Committee for the Study of Nursing Education. New York: The Macmillan Co., 1923.

Goostray, S. "Mary Adelaide Nutting." *American Journal of Nursing* 58 (1958): 1524–1529.

Goostray, S. *Memoirs: Half a Century in Nursing*. Boston: Nursing Archive, Boston University Mugar Memorial Library, 1969.

Kalisch, B., and Kalisch, P. "Heroine Out of Focus: Media Images of Florence Nightingale." *Nursing and Health Care* 4 (1983): 270–278.

Kalisch, P., and Kalisch, B. *The Advance of American Nursing*. Boston: Little, Brown and Co., 1978.

Kelly, L. *Dimensions of Professional Nursing*. New York: Macmillan Publishing Co., 1981.

Lysaught, J. P. *Action in Affirmation: Toward an Unambiguous Profession of Nursing*. New York: McGraw-Hill Co., 1981.

Lysaught, J. P. *From Abstract into Action*. New York: McGraw-Hill Co., 1973.

Lysaught, J. P. *An Abstract for Action*. Report of the National Commission for the Study of Nursing and Nursing Education. New York: McGraw-Hill Co., 1970.

Montag, M. *Community College Education for Nursing*. New York: McGraw-Hill Co., 1959.

National League for Nursing. *NLN Position Statement on Nursing Roles—Scope and Preparation*. New York: National League for Nursing, 1982.

National League for Nursing. *NLN Criteria for the Appraisal of Baccalaureate and Higher Degree Programs in Nursing*. New York: National League for Nursing, 1977.

Palmer, I. "Nightingale Revisited." *Nursing Outlook* 31 (1983): 229–233.

Richards, L. "Early Days in the First American Training School for Nurses." *American Journal of Nursing* 16 (1915): 173–175.

Roberts, M. "Lavinia Lloyd Dock—Nurse, Feminist, Internationalist." *American Journal of Nursing* 56 (1956): 176–179.

Russell, J., Nevins, G., Wald, L., and Stewart, I. "M. Adelaide Nutting as Known by Friends, Students and Coworkers." *American Journal of Nursing* 15 (1915): 445–454.

West, M., and Hawkins, C. *Nursing Schools at the Mid-Century.* New York: National Committee for the Improvement of Nursing Service, 1950.

Woodham-Smith, C. *Florence Nightingale.* New York: McGraw-Hill Co., 1951.

4

Development of nursing education

To conceptualize anyone functioning in a position of responsibility in today's complex health care system without years of preparation is difficult. Yet just over 120 years ago the only nurses who received preparation were members of religious orders. Educational programs to prepare nurses changed considerably over the years. During this time, nursing educators have attempted to organize nursing content in many ways. This chapter will trace the development of nursing education during these years with an emphasis on two aspects of the development: How did the schools grow and develop and what did they teach? At the completion of the chapter the reader will be able to

1. Describe the development of schools for nursing education from 1860 to the present.
2. Describe the curricular design in these nursing schools.
3. Identify the essential elements of a conceptual framework.
4. Describe the relationship of conceptual frameworks to current curricular designs.

THE ENGLISH INFLUENCE

The development of nursing as a field of study began with one person, Florence Nightingale. Nightingale believed that a prepared practitioner of nursing could influence the health of patients. She demonstrated this belief in two ways: through research and education. Her research documented that as nursing care improved, the death rate of the soldiers decreased dramatically. As a result of her assistance to the British soldiers, funds were made available to begin the school she so firmly believed was necessary for nursing. The Nightingale Training School for Nurses opened in June 1860 with fifteen probationers.

This first secular school of nursing was based on three principles which have since become known as the Nightingale principles of nursing education

1. The school should be associated with a teaching hospital; however, they should have their own endowment and be independent of the hospital's nursing service.
2. The matron (director) of the school must have final authority for the entire program, both the instruction and the living environment.
3. The nursing environment or nursing home should be a place to develop discipline and character.

These principles guided the structure and organization of the school. The formal curriculum was structured to train "sick nurses" and "health nurses" as well as matrons and sisters who were "trained to train" (Notter & Spalding, 1976). Students within the school received one year's training followed by two to three years of supervised practice.

Curricula patterned after the Nightingale model included courses in three areas of study (Anderson, 1981; Roberts, 1954). These three areas of study included courses about technical skills and procedures, rules and principles related to hygiene and sanitation, and a philosophy of nursing. The specific courses within these three broad areas were designed to explain the why, how, and when of nursing. Many of the lectures were given by physicians (Watson, 1977). Missing from this type of program was the process of questioning, conceptualizing, testing, and revising nursing knowledge (Newman, 1979). These three areas of study remain in today's programs but are integrated or disguised in some manner, i.e., hygiene and sanitation could be taught in courses called Nursing I, Epidemiology, or Microbiology. The Nightingale model was the first attempt at organizing nursing's knowledge.

EARLY AMERICAN SCHOOLS

In the United States the Civil War demonstrated the need for skilled nurses, and Nightingale demonstrated how they could be prepared. Against this background, the American Medical Association Committee on Training Nurses, in 1869, recommended that every large well-organized hospital have a school. In 1872, the first training school, New England Hospital for Women and Children, was established. In 1873, three more schools (Bellevue Training School, Connecticut Training School, and Massachusetts General Training School) were opened. Most of these initial schools were founded by courageous physicians who dealt with physician biases against educating nurses. By 1900, over 400 hospital schools had been established (Anderson, 1981; Roberts, 1954).

Many of the beginning schools tried to follow the Nightingale principles but without an independent endowment. Without this money, these schools were soon a part of the hospital organization. In most cases, hospitals found a new source of free or cheap labor. Other hospitals saw this and began creating and conducting schools to serve their needs. The education of the nurse became a by-product of her service to the hospital. Each program had been developed to meet the particular needs of the hospital. There were no standard admission criteria or curriculum guidelines. In fact, in many schools students could be admitted at any time.

Although programs varied in length from one to three years, by 1905 most schools were three years in length. The added time was an economic advantage to the schools. Usually there were small student bodies and no formal faculty. Therefore, clinical instruction, other than that done by the senior student, was the responsibility of the nursing supervisors. This teaching was not planned clinical instruction but rather a part of their supervisory responsibilities. In many of the hospitals, these supervisors consisted of the superintendent, a surgical supervisor, and a night superintendent.

Students usually began their program as probies, a term reserved for the beginning student who may be dismissed for any number of reasons. They were under the close supervision of the head nurse (usually a senior student) and, in some of the better schools, did attend a planned program of classes. If they were successful in making the adjustment to the highly authoritarian atmosphere and long hours of task-oriented practice, they became freshmen for the second half of the first year. Much of the junior year consisted of staff nursing under the direction of the senior nurse. Staff nursing involved not only the direct care of patients but also cooking, cleaning, and almost any other task which might need to be done. Senior students were given increasing responsibilities for the functioning of the unit, including the role of head nurses (Kalisch & Kalisch, 1978).

Theory classes, if they were given, began to use a local pathology approach. Nursing programs using the local pathology approach generally superimposed them on the Nightingale model. Students took courses first in fundamentals (skills and procedures), sciences, and professional nursing and then proceeded to courses about specific diseases such as tuberculosis and polio. Nursing care concepts were tucked in these courses. Since nursing students were being prepared to function in specific institutions, the specific diseases covered varied from school to school. The major problem stemming from this approach seemed to be ignoring the patient. Emphasis was on the disease, not the patient. Other problems arose when the number of identified diseases increased and when social sciences began to identify aspects of man which were important to patients' health but were not disease related.

The rapid expansion of these schools which varied greatly in quality resulted in increased concern among the nurses and public regarding the quality of care being given. Many nursing leaders began to look for ways to provide better and more effective education for future nurses.

Nursing's search for help in improving schools of nursing through improvement of the curricula led to the publication of a *Standard Curriculum for Schools of Nursing* (NLN, 1918). In this standard, it was noted that the major weakness in nursing programs related to the lack of a theoretical foundation on which to build good nursing practice. This curriculum guide became a standard adopted by many schools of nursing. Some interesting points from this guide are presented below

1. The class day should not exceed ten hours.
2. All students should have a probationary period of at least four months.
3. Specific courses and organization should include basic sciences, elementary nursing, history of nursing, pathology, medical nursing, surgical nursing, infant and child nursing, communicable disease nursing, obstetrical nursing, psychiatric nursing, public sanitation, modern social conditions, and professional problems.

Many schools followed this guide as well as the subsequent guides developed (NLN, 1927; NLN, 1937). The approach used by many schools of nursing in revising their curricula was the patchwork approach. Since these guides did not dictate the arrangement or sequences of courses, the schools could organize the content in any manner. The NLN guide reflected, among other things, nursing's attempt to deal with the need for an organizational structure for the curriculum. The approach suggested in this guide has been referred to as the patient care areas approach.

The patient care areas approach was an attempt by many nursing educators to organize some of the diseases together by the way they were arranged clinically. Since this approach seemed to work for medicine, many believed it would be equally effective for nursing. The curriculum included studying diseases, which were taught in courses titled medical nursing, surgical nursing, pediatric nursing, obstetrical nursing, and psychiatric nursing. Many residuals of this approach exist today as evidenced by achievement tests, graduate school departments, and certification areas. Specific problems with this approach included scheduling rotations, duplication of diseases covered, focus on illness rather than nursing care, and compartmentalization of care. Many programs attempted to deal with some of these problems by adding the body systems approach to the patient care area approach.

The body systems approach attempted to decrease the duplication of diseases taught by organizing them according to body systems. It was believed that since systems respond similarly to disruptions, diseases could be grouped. However, this approach did not eliminate the problems related to illness orientation, lack of focus on nursing care, or schedule rotations. Additional problems included losing sight of the whole person and the overlapping nature of some systems.

What seemed to be missing from these three approaches was lack of emphasis on nursing and the patient. Emphasis was on the disease process. The amount of knowledge specifically related to nursing was increasing, but was not being included in the nursing courses. The lectures covered etiology, pathology, diagnosis, medical treatment, and, lastly, nursing care. Many lectures were given by physicians, and many times no time was left for presenting nursing care. These curricular designs and the related problems continued to plague nursing into the 1950s and 1960s.

Although these curricula continued to evolve and were an improvement over what was, one of the reasons that attempts to improve the quality of nursing education became severely limited was due to the rapid growth in hospital schools of nursing. This rapid growth of nursing schools of limited quality came to an end with the Great Depression. In 1929, there were 1,885 schools; by 1941, this had decreased to 1,311 (Bullough & Bullough, 1978). The increased emphasis on quality education, along with the move of nurses into the hospitals, made the schools more expensive and less a source of cheap labor for the hospitals.

Much of the documentation for the increased emphasis on quality education came from the Committee on Grading of Nursing Schools. The final report of the Committee's eight year study, *Nursing Schools Today and Tomorrow*, went into great detail on the problems involved in nursing education. The practical results of this study was a smaller number of better schools. The schools were further guided towards improvement by the third of the National League of Nursing Education's curricular guides. The guide, issued in 1937 and titled *A Curriculum Guide for Schools of Nursing*, called for a broader and enriched presentation of scientific and nursing content (Dolan, Fitzpatrick, & Herrmann, 1983).

UNIVERSITY EDUCATION

Although the just described hospital-based diploma programs were declining in the 1930s, university programs were showing a steady pattern of growth. University programs had their beginning at Teachers College, Columbia University in 1899. This first program, which did not offer a degree but a certificate, existed to prepare graduate nurses for administrative or teaching positions.

It was not until 1909 that a lasting basic nursing program affiliated with a university was established. This program, at the University of Minnesota, was initially a diploma program. Students had to meet university admission standards but were graduated in three years with a diploma and not a degree. The first degree option was made available to basic nursing students in 1916 at the University of Cincinnati and Columbia Teachers College (Anderson, 1981). By 1939, there were seventy-five basic nursing programs in universities (ANA, 1943). Most of these programs were five years in length: three years of nursing and two years of liberal arts. The purpose of these basic nursing programs was to prepare leaders. Graduates were expected to function in supervisory or teaching positions. Graduate education had its beginning in 1932 when Catholic University offered graduate courses for nurses. In 1935, their program was approved as a master's degree in nursing education (Grippando, 1977). However, Catholic University was not the first to offer a graduate degree. Yale and Western Reserve University had both established their master's program a year earlier. When these initial graduate programs opened, a great deal of controversy existed concerning their purpose. Visionary nursing leaders believed that the beginning practitioner of nursing should be prepared at the baccalaureate level and that nursing leaders should be prepared at the graduate level.

MID CENTURY

By mid century, a number of trends can be identified. While diploma schools were decreasing, university programs, both basic and graduate, were growing (see Table 4–1). The significance of these events is that nursing education had truly begun its move out of the hospitals and into the universities. Schools of practical nursing, which had existed since the turn of the century, proliferated after World War II. In turn by 1960, all states had licensure laws regulating the practice of the practical nurse (Bullough & Bullough, 1978).

While the practical nurse movement increased the number of bedside nurses, it was not sufficient to meet the overall demand for hospital nurses. In 1952, the associate degree nurse came into being. The associate degree movement began as a national research project under the direction of Mildred Montag, EdD. The purpose of the project was to develop and test an educational program for preparing bedside nurses for general duty in two-year colleges. The project proved successful, and, by 1956, there were twenty-five state-approved programs in existence (Grippando, 1977). Twenty years later,

TABLE 4–1
Number and types of nursing schools 1872–1951

Diploma		Baccalaureate	
YEAR	NUMBER	YEAR	NUMBER
1872	1	1916	2
1900	432	1939	75
1910	1,105	1943	120
1920	1,755	1945	138
1931	1,844	1950	195
1941	1,303		
1951	1,170		

From: Lysaught, J. P. *An Abstract for Action.* New York: McGraw-Hill, 1970.
American Nurses' Association. *1939, 1943, 1951, Facts about Nursing.* New York: American Nurses' Association. 1939, 1943, 1951.

TABLE 4-2
Number and type of nursing programs since 1962

	NUMBER OF NURSING PROGRAMS			
YEAR	DIPLOMA	ASSOCIATE DEGREE	BACCALAUREATE DEGREE	TOTAL
1962	866	84	177	1,127
1972	540	532	290	1,362
1981	303	715	383	1,401

From: National League for Nursing. *Nursing Data Book 1982: Statistical Information on Nursing Education and Newly Licensed Nurses.* New York: National League for Nursing, 1983.

over half of the graduating nurses came from associate degree programs. Table 4-2 shows the changing trends in the setting for nursing education. Not only did the educational setting change, but the curriculum format also changed.

In the 1950s and 1960s the person-centered approach to learning nursing seemed to gain prominence. Within this framework courses were organized around patient concepts such as problems, needs, commonalities, and developmental phases. Four or five major themes were identified and courses developed around them. A commonly used term during this time was "integration" (Heidgerken, 1965). What this meant was that courses were developed around the major themes. Frequently traditional content, such as anatomy, nutrition, and pharmacology, was taught as it applied to the major theme. In these frameworks, each theme included integrated content while the clinical experiences were organized around patient care areas of medicine, surgery, obstetrics, pediatrics, and psychiatry (Allen, 1953).

Many schools of nursing attempted to utilize in one curriculum the best from several of these approaches (Botsford & Hunter, 1953; Jones, 1956). Courses included titles such as Nursing I, II, III; geriatric nursing; industrial nursing; and disaster nursing. The major problem with these approaches to curriculum were insecurity with possible omissions of content, the emphasis of some integrated content over others, and student confusion in learning and applying nursing knowledge.

These problems, along with rapidly expanding nursing knowledge, stimulated nurse educators to search for other ways of organizing nursing curricula. The idea of using conceptual frameworks began to emerge by the 1970s. An additional impetus for the development of conceptual frameworks came in 1972. In 1972, the National League for Nursing stated in its accrediting criteria that all accredited baccalaureate schools of nursing will base their curricula on a conceptual framework. Although the criteria did not specify what conceptual framework, it did state a conceptual framework. Since nursing curricula in most baccalaureate, associate degree, and diploma programs are based on conceptual frameworks, we need to explore this organization of nursing content.

CONCEPTUAL FRAMEWORK

Conceptual frameworks are defined as the structures which hold together the concepts and seek to provide a perception of the reality of nursing practice (Riehl & Roy, 1980). They serve as a guide to the learning and practice of nursing. Conceptual frameworks identify the goals of nursing, the theories, concepts, roles, skills, and functions needed to practice; the settings for practice; the nature of the clients and their needs; the role relationships; and the levels of interventions required to practice.

Elements of Conceptual Frameworks

Since conceptual frameworks identify the essential components of nursing practice as well as the theoretical basis for these components, the underlying assumptions and values must be clearly stated. Concepts utilized in the conceptual framework must be clearly defined and internally consistent. Beyond identification of these assumptions, values, and definitions, there are basically five key elements which should be contained in conceptual frameworks (Peterson, 1977; Riehl & Roy, 1980; Stevens, 1984). These key elements are goal, recipient, nurses' role, source of difficulty, and consequences. Each of these will be briefly described. (See Figure 4-1 for an illustration of how these elements interact.)

Goal. The goal of nursing is expressed as the end product or outcome of the services provided. In other words, the conceptual framework should provide the answer to these questions: Why is the nurse intervening? What does

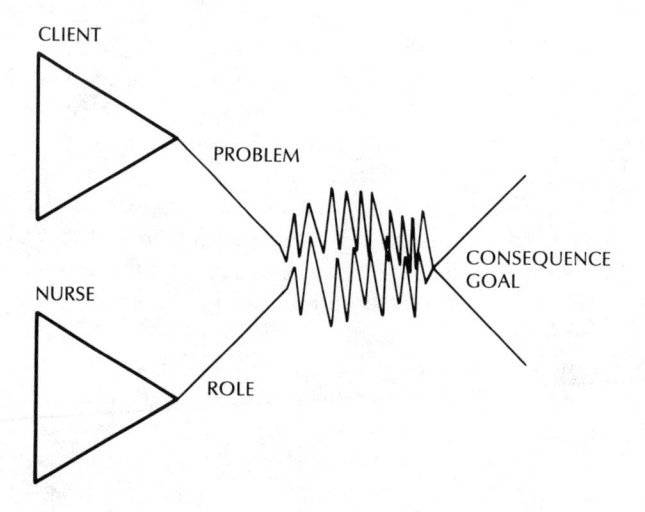

Figure 4-1 Interaction of Elements of Conceptual Framework.

nursing hope to accomplish in working with clients? In most conceptual frameworks this is stated as the ideal, not reality. For example, in the Orem model, nursing intervenes in order to increase the self-sufficiency of clients. Obviously not all clients can reach this ideal goal; however, clients can increase their independence. The goal of nursing using Neuman's model is to reduce stress and enhance adaptation. The conceptual framework sets the goal for nursing in general. It is the guidepost by which specific individual client goals are then written. For example, Orem's goal of self-sufficiency would be too general to apply to a specific client. However, it does influence how the individual client's goal is written. The client's goal might read, "Mrs. J. will walk unassisted 300 feet one time per day."

Recipient. The second key element in conceptual frameworks is recipient, i.e., the target of nursing action. In other words, who is the client and how is he described? Is the client described as an individual, as a family, and/or as a community with health care needs. A particular conceptual framework may include all of these or any one of these. Once identified, the client is described. For example, in the Roy model, the client is described as a bio-psychosocial being who receives stimuli from the environment which requires adaptation. In the Neuman model the client is described as an open system interacting with real or potential stressors in the environment.

Nurse's Role. The conceptual framework describes the role of the nurse in working with the client. How is the nurse viewed and what are the nurse's roles? What behaviors are expected of the nurse? In the Neuman model the nurse's role is described as preventing health problems through manipulation of stressors and adaptation mechanisms, assisting in treating the client who has experienced stressors, and assisting the client to prevent recurrence of stressors.

Source of Difficulty. The fourth element in conceptual frameworks is the source of difficulty: Why does the client need the services provided by nursing? Why does the client need help? What health problems is the client at risk of developing or what health problems has he already developed? In the Neuman model the client needs assistance to prevent or reduce the effects of stressors. In the Roy model the client needs assistance because of inadequate coping mechanisms.

Consequences. Consequences are the last key element in conceptual frameworks. Consequences are defined in terms of intended and unintended. Intended consequences are those desired outcomes of the nurse's actions; unintended consequences are those not planned for, usually negative in nature. The consequences should tie into the goals addressed earlier in this section. Questions generally answered under consequences include how is health defined, i.e., as satisfied needs, adaptation, high-level wellness, continuum, balance, and/or stability? In the Neuman model the intended consequence is maximum level of total wellness and the unintended consequence is unstimulated system. In the Roy model the intended consequence is high-level wellness and the unintended consequence is assumption of too much responsibility on the part of the nurse.

Relationship to Practice

Students enrolled in NLN-accredited nursing schools will learn a conceptual framework that will guide their clinical nursing practice. Students frequently ask questions about the usefulness of such conceptual frameworks as they attempt to organize their thinking and learning. Questions asked include: How will this help me be a better nurse? Will it help me function in the clinical setting? Will I use it when I graduate? When will I learn all the psychomotor skills if I have to spend my time learning this theory?

At present the conceptual framework you will be learning will facilitate your nursing practice by providing a guide for data collection, data analysis, planning, implementing, and evaluating of the care you give. It will help you focus on those areas of need which have implications for nursing care.

Students of nursing must be prepared to function in the now as well as in the future. Conceptual frameworks will help prepare students to function in the future by focusing on concepts and processes. They provide a structure into which you will be able to fit new facts and skills as they develop. Conceptual frameworks help you handle the explosion of knowledge by providing you with a way to organize it. The advances of new treatments and research will place new and different responsibilities on the nurse. New roles will develop that will enlarge the opportunities and scope of responsibilities to nurses. There will be increasing demands for nurse researchers and advocates for better client care. The point to remember is that the conceptual framework you are currently learning may not be the only one you ever use. You may need to learn new conceptual frameworks in the future.

SUMMARY

This chapter has moved from the beginning of formal schools in nursing to the current status of those schools. The focus has been on trends. The three major trends which are identified are the growth of the schools of nursing, the changing settings in which this change occurred, and, finally, how nursing knowledge has been and is organized. Conceptual framework has been defined, and the essential elements of the framework have been provided. Lastly, the relationship of conceptual frameworks to professional nursing practice and the future were described.

Key points to remember are

1. The development of nursing education has shown a consistent pattern of increasing quality.
2. Nursing organization of knowledge has undergone many forms, the most current being the conceptual framework.
3. The essential elements of a conceptual framework are goal, recipient, nurse's role, source of difficulty, and consequences.

REFERENCES

Allen, D. E. "Core Content in the Basic Curriculum." *Nursing Outlook* 1 (1953): 286-288.

American Nurses' Association. *1939, 1943, 1951, Facts about Nursing*. New York: American Nurses' Association, 1939, 1943, 1951.

Anderson, N. E. "The Historical Development of American Nursing Education." *Journal of Nursing Education* 20 (1981): 18-36.

Botsford, E. R., and Hunter, E. "A Four-Year Collegiate Basic Program." *Nursing Outlook* 1 (1953): 136-139.

Bullough, V., and Bullough, B. *The Care of the Sick: The Emergence of Modern Nursing*. New York: Prodist, 1978.

Committee on the Grading of Nursing Schools. *Nursing Schools Today and Tomorrow*. New York: National League for Nursing Education, 1934.

DeYoung, L. *Dynamics of Nursing*. St Louis: The C. V. Mosby Co., 1981.

Deloughery, G. S. *History and Trends of Professional Nursing*. St. Louis: The C. V. Mosby Co., 1977.

Dolan, J., Fitzpatrick, M., and Herrmann, E. *Nursing in Society: A Historical Perspective*. Philadelphia: W. B. Saunders, 1983.

Fitzpatrick, M. L. *Prologue to Professionalism*. Bowie, MD: Robert J. Brady Co., 1983.

Grippando, G. *Nursing Perspectives and Issues*. Albany: Delmar Publishers, 1977.

Hardy, M. E. "Theories: Components, Developments, Evaluation." *Nursing Research* 23 (1974): 100-107.

Heidgerken, L. E. *Teaching and Learning in Schools of Nursing*. Philadelphia: J. B. Lippincott Co., 1965.

Jacox, A. "Theory Construction in Nursing." *Nursing Research* 23 (1974): 4-13.

Jones, V. A. "Establishing a Basic Professional Nursing Program." *Nursing Outlook* 4 (1956): 383-386.

Kalisch, P., and Kalisch, B. *The Advance of American Nursing*. Boston: Little, Brown and Co., 1978.

Longway, I. M. "Curriculum Concepts—An Historical Analysis." *Nursing Outlook* 30 (1972): 116-120.

Lysaught, J. P. *An Abstract for Action*. New York: McGraw-Hill Co., 1970.

National League of Nursing Education, Committee on Education. *A Standard Curriculum for Schools of Nursing*. Baltimore: Waverly Press, 1918.

National League of Nursing Education, Committee on Education. *A Curriculum for Schools of Nursing.* New York: National League of Nursing Education, 1927.

National League of Nursing Education, Committee on Education. *A Curriculum Guide for Schools of Nursing.* New York: National League of Nursing Education, 1937.

National League for Nursing. *Conceptual Framework—Its Meaning and Function.* New York: National League for Nursing, 1975.

National League for Nursing. *Criteria for the Appraisal of Baccalaureate and Higher Degree Programs in Nursing.* New York: National League for Nursing, 1972, 1982.

National League for Nursing. *Criteria for Evaluation of Associate Degree Programs in Nursing.* New York: National League for Nursing, 1982.

Neuman, B. *Neuman Systems Model: Application to Nursing Education and Practice.* Norwalk, CN: Appleton-Century-Crofts, 1982.

Newman, M. *Theory Development in Nursing.* Philadelphia: F. A. Davis Co., 1979.

Notter, L. E., and Spalding, E. E. *Professional Nursing: Foundations, Perspectives and Relationships.* Philadelphia: J. B. Lippincott Co., 1976.

Orem, D. *Nursing: Concepts of Practice.* New York: McGraw-Hill Co., 1971.

Peterson, C. J. "Questions Frequently Asked about the Development of a Conceptual Framework." *Journal of Nursing Education* 16 (4) [1977]: 22-32.

Riehl, J. P., and Roy, C. *Conceptual Models for Nursing Practice.* New York: Appleton-Century-Crofts, 1980.

Roberts, M. M. *American Nursing: History and Interpretation.* New York: The American Journal of Nursing Company, 1954.

Roy, C. *Introduction to Nursing: An Adaptation Model.* Englewood Cliffs, NJ: Prentice-Hall, Inc., 1976.

Roy, C. "Relating Nursing Theory to Education: A New Era." *Nurse Educator* 4 (2) [1979]: 16-21.

Stevens, B. J. *Nursing Theory: Analysis, Application, Evaluation.* Boston: Little, Brown and Co., 1984.

Tschudin, M. S. "Educational Preparation Needed by the Nurse in the Future." *Nursing Outlook* 12 (1964): 32-35.

Watson, J. "The Evolution of Nursing Education in the United States: 100 Years of a Profession for Women." *Journal of Nursing Education* 16 (7) [1977]: 31-38.

Yura, H., and Torres, G. "Educational Trends Which Influenced the Development of the Conceptual Framework Within the Curriculum." In *National League for Nursing, Department of Baccalaureate and Higher Degree Programs, Conceptual Framework: Its Meaning and Function.* New York: National League for Nursing, 1975.

UNIT II

SELECTED THEORIES UTILIZED IN NURSING

Man as a rational being constantly strives to explain the happenings of his world. Why is the grass green? Why do people get sick? Why do some people learn so much easier than others? Why do the tides move? The list of questions is endless. As we search for answers to these questions we frequently explore how these events occur. How does a plant develop and use chlorophyll? How do people get sick? How do people learn? A theory is a scientifically acceptable explanation of observed phenomena. In other words, man develops theories through systematic study and experimentation to explain phenomena he observes in his world. Theories explain how things operate, how they work. They explain why phenomena occur in the manner that they occur. But why is it important to understand how things work? Through this understanding man gains control of his world. If, for example, we can understand how people become ill it may be possible to intervene and prevent this illness. Needless to say, some of our explanations or our theories are better than others. But how does one judge the quality of a theory?

According to the National League for Nursing (1975), a theory should meet the following criteria:

1. It should include a set of postulates and definitions of the terms involved in these postulates.
2. It should be explicit in its boundaries and its concerns and limitations.
3. It must be internally consistent and its concepts must have a logical set of interrelationships.
4. It should be congruent with empirical data.
5. It should be capable of generating hypotheses.
6. It must contain generalizations which go beyond the data.
7. It must be verifiable and must be stated in such a way that it is possible to collect data to prove or disprove it.
8. It must explain past events and predict future ones.
9. Its propositions should be properly derived from the data (pp. 5-6).

What is interesting to note in these criteria is the difference between the use of should and must. Since there are levels of theories as there are levels of concepts, to meet the lowest level theory, the theory being analyzed would have to meet all the "must" criteria. The more of the "should" criteria it meets, the higher the level of the theory.

In analyzing a theory at its lowest level, you would ask specific questions such as: Are the basic assumptions, postulates, and definitions logical? Consistent? Are the definitions operational, i.e., can they be tested? Is the theory general enough to be useful or is it so specific it applies to a very narrow population or phenomena? Does it predict?

In this unit six theories have been selected to help explain the phenomenon of man. Man is the focus of nursing. Each theory which adds to our understanding of man adds to the effectiveness of nursing. Each of the theories in this unit interrelates and overlaps. This is true because each theory is an attempt to explain the phenomenon of man.

Chapter 5 presents systems theory. Systems theory provides a mechanism for understanding the interrelationship of individuals, families, and communities. Chapter 6 presents stress theory. Stress theory explains how man interacts and adapts to the stressors of his environment. Chapter 7 presents learning theory. Learning theory explains how man takes in new information and uses that information to modify his behavior. Chapter 8 presents communication theory. Communication theory explains how man goes about the process of sharing information about himself and his world. Chapter 9 presents change theory. Change theory explains how man produces change and reacts to change as he lives in a world of constant change. Chapter 10 presents role theory. Role theory explains how man can pattern his behavior to influence interactions within positions.

Each of the chapters in Unit II is presented with a different framework from that used for Units I and III. Theories by their very nature are more abstract, yet they are an attempt to understand reality. As a result many new terms are introduced within each chapter. To assist the learner in learning these terms, each chapter begins with a list of terms and definitions. This list of terms and definitions is then followed by a situation. The situation reflects the phenomena described by the theory.

REFERENCE

National League for Nursing. *Conceptual Framework—Its Meaning and Function.* New York: National League for Nursing, 1975.

5

Systems theory

DEFINITION OF TERMS

Adaptation   The critical process of change or adjustment of a system in an attempt to deal with internal or external changes.

Attributes   The properties of the parts, components, or subsystems of an open system.

Boundary   The barrier or area of demarcation that makes the system distinct from its environment.

Decision Making   The critical process of choosing which alternative action to use in functioning.

Dynamic Homeostasis   A state of equilibrium in a system produced by the effective functioning of the system.

Energy   The ability to do work. May exist as actual or potential energy.

Entropy   A measure of the randomness or disorder in a system.

Environment   The set of all objects, a change in whose attributes affects the system and also those objects whose attributes are changed by the behavior of the system. (Adapted from Hall & Fagen, p. 22.)

Equifinality   The tendency of open systems to reach a characteristic final state from different initial conditions and in different ways.

Feedback   The process whereby a part of the system's output is returned to the system as input. This input is used for adaptation.

Function   The performance of work or activities.

Heap or Complex   A set of parts which are mutually independent.

Information   The degree of freedom that exists to choose among signals, symbols, or messages.

Input   The process of taking into a system energy, matter, and information.

Integration   The critical process of organizing the various functions of the subsystems to perform the functions of the system.

Leading Part A centralized subsystem which plays a major or dominant role in the operation of the system.

Matter Anything that has mass.

Negentropy A measure of the energy which can be used by the system for maintenance and growth; a tendency toward increased order in the system.

Output The process by which a system discharges matter, energy, and information.

Reverberation The process whereby a change in one part of the system produces responding changes throughout the system.

Steady State See dynamic homeostasis.

Structure An arrangement of units, components, or parts to form the whole of any item.

System A set of interrelated components or units within a boundary.

    Closed A set of interrelated components or units which is sealed off from its environment.

    Open A set of interacting, interrelated units or components within a boundary which filters both the kind and the rate of inputs and outputs to and from the system.

Throughput The process by which a system uses and in turn transforms matter, energy, and information.

Wholism A concept referring to a system being greater than and different from the sum of its parts.

When the letter arrived Pat was euphoric. She had had no idea how the college would react to her application. Pat had not decided to attend college until her junior year in high school. Her decision had been a turning point which her grades clearly reflected. Although her overall grade average was not that high, her senior year grades were mostly A's. Now she knew and while she was excited, Pat realized she was also nervous.

Pat would be leaving family and friends behind and moving into a whole new world. As Pat sat looking at the letter she began thinking of all the things she would be leaving behind—mainly her family and friends. As the oldest of four, she wondered how the family would adjust without her. How would her brother and two sisters manage after school until her mother came home from work? Who would drive them to their various activities? She had tried talking to her parents about some of these problems but they both said not to worry; they would manage. It was true they always seemed to find some way, like the time Tommy was sick with rheumatic fever. Her father had found through a church a grandmother-type person to temporarily care for Tommy.

Not only would there be changes in her family but there would also be changes with her many friends. Most of them were also going away to school. She realized that as each went their own way things would never again be the same.

Systems Theory   81

She began wondering what her future would hold—how she would adapt to this whole new world she would be entering. Clifton was a large school with 15,000 students, and she did not really understand how things worked there. With her acceptance letter came many materials, which did more to confuse Pat than answer her questions. The letter itself listed three people she was to contact—the registrar, an academic counselor, and the housing director. Pat was not really sure who these people were or why she was to see them. Pat, like many of you, was leaving the security of a familiar environment and moving into a whole new system. But what is a system?

You are a system. The health care *system*, the government, the educational *system*, the family, the social *system*, and the system we all can't beat are systems. We are systems which live and die within systems. Yet we are like the fish who lives and dies in water, never knowing it was there. The fish is unaware his world exists in water because he has never seen a world without water. Many times we are as unaware of the systems within and around us because we have never known any other kind of world. The purpose of this chapter is to change that unawareness and increase our understanding of ourselves and the world in which we live.

At the completion of this chapter the reader will be able to

1. Explain and define systems.
2. Identify and describe the four structural characteristics of a system.
3. Recognize key concepts in systems' functioning.
4. Recognize five characteristics of systems changing over time.
5. Describe the concept of purpose as it relates to open systems.

SYSTEM DEFINED

Although several systems have been identified, we have not defined or explained why these are systems. As we state the common elements of systems in scientific terms, do not be concerned if you feel you don't clearly understand some of the ideas. You will understand enough to begin an analysis of the characteristics of systems. Later in the chapter you will be asked to return and reread this section. At that point you will read with a different level of understanding.

Ludwig Von Bertalanffy, the father of general systems theory, considered a system a complex of elements in interaction (Von Bertalanffy, 1975). Hall and Fagen enlarged on this definition in an attempt to deal with the many colloquial meanings the word *system* has. They presented the following definition: "A system is a set of objects together with relationships between the objects and between their attributes" (Hall & Fagen, 1968, p. 81).

In both of these definitions there are two types of interactions. First, there are the interactions which occur within the system and second, there are the interactions which occur between the system and its environment.

If we focus first on the interactions within a system we have the basis for contrasting a system with a nonsystem. The difference between a system and a nonsystem can be seen in summing the parts. A system is more than the sum of the parts, and a nonsystem is the sum of its parts. This difference evolves because within a system there is interaction between the parts. This interaction between the parts produces behaviors which are more than and different from the behaviors of any of the parts. Take, for example, the human body. There is no part of the human body which in and of itself can run; yet in many cases it runs well (Ackoff, 1974).

In contrast to a system a nonsystem has been described as a "heap" or "complex." A **heap** or **complex** is a set of parts which are mutually independent. In a heap a change in any part of the heap has no effect on any other part and the total is equal to the sum of the parts (Hall & Fagen, 1968). Since all things have the potential of a relationship there is in reality no nonsystem. Nonsystem is a theoretical construct. In contrast a **system** is a set of interrelated components or units within a boundary.

The interaction which occurs between a system and its environment provides the basis for defining the two types of systems. As already implied, more than one type of system exists. The two types of systems which are usually identified are open and closed. A **closed system** is a set of interrelated components or units which are sealed off from its environment. No interaction with the surroundings of the system occurs. The most common example of a closed system is a chemical reaction taking place in a sealed, insulated container. This lack of interaction with the surrounding environment is what differentiates a closed system from an open system.

An **open system** is a set of interacting, interrelated units or components within a boundary which filters both the kind and the rate of what comes into and goes out of the system (Hall & Weaver, 1977). A key difference between an open and closed system is its relationship with the environment. One way to conceptualize this difference is to think of an open system as having a semipermeable membrane and a closed system as having an impermeable membrane.

While the definitions of open and closed systems are presented as an either/or proposition, this is not the case when dealing with systems we encounter in real life. More realistically open and closed systems can be thought of as end points on a continuum. (See Figure 5-1.) Some systems are more open or more closed than others. Living systems in general tend to be more open than inanimate systems.

For example, you (living system) could be expected to have more interaction with your environment than your car (inanimate system) would have with its environment. Yet both you and your car have inputs from the environment and outputs into the environment. Although living systems tend

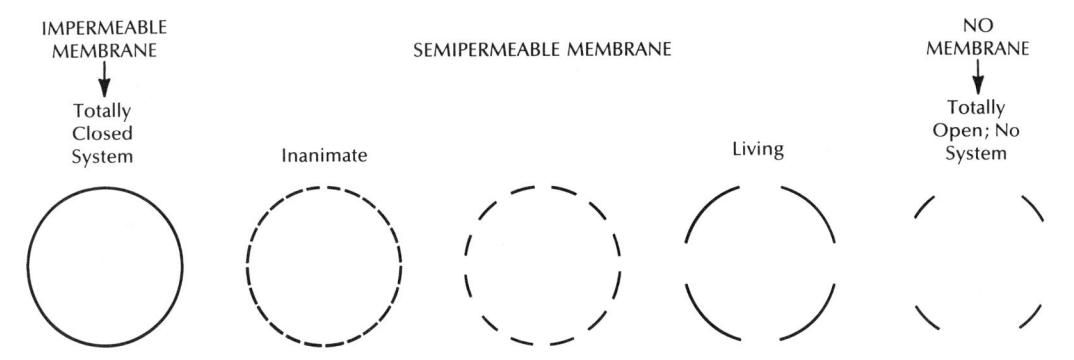

Figure 5-1 System Continuum. Systems can be conceptualized as existing on a continuum. A totally closed system would have no interaction with the environment. A totally open system would no longer have a membrane and, therefore, would not be a system, since it could not control inputs or outputs. Most systems exist between these two extremes. In other words, there is a great deal of variation in how permeable a semipermeable membrane is.

to be more open than inanimate systems, living and inanimate systems do vary. For example, some forms of government are more open to inputs from the populace than others. Did you notice the number and variation of systems in the earlier situation with Pat?

Though closed systems are characterized by their lack of interaction with the environment, open systems are characterized by their structure, function, purpose, and how these change over time as they interact with their environment. In nursing our concern is with systems and more specifically with living systems. The rest of this chapter focuses on the characteristics of open systems. Characteristics are facts which are true of all open systems. For purposes of discussions as well as understanding, characteristics of open systems will be classified here under the concepts of structure, function, purpose, and change through time. (See Table 5-1.)

STRUCTURE IN AN OPEN SYSTEM

Structure is the arrangement of the units, components, or parts of an item to form the whole. If the item being discussed is an open system, its structure will demonstrate four key characteristics.

First, the structure will include a **boundary**, an area of demarcation or barrier that makes the system distinct from its environment. The degree of permeability of this boundary defines how opened or closed a system is. The boundary of any given system is subjective. It depends on who is analyzing the system and for what reason (Hazzard, 1971). For example, the skin of a person might be considered his boundary. Everything that is within the skin is within the system. Everything that is outside of the skin is outside of the

84 SELECTED THEORIES UTILIZED IN NURSING

TABLE 5-1
Key characteristics of an open system

STRUCTURE
Boundary
Environment
Hierarchical Order
Attributes
FUNCTION
BOUNDARY FUNCTION
Taking In
Keeping Out
Keeping In
Putting Out
CRITICAL PROCESSES
Adaptation
Integration
Decision Making
CHANGE
Dynamic Homeostasis
Entropy
Negentropy
Reverberation
Equifinality
PURPOSE

system. But does the personality of an individual exist within his skin or is there another boundary?

Since all systems have a boundary which delineates the inside from the outside of the system, the second key structural characteristic of systems is **environment**. This environment is the world outside of the boundary. Hall and Fagen have defined environment as follows:

> For a given system, the environment is the set of all objects a change in whose attributes affect the system and also those objects whose attributes are changed by the behavior of the system. (1968, p. 83)

Since systems consist of interacting parts and systems affect and are affected by their environment, can we not now apply these ideas to our situation with Pat? Pat is about to experience a major change in her environment. She will be moving from a familiar environment—the family—to an unfamiliar environment—the college. Not only will this change affect Pat, but

Pat will also affect the new and old environments. For instance, she will bring to the college environment some of her family's ideas and beliefs; in turn, when she returns home she will bring to the family new ideas, values, and beliefs. As a result of these interactions, the college, Pat, and her family will all have experienced change.

Once the boundary and the environment of a system are identified, the next question becomes how are the parts arranged within the system? Within an open system the arrangement of the parts has a hierarchical order. Within any system are subsystems which make up the parts of the system. For example, in our human system are the body systems (e.g., cardiovascular, neurological, and gynecological). These systems, in turn, consist of cells which are subsystems of the body system. While any one system can be conceptualized as having subsystems it can also be seen as a subsystem of a greater system. This greater system is referred to as the suprasystem. An example of the suprasystem for our human system could be the family. Note in Figure 5-2 how the concept of hierarchical arrangement can be applied to Pat.

Within any situation, what is defined as the subsystem and suprasystem depends on what is the focus or target system. For example, in Figure 5-2 Pat is the focus or target system. If, however, the target system were to become the family, then Pat becomes a subsystem and the community becomes a suprasystem.

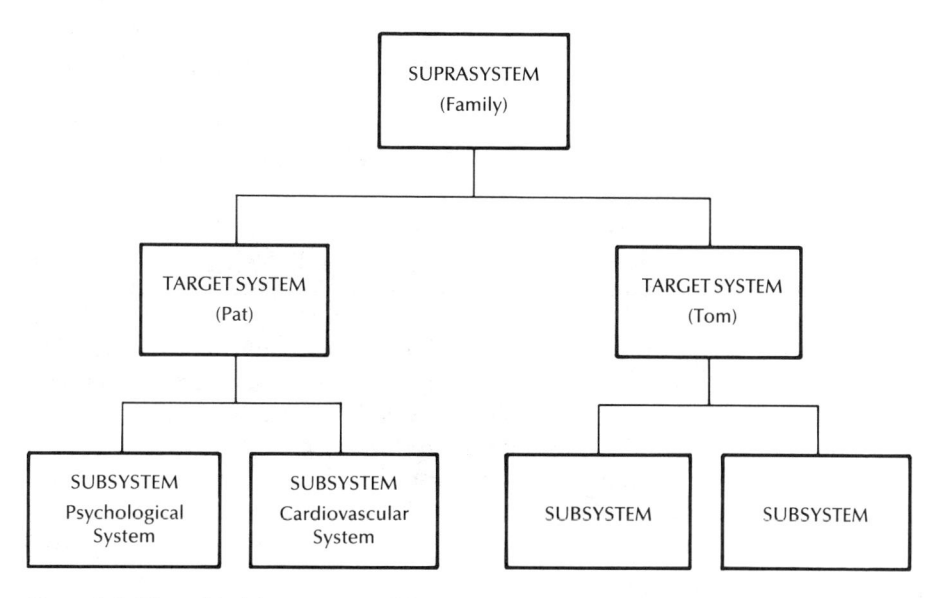

Figure 5-2 Hierarchical Arrangement of Systems.

This characteristic, hierarchical arrangement, like boundary and environment, is subject to interpretation. What is the system, the subsystem, and the suprasystem depends on the perspective of the individual who is analyzing the system. These three characteristics, boundary, environment, and hierarchical arrangement, are also interrelated. What is inside the boundary are the parts of the system or the subsystems. What is outside the system or in its environment is the suprasystem.

The final structural characteristic of open systems is termed attributes. **Attributes** are the properties of the parts, components, or subsystems of the system. Attributes of any system can be extensive in that they are frequently those factors used to describe. For example, if your hair is red, this is one of the properties of your subsystem hair. Much of the data nurses collect in working with clients are really attributes of individuals. The data they collect about sex, race, age, and religion are all properties or attributes used to describe. Social systems also have attributes. For example, when collecting data about leadership styles and communication networks, researchers can use the terms autocratic, bureaucratic, and democratic to describe the properties or attributes of social systems.

FUNCTION IN AN OPEN SYSTEM

Function is what an open system does—the work, activities, and actions which are performed by the system in order to survive and grow. For example, the functions of the health care system or of the educational system are the work or tasks engaged in by these systems. Function is different from purpose. Purpose is why the activities are performed and will be discussed later under the heading "Purpose."

All functions require energy. Therefore, to carry out functions, energy is taken into the system. However, energy exists only in combination with matter and information. Although energy, matter, and information exist together, each emphasizes a different aspect of what is taken into the system. This idea can be analogous to taking pictures of something from different angles. Each picture is of the same thing, yet each picture will show a different aspect. **Energy** is the ability to do work. It exists as actual or potential energy. **Matter** is anything that has mass and occupies space. **Information** is the degree of freedom that exists to choose among signals, symbols, or messages and is demonstrated in the meaning or significance of the information to the processing system (Miller, 1965).

A specific example of intake as energy, information, and matter is food. Food is potential energy which when taken into the system may be converted to actual energy. It has mass or occupies space, and certainly there is a variety of meanings attached to food.

The process of taking energy, matter, and information into the system is called **input**. The process by which the system uses this energy, matter, and information is called **throughput.** Some of the energy, information, and matter is retained by the system. Unretained energy, matter, and information is discharged and is called **output.** Therefore, all living systems in order to survive are involved in a dynamic exchange of energy, matter, and information with the environment. In living systems, seven specific functions involving this dynamic exchange have been identified. Four of these functions are termed boundary functions, while the other three are called critical functions.

Boundary Functions

The term *boundary functions* implies that the boundaries of the system work. They perform functions which require the use of energy. These functions or tasks have been implied in the discussion of input and output.

The first boundary function is *taking in*. Taking in is a selective process. Everything presented at the system's boundary will not be taken in. For example, one does not eat everything in the environment nor does the digestive track absorb everything taken in. The process of keeping some things out is the second function of the boundary. *Keeping out*, like taking in, requires the system to utilize energy. For example, in the cleaning and preparing of food, work is required to keep certain things out. Therefore, the process of input involves two boundary functions—taking in and keeping out.

Once matter, energy, and information are taken into the system, the two final boundary functions are *keeping in* and *putting out*. To continue on with the example of eating, some of the food consumed and processed will be put out or eliminated from the system. Not everything consumed will be put out or kept in if the system is to continue. The system must hold in sufficient fluid, electrolytes, and nutrients to meet its energy needs. For example, if an individual has diarrhea, he will be eliminating energy he needs to keep in the system. There is a limit to how long this diarrhea can continue before it becomes fatal. The time limit depends on the resources of the individual. In the case of an infant this can be a fairly short time period. On the other hand, excessive fluids, electrolytes, and the end products of metabolism must be eliminated. For example, a patient with kidney failure becomes ill because he cannot put out the excessive fluids, electrolytes, and the end products of metabolism.

Critical Processes

Along with the four tasks or functions of the boundary, three other functions are performed by open systems. These functions, usually called critical processes, involve input, throughput, and output processes. Critical processes are necessary for survival and growth. These three functions are **adaptation, integration,** and **decision making** (Hall & Weaver, 1977). These three functions are different aspects of how the system uses energy.

Systems experience change within their boundaries and within their environments. This constant change is dealt with through the process of adapting, which is changing to deal with change. Adapting occurs in two ways: The system may change itself or it may change the environment. Usually the process of adaptation involves both types of change.

For example, you, as an open system, may be cold as a result of a change in the temperature. Your body may increase the amount of heat it is producing by shivering. At the same time you may also build a fire to increase the temperature in the environment. In both of these changes, adaptation required energy to deal with change.

The process of adaptation requires the system to integrate the various functions of the subsystems to produce those behaviors of which only the system is capable. Integration is defined as the critical process of organizing the various activities of the subsystems to perform the functions of the system. For example, to build the fire and/or shiver is impossible without the various subsystems working together or integrating their activities. The process of integration is work and requires a complex organization and communication scheme. You refer to this process of integrating when you say someone or something (e.g., the health care system) is poorly or well organized.

While integrating the various functions of the subsystems to adapt to change, a system must always deal with a variety of possible actions. The critical process of choosing which alternative action to use is decision making. In the example of being cold, a fire could be built. But, where the fire is built, what materials are used, and how the fire is started are all decisions which must be made before integration can occur. Although the example given is of a conscious decision, systems do not always make decisions on a conscious level. For example, as the oxygen level in your blood stream drops you make an unconscious decision to breathe. Not only do individuals make unconscious decisions, but large social systems also make these kinds of decisions.

These three processes or critical functions interact together so that the system can deal with the constant changes which occur both within the system and within its environment. To react to change, the system must be aware of the change. This awareness occurs through a process called **feedback**. In feedback a part of the system's output is returned to the system as input. Adjustments based on this input are then made. Looking at the previous example, as a change in temperature is experienced, a feeling of warmth becomes new input to the system. Changes will now be made based on this input. You might stop shivering.

Looking back over the information on boundary functions and critical processes, can you now apply some of these ideas to Pat and her situation? She will be experiencing a variety of changes as she moves from her current environment to a new environment. How will her boundary functions be influenced by the changes in her environment? For example, how will Pat's eating habits and ultimately her energy level be influenced by not having access to her mother's home cooking? Can you think of other examples? How will her critical processes be influenced by the changes in her environment? For example, how will she handle the variety of course requirements? What decisions will she face as she organizes her time? How well she performs the boundary and critical processes functions will determine her success in adjusting to college life. If her initial adjustment is successful, Pat will discover she has increased energy and time. Can you explain why this would be true? Can you explain how this relates to your client?

CHANGE IN AN OPEN SYSTEM

Systems and the environments in which they exist are constantly changing. Systems exist in the dimension of time. The influence of the time dimension is demonstrated by five characteristics of systems.

The first of these five change characteristics is referred to as homeostasis, **dynamic homeostasis**, or steady state. These terms refer to the fact that open systems are constantly working or changing in order to maintain themselves within the limits of survival. For example, you are constantly breathing in order to maintain your oxygen level. While this is an easy example, you must not forget that large social systems constantly work to maintain the status quo.

Entropy is the tendency of a system to break down, to increase its disorder. Living systems, unlike closed, are able to counteract the effects of entropy because they are able to work to maintain a steady state. Entropy is a measure of the randomness or disorder in a system. In closed systems there is a tendency for the system to break down or go to complete disorder. The effects of entropy can be seen in the tendency of a mountain to get smaller. It will wear away with time. Though open systems can counteract the effects of entropy, it is always present in the system as bound energy. This presence of entropy and in turn the tendency of the system to break down and finally to die is the second characteristic of how systems change over time.

The third characteristic of change over time is the tendency of the system to counteract the effects of entropy—negentropy. **Negentropy** is a measure of the energy which can be utilized by the system for maintenance as well as growth. All living systems have a tendency toward growth and increased organization. As systems grow, there are increased divisions into subsystems and subsubsystems. The subsystems differentiate and specialize. An excellent example of this is the increased differentiation and specialization in nursing as the nursing role has grown.

As the system grows, differentiates, and specializes, there emerges a centralized system in which one element or subsystem plays a major dominant role in the operation of the system. This subsystem is called the **leading part,** and the system is centered around this part. For example, in the human the central nervous system is a leading part. In a nursing service organization the director of nursing could be the leading part. A change in this leading part is reflected in considerable change throughout the total system (Hall & Fagen, 1968).

Although a change in the leading part is amplified throughout the system, any change in any part will produce some effect throughout. The process of change throughout the system in response to a change in one part is called **reverberation**. For example, if the director of nursing is fired there will be an effect throughout the whole nursing system. Reverberation is the fourth characteristic of how the time dimension influences systems.

The degree or amount of reverberation which occurs is influenced not only by the part which is changed but also by the degree of interrelatedness which exists within the system. This degree of interrelatedness can be seen on a continuum. At one end of the continuum would be 100 percent wholeness or coherence of the parts. At the other end would be 100 percent independence—a heap or complex (Hall & Fagen, 1968). For example, in looking at a hospital organization, if the individual fired is in the physical therapy department it may not reverberate to the nursing department in the same degree as if he were part of nursing service. Two factors influence the amplitude of the change which occurs through the process of reverberation. The first factor is the centralization of the part which is changed. The second factor is the degree of wholeness within the system.

The final change characteristic of open systems is equifinality. **Equifinality** is the tendency of open systems to reach a characteristic final state from different initial conditions and in different ways. This is in contrast to closed systems where if either the initial conditions or the process is altered the final state will also be changed (Von Bertalanffy, 1975). An interesting example of equifinality can be seen in the development of a normal human from an ovum. A normal human being can be the final result of a complete ovum or from each half of a divided ovum, in the case of twins.

At this point in the chapter, you may be wondering why you are learning so many new ideas. It may be difficult for you to see the relationship of concepts like negentropy to nursing. Yet nursing is more than doing things to patients to help them recover from illness. Nursing requires an understanding of how man progresses through his life cycle; it requires you to work with people to help them help themselves. To do this requires the ability to anticipate change, as well as to plan for change. You will use these concepts as you live with, work with, and plan for change in your clients and in the systems in which you function. Now that you have analyzed the characteristics of an open system, you are ready to appreciate the definition of a system on a more sophisticated level. Go back to the first part of this chapter and read again the information under the heading "System Defined." Don't yield to the temptation to skip this reading. It really will help your comprehension.

PURPOSE OF AN OPEN SYSTEM

The purpose of an open system involves the reason(s) for its existence. Purpose and function are often confused. Function is what the system does and purpose is why it performs these functions. For example, the expressed purpose of the health care system is to provide for the improvement of health. A number of tasks or functions are needed to achieve this purpose.

To understand an open system, it is necessary to have a clear statement of its purpose; however, purpose(s) is not always clearly defined or agreed upon. In the example above, the purpose of the health care system is to improve health, but does this mean (1) to prevent illness; (2) to cure when illness occurs; (3) to treat when illness occurs; (4) to prevent recurrences, or (5) could it mean all this and even more? This lack of an agreement of purpose is one of the major problems in the health care system.

Another area to examine is how the structure and function support the purpose. What happens in many cases is that systems evolve through time. As a result the structure and functions of a system are not always the best ways to achieve the purposes of that system.

In analyzing systems, the relationship between function and purpose is often an area of confusion. Systems can become so involved in performing their functions that the functions become ends in themselves. For example, it has been recommended that individuals have yearly physicals for early detection of disease. However, one can become so involved in doing the best physicals possible that the reason for doing the yearly physicals is forgotten. As a result, improved ways of doing physicals are emphasized rather than improved ways of doing mass screening for early detection of disease.

So far, the discussion of purpose has centered around social systems. Individuals are also open systems and, therefore, exist for a purpose. What this purpose is has been the concern of many fields of study from religion to art to philosophy. It is interesting to note that the father of general systems theory was motivated to develop this theory because of his concerns with the purpose of life

> As a biologist, I reject a biologistic concept of man, i.e., the attempt to reduce human behavior and human values to simple biological factors, to mere usefulness and adjustment for the individuals and to an advantage for the species in the struggle for existence. How could one reduce human culture, science, art, ethics, and religion to such biological factors. (Von Bertalanffy, 1975, p. 49)

SUMMARY

In the beginning of the chapter, five objectives were identified. These objectives provide a basis for summarizing this chapter. First, systems were defined and explained. For our purposes, emphasis was on open systems. The concepts of structure, function, change, and purpose were used as a framework for identifying the characteristics of all open systems. The structural characteristics identified were boundary, environment, hierarchical order, and attributes. The functional characteristics considered boundary functions and critical processes. Dynamic homeostasis, entropy, negentropy, reverberation, and equifinality were the five change characteristics discussed. Finally, the purpose of the system was identified as the rationale or reason for the system's existence.

Some key points to remember as you use systems theory in nursing are

1. Every living thing is an open system interacting in a world of open systems.
2. All systems are constantly changing as they live in a world of change.
3. All systems require energy to function.
4. The efficiency of a system is dependent upon the relationships that exist among structure, function, and purpose.

REFERENCES

Ackoff, R. *Redesigning the Future: A Systems Approach to Societal Problems.* New York: John Wiley and Sons, 1974.

Buckley, W., ed. *Modern Systems Research for the Behavior Scientist: A Sourcebook.* Chicago: Aldine Publishing Co., 1968.

Capelle, R. *Changing Human Systems.* Toronto: International Human Systems Institute, 1979.

Chapman, G. P. *Human and Environmental Systems: A Geographer's Appraisal.* New York: Academic Press, 1977.

Cleland, D., and King, W. R. *Systems Analysis and Project Management.* 2nd ed. New York: McGraw Hill Co., 1975.

Hall, A. D., and Fagen, R. E. "Definition of System." In *Modern Systems Research for the Behavior Scientist*, edited by W. Buckley. Chicago: Aldine Publishing Co., 1968.

Hall, J. E., and Weaver, B. R., eds. *Distributive Nursing Practice: A Systems Approach to Community Health.* Philadelphia: J. B. Lippincott Co., 1977.

Hazzard, M. E. "An Overview of Systems Theory." *Nursing Clinics of North America* 6 (1971): 385–394.

Maurer, J. *Readings in Organizational Theory: Open System Approaches.* New York: Random House, 1971.

Miller, J. G. *System Theory.* New York: McGraw Hill Co., 1978.

Miller, J. G. "Living Systems: Basic Concepts." *Behavioral Science* 10 (1965): 193–237.

Phillips, D. C. *Holistic Thought in Social Science.* Stanford, CA: Stanford University Press, 1976.

Putt, A. *General Systems Theory Applied to Nursing.* Boston: Little, Brown and Co., 1978.

Ruben, B. D., and Kim, J. Y., eds. *General Systems Theory and Human Communication.* Rochelle Park, N.J.: Hayden Book Company, Inc., 1975.

Von Bertalanffy, L. *Perspectives on General Systems Theory.* Edited by Edgar Toschdjian. New York: George Braziller, 1975.

Von Bertalanffy, L. "General Systems Theory." In *General Systems Theory and Human Communication,* edited by B. D. Ruben and J. Y. Kim. Rochelle Park, N.J.: Hayden Book Company, Inc., 1975.

6

Stress-adaptation theory

DEFINITION OF TERMS

Adaptation A response of the system to change involving new creative behavior and problem solving. Some use of the term *adaptation* includes maladaptation, i.e., the system adapts self-destructively.

Coping Refers to a successful adaptation to stressors, usually with the aid of psychological means.

Defense Measures that shield the system from perceived dangers and occur unconsciously. *Defense* has been described extensively in psychoanalytic writings.

Pressure The demands that force the system to speed up efforts. These are often inner forces.

Stress An energy state set into motion in man as a response to exposure from challenging or demanding stimuli.

Stressor The causative agent of stress. Term originated by Selye.

As she sat in her dorm room, Jenny tried hard to study for her finals but her mind kept drifting. She couldn't make herself stay with the topic even though she knew she had to. Her grades in college were riding on the final exams. She mused how different she and her roommate Doris were. Doris was lucky. Her private high school had prepared her much better for the college experience. Jenny, on the other hand, seemed to go through high school with very little effort. It was so much fun then but now things were different. Maybe it wouldn't be so hard if the teachers had used more quizzes. After all, these were difficult courses. Why put everything on the student to figure out? In fact, the more Jenny thought about how unfair everything was, the more she needed another candy bar. She tried talking to Doris about her fears. But Doris, in her organized manner, was only willing to spend so much time listening. It was irritating to have a roommate who had adjusted in college with so little effort. Doris had been away from home before. Each summer, she had spent a month at camp. She was used to living with a group of girls and not with her family. The pressure was really on Jenny. The candy bar now felt like a rock in her stomach. She was tired yet too keyed up to sleep. She just knew when they handed the test to her tomorrow her heart would start to pound and she would have trouble breathing again. How could she ever adjust to all this?

What Jenny is experiencing is commonly referred to as stress. Stress is an aspect of life that all people must deal with. Hans Selye, a pioneer in stress theory, summed up in one sentence how Jenny and all of us should deal with stress.

> Try to establish what you consider to be the purpose of your life and fight for it ardently, at the same time avoiding all efforts to achieve what is outside the limits of your capacity. (Selye, 1977, p. 42)

This sounds like a clear task, but the nature of stress with all its complexities can present a puzzling and confusing picture. For the nurse, learning about stress adaptation theory enhances understanding of man in his attempt to stay healthy or to recapture health following a stressful experience.

Systems theory can be used as a frame of reference when looking at stress involvement. Agents of stress, that is, stressors, are viewed as inputs into the system of man. Stressors produce change that requires adaptation. How man adapts to these changes is demonstrated by his behavior, output. This way of thinking about stress organizes and facilitates later application of appropriate measures through the nursing process.

At the completion of the chapter the reader will be able to

1. Identify characteristics of stress and stressors.
2. Classify stressors according to three dimensions of man.
3. Identify key characteristics of how man adapts.
4. Relate stress adaptation theory to systems theory.
5. Identify areas for assessment of stress.
6. Identify strategies for stress reduction.

The following information about stress is eclectic in nature, drawing from a variety of sources; however, ideas from Hans Selye (1977, 1965, 1956) permeate throughout.

STRESS DEFINED

Stress as a concept is discussed in the literature along a number of parameters. Stress is defined as an energy state set into motion in man as a response to exposure from challenging or demanding stimuli called **stressors.** Using this definition, five characteristics have been identified.

The first characteristic is that stress is a hypothetical abstraction which possesses no independent existence. It can be identified only when changes in the system are manifested. This means that stress cannot be observed in and of itself, only the responses to stress can be detected. When in contact with a stressor, the system reacts. An example is seen when an older child in the family meets the new baby. An increased tension in the older child is not directly observable. However, tension can be inferred by the child's behavior. The part that is not observed is the hypothetical abstraction.

While the stress state intensifies when man is confronted with a change or threat, stress always exists in man. This is the second characteristic. Even when man lacks awareness of his ongoing stress status, stress is operating in the system. Respiratory cells taking in oxygen, receiving a phone call from a friend, measuring summer growth, and viewing a travelogue film all represent instances in which stress is possible. The system responds to these events, sometimes in the form of stress.

Recognizing that stress always exists leads to a third characteristic: Stress is essential for life. Adequate development depends on a select amount of stress for a given individual. Without exposure to stressors and a resultant stress response, man's system would be in a precarious state; in fact, dead. Without the opportunity to exercise its skills and experience the rich challenges of life the system cannot develop.

The fourth characteristic of stress concerns input needs. When the input needs of man's system are not satisfied, stress results. For example, man has an input need for food. When he does not have this input he experiences hunger, which is an intensification of the stress state. Input needs are not only physical but include all the needs of man.

The final characteristic is that stress can result from both pleasant and unpleasant experiences. For example, consider the surprise birthday party. The happiness and joy that floods the delighted guest of honor produces stress within the system. This type of stress is sometimes called eustress or stress resulting from happy or pleasant experiences. Likewise, the individuals arranging the surprise are stressed. Any person who really did not want to attend may be experiencing unpleasing stress, or distress.

FACTORS INFLUENCING STRESS

Stressors are stimuli which increase the stress state of man. Some stressors are barely noticeable on a conscious level, and it isn't until a combination of events trips them off that they leave their latent status and become observable. Whether latent or obvious in impact, stressor inputs challenge the adaptive capacities of the system. This challenge can be understood by reviewing the nature of stressors.

The nature of the stressor influences the amount of energy needed to maintain balance in the system. The nature of stressors includes type, intensity, scope, and meaning.

Type describes the actual content of the stressor. For example, hunger, pain, or a failing grade are types of stressors. Knowing the type helps to determine if the stressor is predictable or not. Identifying predictable stressors can assist in planning for **coping** strategies. If the death of a loved one is expected, a person can prepare his adjustment to it. Certain responses to the death of a loved one are known to be different when the death is sudden. Some references will use type as the basis of a classification such as chemical, physical, emotional, or environmental stressors.

The intensity of the stressor refers to the magnitude of the stressor on the system. Failure on a test within a series of tests in a course is viewed as less intense than failure in the course. Pain from a small cut on the finger is less intense than pain from a burn over two-thirds of the body.

The scope of the stressor reflects the extent of investment of the system. Stressors at the point where the system has a strong investment to satisfy needs or remain viable can constitute a sweeping scope. Loss of oxygen in the system due to a respiratory impairment suggests an extensive scope threatening the viability of the system attempting to meet basic physiological needs. There is usually a parallel between scope and intensity. When one increases, the other often increases.

The meaning of a stressor is a reflection of the importance of the stressor to the life of that system. It will vary from individual to individual depending upon the beliefs and values in operation. For example, if Jenny fails her final examinations, this failure would probably be much more important than if she would fail to complete an informal sewing course. However, Doris may place an even higher value on her course work and be more severely stressed by a failure in final examinations.

Though the nature of the stressor helps us to understand the concept of stressor, no discussion of stressors would be complete without a more structured classification. As we can see from this discussion of stressors, potentially anything can be a stressor. The nature of a stressor provides the beginning basis for identifying specific stressors experienced by man. However, a classification system is necessary if the identification of stressors is to be done systematically.

CLASSIFICATION OF STRESSORS

There are many ways to classify stressors. One way is from a standpoint of environmental origin, i.e., intrapersonal—from within—and extrapersonal —between individual and outside force(s). Stressors can also be viewed in terms of how the person perceives them, such as favorable, unfavorable, positive, and negative. Some classifications of stressors have used needs of man or broad concepts to organize stressor information. The following classification organizes stressors according to three dimensions of man: physiological, psychological, and sociocultural.

Physiological stressors follow the physiological dimension of man. This dimension consists of man's physical being and all of his physiological regulatory mechanisms. The dimension may be considered on a cellular level, an organ level, or by networks within the whole person level. Two types of physiological stressors are physical and chemical stressors. Physical stressors are generated by many stimuli affecting the senses such as light, darkness, sounds, heat, cold, pressures, and textures. Chemical stressors include a host of known substances containing chemicals and are provided in toxic and nontoxic forms such as food, drugs, and gases. Some stressors are combinations of chemical and physical stressors, such as pollutants with noxious gases and particulate matter.

Psychological stressors follow the psychological dimension of man. The psychological dimension involves man's mental state of well-being, his emotions, personal feelings, and his self-concept. Stressors in this area would evoke a changed mental or feeling state. Loss and conflict are seen as major themes. For example, having to take an examination, moving away from home, having a fight with a friend, attending a job interview, getting married, and retiring all represent psychological stressors.

The sociocultural stressors follow the sociocultural dimension. This dimension includes man's values, customs, and norms. Any stressor in these areas would be sociocultural. Reich (1970) has brought into focus a number of sociocultural stressors that face man today. He has emphasized the threatening nature of changes going on in America. He identified lawlessness, poverty, uncontrolled technology, powerlessness, meaningless work, absence of community feeling, and loss of self as major social issues with which we must deal. He envisioned a revolution in human values surpassing values associated with impersonalized pressures of today's society. He cited the Vietnam War, for example, as an event which stripped the self-concept and fired rapid changes into the thinking of the young.

This classification system is simple yet provides a frame for a viewing of stressors. It closely follows many assessment guides. For example, many assessment guides have a section on mental status reflecting the psychological dimensions, a section on review of systems reflecting the physiological, and a section on values, work, family, and religion reflecting a sociocultural dimension.

Although we have classified stressors by dimensions, man reacts as a whole. All his dimensions are involved in his response to stressors. One clear example is demonstrated by stressors along a developmental continuum. The developmental continuum is viewed from the standpoint of time, i.e., conception to death. Saxton and Hyland (1979) have provided insights about stressors occurring over the life of man with a focus on development. One may consider the developmental tasks which have been identified for a period of life and then analyze the tasks in relationship to a life context of a given individual noting perceptions concerning stress and life events.

Examples of developmental tasks which are stressful to the young include toilet training, being told "no" when exploring, and separation from a parent. Examples of stressful adult developmental tasks include marriage, childbearing, and relocations associated with employment requirements. In each of these examples of stressful developmental events, man will function as a whole involving and utilizing each of his dimensions.

STRESS RESPONSE

When in contact with a stress producing agent, the system must respond. If a person is healthy, responding to a stressor might alter his functioning in some way but not necessarily make him sick. If he has a disease, it could accelerate the disease process. In looking at how man responds to stress one needs to first identify factors that influence that response and, secondly, to identify the adaptive responses man can demonstrate.

Factors Influencing Stress Response

Several factors have been identified as influencing the extent and type of response man will demonstrate to stressors. As we discuss each of these factors remember that each man is unique so that the specific effect of these factors will be unique. For our purposes we will focus on five major factors that influence this response (Byrne & Thompson, 1978). These factors are nature of stressor, duration of exposure to the stressor, number of stressors, previous experience with similar stressors, and limitations of the system.

The first factor influencing the stress response is the nature of the stressor. The nature of the stressor is the specific stressor with which the system is interacting and includes type, intensity, scope, and meaning. While nature influences the response, nature by itself does not determine the response. How long the stressor interacts with the system or its duration is the second influencing factor. The longer the duration, the greater the extent of energy expended. For example, severe pain is tolerable if its duration is short. On the other hand, less severe pain of long duration may deplete energy reserves. Can you think of a time when your tolerance to pain was influenced by the anticipated duration of that pain?

Your tolerance to this pain was also influenced by the number of other problems you were experiencing at the same time. When many stressors occur at one time, it becomes more difficult for the system to deal favorably with them. If a job is lost at the same time that dental repair must be done and a crisis develops in a relationship with a friend, you are stressed to a far greater extent than if any one of these events had occurred alone.

In each of the examples or situations described above, the individual's response is influenced by previous experience with comparable stressors. Through contact with stressors, man learns about both the nature of stressors and his response to them. Based on this learning, man then avoids, approaches, or attempts new responses to those current stressors encountered. His approach to each stressor is influenced by the unique limits of his own system. These limits are of two types. The first are limitations which are true for all systems of that type. For example, an octopus can regenerate a lost tentacle where man cannot regenerate a new arm. The second type of limitation is unique to individuals. For example, an individual with a low IQ will deal with learning limitations. Individuals with high IQ's will not experience the same limitations.

These five factors which influence how a system responds to stress can be used to consider Jenny's situation. The nature of her stressor is final exams. The duration of the stressor will be until she receives results of the exams. The number of stressors includes all other personal stressors she is experiencing, i.e., the number of exams she needs to take and the number she must take in any one day. Past experience considers not only her previous experience with final exams but also her response to testing situations. In this case, she has experienced shortness of breath and good grades in high school. Her limits include the fact that only so much time is left for learning before the final. In looking at this situation, we are considering factors that influence her response but have not yet looked at how she would respond.

Adaptive Responses

Man responds to stress as a whole. The dimensions of man do not operate autonomously, but actually in concert with each other as parts of a total system. When any type of stressor is contacted, the response on the part of man would not be pure in any one dimension. This is one reason why stress research is difficult. The variables become muddied with the different dimensions coming into play (Rahe & Ransom, 1978). Even though the dimensions do not operate independently, to understand stress response one must examine the adaptive capacity of each dimension separately. Once the adaptive capacities of each dimension are considered, then one can examine the interaction of the dimensions in producing man's responses to stressors.

Physiological Adaptation. Physiological adaptation is the ability to maintain a balance or steady state in the system with respect to the structure and function of tissues, organs, body parts, and regulatory mechanisms. Selye identified physiological capacity for **adaptation** by using the categories: local adaptation syndrome (LAS) and general adaptation syndrome (GAS).

The body's initial effort to combat a physiological stressor consists of a local inflammatory response. This local response is referred to as the local adaptation syndrome. The LAS demonstrates that the system attempts to adapt initially by using the least energy. This characteristic helps to conserve energy. If LAS is ineffective in walling off the stressor, a more general adjustive response occurs. The system must expend more energy to initiate this response. General adaptation syndrome (GAS) amplifies essential body functions while suppressing the less essential. Three phases—alarm, resistance, and exhaustion—are identified in the general adaptation syndrome.

The alarm stage is an immediate trigger phase. At this time the stressor is perceived and the body is prepared to act. Goodwin (1980) observed that body changes occurring during the alarm stage represent a survival mechanism and harkens back to early man who constantly faced immense dangers. The alarm stage is also referred to as "the flight or fight syndrome," an observation credited to Walter Cannon, an early pioneer in the stress field (Dubos, 1965). The flight or fight response is the result primarily of autonomic nervous system activity. Many neurological and hormonal signals help to mediate the stress response. For a breakdown of these events see Figure 6-1.

The stage of resistance is the body's effort to adapt. The body attempts to bring about a successful resolution to the stressful situation. An adrenocortical response results from stressor impact, which, in turn, accelerates the body's energy expenditure. Hormones begin secreting and blood levels are altered to sustain an intense reaction. In a normal situation, this process is eventually diminished back to base line levels. However, if the stressor continues, the next stage appears.

The stage of exhaustion occurs when the system's energy resources are depleted. Disease and/or death can result if this stage persists. For an overview of the major body changes during the GAS see Figure 6-2.

The physiological adaptive response can be initiated from contact with any type of stressor. For example, jogging, a physiological stressor; phobia, a psychological stressor; and peer pressure, a sociocultural stressor, can all stimulate the physiological adaptive capacities of man. Note the physical symptoms Jenny demonstrated in response to a psychological stressor—fear of not doing well on an exam.

Psychological Adaptation. Psychological adaptation achieves balance or a steady state in the system by using mental strategies and operational patterns of behavior that have succeeded in the past. Psychological adaptation usually begins unconsciously, but individuals can become conscious of their adaptation, e.g., "I might be rationalizing, but I think I worked hard enough and it's time to take a break." Psychological adaptation consists of three coping patterns: built-in defense and damage repair mechanisms, defense-oriented mechanisms, and task-oriented mechanisms.

The first coping pattern, built-in defense and damage repair, refers

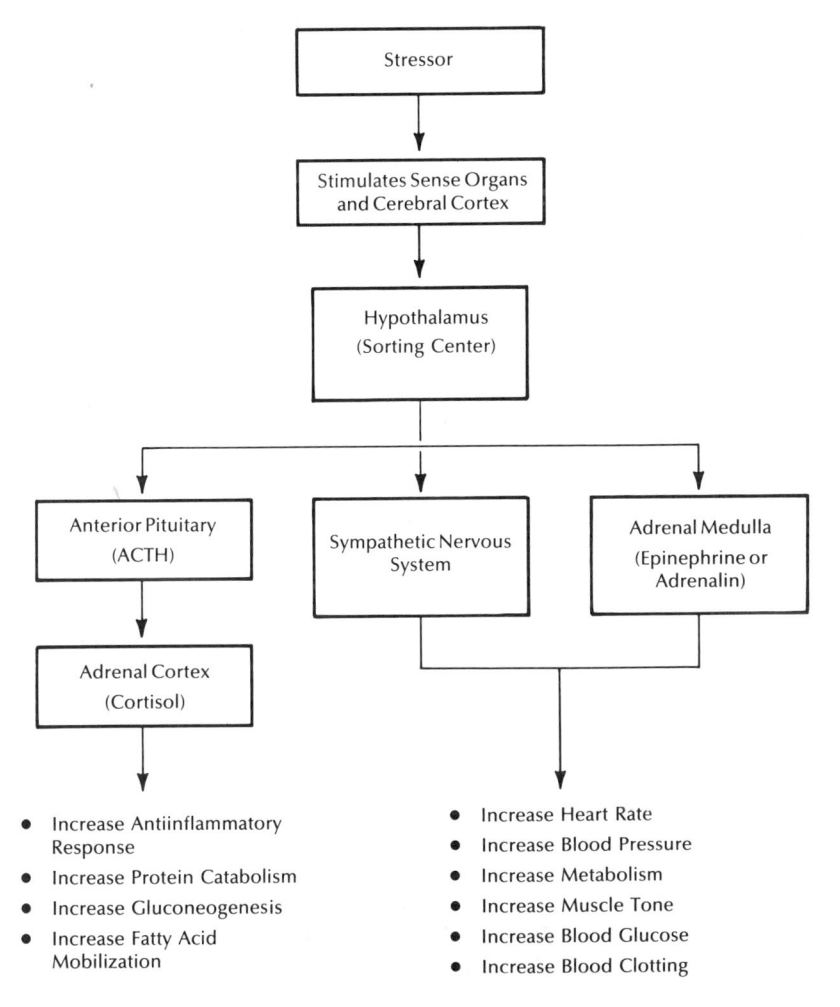

```
                    ┌─────────────┐
                    │   Stressor  │
                    └──────┬──────┘
                           ▼
              ┌────────────────────────┐
              │ Stimulates Sense Organs│
              │   and Cerebral Cortex  │
              └───────────┬────────────┘
                          ▼
              ┌────────────────────────┐
              │      Hypothalamus      │
              │    (Sorting Center)    │
              └───────────┬────────────┘
```

| Anterior Pituitary (ACTH) | Sympathetic Nervous System | Adrenal Medulla (Epinephrine or Adrenalin) |

Adrenal Cortex (Cortisol)

- Increase Antiinflammatory Response
- Increase Protein Catabolism
- Increase Gluconeogenesis
- Increase Fatty Acid Mobilization

- Increase Heart Rate
- Increase Blood Pressure
- Increase Metabolism
- Increase Muscle Tone
- Increase Blood Glucose
- Increase Blood Clotting

Figure 6-1 Stress Reaction.

to the shock-depression-adaptation process which helps the system work through strong feelings. Lawrence and Lawrence (1979) have developed a model of adaptation directed toward repair and the working through of feelings. They have included shock and disbelief, developing awareness, and a resolution of the loss in their model. Depression is also a hallmark of repairing defenses. An illustration of this is a person involved in an auto accident who may be in such psychological shock that he does not realize he is hurt. This shock serves to numb the mind and body and prevent additional stressors from impinging upon a system already overloaded. Later he becomes depressed about the accident and all that is involved. This is the body's attempt at providing time for adapting. He musters together his coping ability and

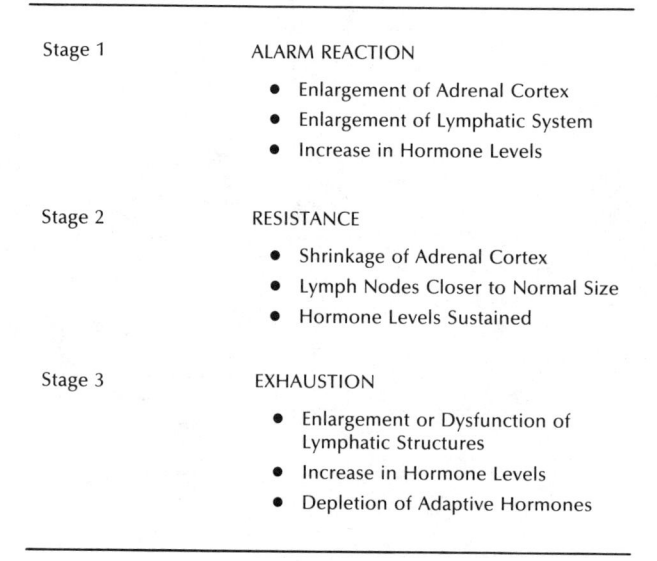

Stage 1	ALARM REACTION
	• Enlargement of Adrenal Cortex
	• Enlargement of Lymphatic System
	• Increase in Hormone Levels
Stage 2	RESISTANCE
	• Shrinkage of Adrenal Cortex
	• Lymph Nodes Closer to Normal Size
	• Hormone Levels Sustained
Stage 3	EXHAUSTION
	• Enlargement or Dysfunction of Lymphatic Structures
	• Increase in Hormone Levels
	• Depletion of Adaptive Hormones

Figure 6-2 General Adaptation Syndrome (GAS). A stress syndrome, termed the general adaptation syndrome (GAS) by Hans Selye, evolves in three stages. Stages 1 and 2 are continuously repeated throughout a lifetime cycle. If resistance cannot be sustained, exhaustion (Stage 3) with its altered psychophysiological functioning occurs. (Smith, M., and Selye, H. "Stress—Reducing the Negative Effects of Stress." *American Journal of Nursing* 79 (1979): 1953–1955.)

begins to handle the details of the auto accident, i.e., filing insurance forms, making arrangements for repair of the car.

The second coping pattern involves **defense** mechanisms that protect the ego and self-concept. These mechanisms are described in various sources of psychoanalytic writing. They include such forms of thinking as denial, projection, and rationalization. They arise from the unconscious automatically when a need for them is stirred. Recall the introductory situation. Can you identify the coping pattern Jenny uses that involves defense mechanisms?

In contrast with the first two coping mechanisms which tend to be unconscious, the third coping pattern occurs on a more conscious level. The third is termed task-oriented coping. This is a heads-on approach to dealing with stressors. This process involves consciously planning activities to deal with specific stressors or problems and is frequently referred to as problem-solving. Can you think of specific strategies or approaches Jenny could utilize if she used the task-oriented coping pattern? For example, could she make an appointment with her instructor to discuss difficult areas of content in the course?

When man uses new psychological adaptive measures successfully there is a feeling of discovery and of being in uncharted waters. With the help of imagination and a feeling for change he moves toward a healthy goal. It is not necessarily a glowing and rosy state but the system moves in the general direction of growth and development. At times there are sharp-edged discoveries that can be turned in favor of the system when creative faculties are brought to bear.

Studies have tended to focus on the physiological or psychological aspects of adaptation, but these aspects are not exclusive of each other and show similar patterns. Systems theory, which deals with the totality of man, also lends itself to a corresponding pattern. This corresponding pattern is demonstrated in Table 6–1.

All of the adaptive patterns roughly consist of five periods including before, during, and after events. The systems theory approach shows how the system responds following contact with a stressor. At that point energy is used and eventually organized and directed to combat the stressor. The results can be effective or ineffective. The GAS shows a forceful response that effectively or ineffectively resists exhausting the individual. In terms of perception, the individual can perceive a stressor as favorable, resulting in effective acceptance of the happy state or nonacceptance, depending on intervening factors. Unfavorably perceived stressors may also be experienced and accepted or not, depending on the important intervening variables.

Sociocultural Adaptation. Sociocultural adaptation works to resolve stressors arising from the social fabric and climate of the culture. This area is vast and hints at many varied sources. Man's system maintains a steady state by adjusting to norms, beliefs, values, and **pressures** from society. As society

TABLE 6–1
Comparison of event-response stress models

Systems Approach	GAS* (Physiological)	Favorably Perceived Stressor (Psychological)	Unfavorably Perceived Stressor (Psychological)
Precontact	Prealarm	Prestimulation	Preinjury
Contact	Alarm	Shock	Shock
Energy Mobilized	Alarm	Happiness Excitement	Anger Depression
Directed Energy or Misdirected Energy Ineffective	Resistance or Exhaustion	Acceptance or Nonacceptance	Acceptance or Nonacceptance

* After Selye.

and the culture change, man's system has to adjust to these changes. Janis (1968) has developed a coping model which could assist decision making for sociocultural adaptation. The model is a five-stage operation beginning with (1) appraising the alternatives (Is the challenge serious enough to bother about?) and moves on to (2) identifying the alternatives, (3) analyzing the alternatives, (4) selecting a new personal policy, and then (5) keeping to the policy.

An example can be seen in the gradually changing social values concerning utilization of world energy resources. A change from industrial values of exploration to conservation in an individual's value system would require some decision making regarding what is to be conserved, how much is possible for one person to conserve, and to what extent resources are needed to maintain life. If the individual decided in the end to conserve electricity by installing a windmill in his backyard and his closest neighbors found the windmill unsightly, could he continue to adhere to his decision despite the negative feedback?

One can see where a number of stressors may enter this situation. However, if man reaches Janis' fifth stage, which adheres to the new policy despite challenges, he has found a means to cope. Being able to keep to the new policy implies strategies that strengthen man in the face of challenges. He can reason through, he can block out, he can counterclaim. Indeed, there is an array of strategies.

Dimensional Interaction. Although each of man's dimensions adds to his adaptive capacity, his response to stress is produced by the interactions within the total system. This response requires the use of energy as adaptive mechanisms are active dynamic processes.

Saxton and Hyland (1979) have described five levels of energy utilization in adaptation. These levels move from least energy draining to the most energy draining. The first level involves simple responses to ordinary stressors that rarely reach awareness. The second level involves stronger responses to handle more complex stressors. This level of energy utilization results in a general awareness that something is wrong. Nonspecific, generalized responses of the system giving rise to symptoms of disease is the third level. In the fourth level, adaptation causes new stressors and irreversible damage can occur. The last level, the most energy draining, interferes with life functions. This level requires outside intervention.

As can be seen from these levels of energy consumption, adaptation may be adaptive or maladaptive. Rahe and Ransom (1978) have devised a model which attempts to identify the events that flow between contact with a stressor and the system's response. Figure 6–3 is a modified version of this model. It shows the potential for a healthy or unhealthy outcome. This model moves from man's contact with an experience in life to deeper and deeper involvement regarding it.

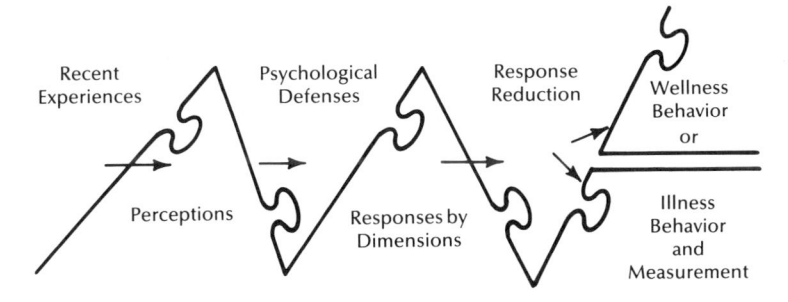

Figure 6-3 Experiences, Intervening Variables, and Outcomes.

Recent experiences are changes that go on; they could include such events as the birth of a new baby, retirement, launching children into the adult world, loss of a job, or inability to achieve according to self-expectations. When the experience occurs it will immediately be influenced by man's perception of the event. The perception reflects past situations and what resulted from them; human and material resources; and any unique qualities that can strengthen a particular individual. From this point psychological defenses come into play, shielding through denial or other means to assist the ego. This is based on psychoanalytic theory.

Next, all the dimensions of man could begin operating, including more psychological aspects. Rahe and Ransom (1978) have focused on a combination of psychological and physiological responses giving rise to mild sensations of not feeling "good." Moodiness, tight muscles, headaches, and certain internal shifts, such as elevated blood pressure, fall into this category of psychophysiological responses. The sociocultural dimension with value and norm concerns also adds to the psychophysiological response. Then the concerned response with mild discomfort could also reflect difficulty with developmental tasks.

Response reduction aims at modifying the course which man's body is taking to handle the stressor input. This acts to reduce the mild discomforts that have arisen. Relaxation techniques, for example, have served the purpose of response reduction. Illness behaviors may be manifested at this time through more intense concentration on the symptoms that have appeared and greater disruption in the normal life style. The person might also begin identifying with the sick role and find his way to a care provider where illness measurements are conducted. Wellness behaviors could result if the response reduction methods are effective. The system then returns to a steady state and energies are normalized.

From exposure to a life experience, a chain of events follows, bringing about a mixture of responses that mean successful adaptation or maladaptation for the system. In the model shown, the events fit together like a puzzle. How these pieces fit together varies from one individual to another, depending on past experiences, overall capacities, and the existing state of health. Man's system is a working system which attempts to adapt to stressors that are encountered. Adaptation may make the system more sensitive to some stimuli than to others, as in the case of the admiring teenager who wants to appear so perfect for his first "heart throb" that he stumbles on a stone as he walks to her front door.

In concluding our discussion on stress reaction, let us look at a specific situation. As you read this situation try to determine the dimensions involved and the levels of adaptation.

A twenty-month-old boy who has cruised down the wrong aisle in the supermarket all of a sudden realizes he is not with Mommy and is exposed to stressors of loss. In addition, he cannot decide which way to go to correct the situation. This brings conflict into the picture. He makes an effort around one corner and bumps into a display stand. His system must deal with the stressor inputs. He cries, he yells, he runs, Mommy finds him. He pushes into her skirt and hugs her legs and breaks into a gleeful laugh, jumping up and down with remnants of tears drying on his face. He is adapting.

STRESS ADAPTATION AND SYSTEMS THEORY

Within the study of man no theory exists in isolation from the study of other theories. One excellent example of theory overlap is stress adaptation and systems theory. Figure 6-4 visually depicts this relationship. By looking at the overlap in these two theories, we can begin to appreciate the interrelatedness of all theories which focus on the phenomena of man. In other words, as

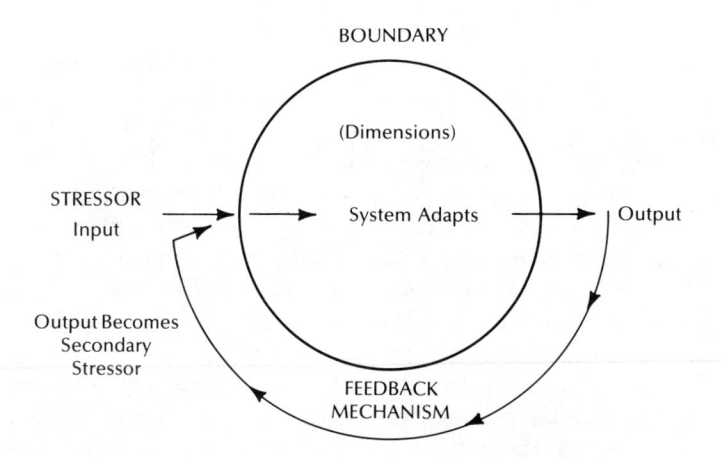

Figure 6-4 A System's Approach to the Stress Adaptation Cycle.

nurses we can appreciate the value of a variety of theories in finding ways to assist man.

All stimuli to which the system is exposed can be considered potential stress inputs or stressors to the system. These stressors can challenge the system constructively or destructively. Constructive inputs are stimulating, aesthetically pleasing, satisfying to needs, and usually enhancing to the system. Constructive inputs are usually perceived by the system favorably. Destructive inputs are just the opposite. These are usually perceived by the system unfavorably. They can lower adaptive efficiency and reduce resistance. In a situation of prolonged exposure, they may bring about irreversible wear and tear and finally termination of the system. The system has a limitation of resources to deal with stressors. Each system can only tolerate so much stimulation and then the situation becomes destructive. The point when stimuli become destructive varies with each system.

The boundaries of the system have some control over the amount of stimuli received. They operate to keep stressors out or to put out those that are destructive. Painful stressors are considered in this category. Conversely, stressors are accepted in and kept in if constructive to the system. Warm, loving relationships are included here.

The process of reverberation explains to some degree the amount of stress produced by the stimuli. Reverberation results from stressor inputs and may be highly visible or not, depending on the particular mix of stressor(s) and the system. A given stressor may have a pounding reverberation into one system but the same stressor may have little consequences reverberating through a second system. A new job, for example, may create an intense rippling effect in the buying habits of a family previously deprived of buying or whose perceptions include feeling strongly deprived. A family without this strong feeling may not alter buying habits in the event of a new job. The meaning and importance of the stressor has an impact on the extent of the reverberation and overall capacity of the system to handle the stressor.

Assessment of the Stress State

According to Hans Selye, one must learn to detect what for oneself and one's client is "overstress," when we have exceeded our limits of adaptability, and "understress," when we have not achieved self-realization. Selye suggests that our main goal is to seek out a balance between overstress and understress and to experience more good stress than bad. He believes that we have a limited amount of energy allocated for coping with stress and if we are under heavy stress, we undergo very rapid wear and tear. So, the main idea would be to seek an adequate means of dealing with stress so that we conserve this valuable energy.

Before dealing with an unhealthy stress state, we must be able to recognize stress. There are many signs of stress which are experienced every day.

For example, you may be quietly sitting, eating dinner at home when you hear announced over the radio that there has been a fatal bus accident close by. You know that your mother was supposed to be on that bus. Moments later, your mother walks through the door, safe and sound, because she caught an earlier bus. You feel just as overwhelmingly happy now as you had felt shocked initially. However, the signs of stress you experienced in both cases are the same. Aggravation, increased pulse, rise in blood pressure ("thumping" in the chest and perspiration)—all these signs are the result of increased hormone secretion or nervous activity.

A number of indices of stress which are not so obvious but which we should monitor throughout our lifetime also exist. Depending on our conditioning, we all respond differently to general demands. But, on the whole, each of us tends to respond particularly with one set of signs caused by the malfunction of whatever happens to be the most vulnerable part of our machinery, and when these signs appear, it is time to stop or change our activity (Selye, 1977). It is important that you are aware of these warning signs of stress in yourself as well as in your clients. The nurse can assess the clients' stress state according to the dimensions of man.

Physiological Dimension of Man. When looking for signs of stress in this dimension, you look for evidence of stimulation of the sympathetic nervous system. Because this system is activated, the client experiences the general adaptation syndrome and therefore you need information about the client's temperature, pulse, blood pressure, appetite, coordination, urine output, and pupil size. All of these signs would be considered evidence of the short-term effects of stress. If stress persists over a period of time, the client may exhibit ulcers, skin disorders, bowel problems, or nervousness. This list is by no means complete, but it gives you some ideas of what overstress can do to a body.

Psychological Dimension of Man. When assessing this area, you look for alterations in a client's behavioral patterns. Some signs of this are

1. *Accentuation of one mode or pattern.* A client may overuse one mode or pattern of behavior. This may be a cue that the person is using more energy than usual in an effort to maintain a steady state. A nurse might observe that a person who ordinarily nibbles at his food suddenly eats constantly due to intensification of stress. A client who laughs inappropriately may also be experiencing the same problem. It can be said that accentuated use of a behavioral pattern may indicate that a person's steady state is threatened.
2. *Alterations in activity patterns.* One way in which clients conserve energy is to decrease activity. Prior to an exam, a student may not perform any household tasks in order to concentrate on it fully. On a hospital unit, a nurse might notice that a client who usually carefully grooms herself has suddenly stopped. This may be an indication of increasing stressors. Other clients may increase activities

as a means of coping. A mother of a child who has cancer may do volunteer work in addition to all her other duties. Therefore, when coping with stressors, an individual may alter his normal routine.

3. *Disorganization.* It is important to know that all people have organized themselves within their own environments. When stressors intensify, the nurse tries to identify clues pointing to disorganization. This state can be identified if you remember that the client's priorities will seem inappropriate and he may give inappropriate attention to detail or any activity which would seem purposeless. A client may exhibit such purposeless activities as eye blinking, lip biting, pacing, and nail biting. You must also be able to make a distinction between stress states and habits. A person may bite his nails regardless of his stress state.

4. *Distortion of reality.* When the stress state increases, a person's thought processes may become so impaired that he can no longer think logically and solve problems. The client might misunderstand events which would seem normal to you and me. A client who is told to turn, cough, and deep breathe after surgery might automatically think she had pneumonia. Distortion of reality can be quite normal under very stressful conditions, and it is very important for you to be aware of its existence in your clients (Byrne & Thompson, 1978). You obtain all of this information by observation of the client and his family. In order to make the most valid observations, you get a base line by asking the client about his eating and sleeping patterns, etc., as well as considering the age appropriateness of the behavior.

Sociocultural Dimension. To assess the stress state in this dimension, you look at the client's and his family's norms, beliefs, and values. You should obtain some valid clues in your interview. For instance, you may learn that a patient is a Jehovah's Witness, a group that strongly forbids blood transfusions. This fact could place untold stress on a client and his family if the person needed to have open heart surgery.

In this day and age of "instant answers," many questionnaires have been devised to measure stress in an individual. One such useful instrument is called the Social Readjustment Rating Scale, which simplifies recognition and prediction of stress-related events. Originally, this scale consisted of 43 events associated with stress that require coping, adaptation, or adjustment. A numerical weight called a Life Change Unit (LCU) was assigned to each event. The greater the degree of impact of the life change, the higher the LCU number. Holmes and Rahe developed this scale for adults, and Coddington adapted it for children and adolescents (Holmes & Rahe, 1967; Coddington, 1972). Many have determined that a score of 200 LCU's or more per year increases an individual's susceptibility to illness. You may want to take a few minutes and look at sample items from these two scales found in Tables 6-2 and 6-3.

People utilize many behavioral maneuvers in order to regain balance; these may be adaptive or maladaptive. If the nurse examines the client's behavior, these changes may be noted and an estimate of the intensity of the

TABLE 6-2
Sample items from social readjustment rating scale (children)

Rank	Life Event	Life Change Unit
1	Getting married	101
2	Unwed pregnancy	92
3	Death of a parent	87
4	Acquiring a visible deformity	81
5	Divorce of parents	77
6	Male partner in pregnancy out of wedlock	77
7	Becoming involved with drugs or alcohol	76
10	Death of a brother or sister	68
12	Pregnancy in unwed teenage sister	64
13	Discovery of being an adopted child	64
14	Marriage of parent to stepparent	63
15	Death of a close friend	63
17	Serious illness requiring hospitalization of child	58
18	Failure of a grade in school	56
19	Move to a new school district	56
21	Serious illness requiring hospitalization of parent	55
23	Breaking up with a boyfriend or girlfriend	53
24	Beginning to date	51
25	Suspension from school	50
29	Loss of job by a parent	46
30	Outstanding personal achievement	46
32	Being accepted at a college of his/her choice	43
33	Beginning senior high school	42
42	Mother beginning to work	26

From: Coddington, R. D. "The Significance of Life Events as Etiological Factors in Disease of Children." *Journal of Psychosomatic Research* 16 (1972): 7.

state of stress as well as the client's ability to use his adaptive capacities can be made.

In addition to looking for these signs and symptoms, the nurse obtains a "history." A history consists of asking the client questions about his past and present state of health. These questions include ones which would give you pertinent information about all of man's dimensions.

When obtaining a history you collect information from the client regarding how stress has been handled in the past. You question the client as to the type, number, and duration of the stressors. Here are two questions which you could ask that would help you obtain this information: (1) What stressors has the client and his family experienced in the past? You may ask what types of major events have occurred in the past; (2) What coping mechanisms does the client and family utilize? You may ask how he and his family coped with the various stress he has identified in the past. After collecting data about the past, you now focus on the present problem.

Identification of actual or potential stressors begins by recognizing those stressors which would commonly be perceived by most people as stressors. Events which present a potential threat to any of man's dimensions are

TABLE 6-3
Sample items from social readjustment rating scale (adult)

Rank	Life Event	Life Change Unit
1	Death of spouse	100
2	Divorce	73
3	Marital separation	65
4	Jail term	63
5	Death of close family member	63
6	Personal injury or illness	53
7	Marriage	50
8	Fired at work	47
9	Marital reconciliation	45
10	Retirement	45
12	Pregnancy	40
13	Sex difficulties	39
16	Change in financial state	38
19	Change in number of arguments with spouse	35
21	Foreclosure of mortgage or loan	30
22	Change in responsibilities at work	29
23	Son or daughter leaving home	29
24	Trouble with in-laws	29
25	Outstanding personal achievement	28
28	Change in living conditions	25
30	Trouble with boss	23
32	Change in residence	20
36	Change in social activities	18
41	Vacation	13
42	Christmas	12

From: Holmes, T., and Rahe, R. N. "The Social Readjustment Rating Scale." *Journal of Psychosomatic Research* 2 (1967): 213.

identified as universal stressors. For example, physical danger, losses, conflict, and change are potential stressors for everyone. Knowing certain events are potential stressors is helpful to the nurse when assessing specific stressors for specific clients. In Table 6-4 are several examples of potential universal

TABLE 6-4
Model for identifying potential and/or existing stressors using major concepts and dimensions of man

Continuum	Physiological	Psychological	Sociological
Infant	Premature delivery	Inadequate touching	Disrupted mother and infant relationship
Child	Casted leg	Feeling isolated	Limited socialization
Young Adult	Drug dependency	Emotional instability	Loss of support systems
Adult 40–60	Myocardial infarction	Fear of dependency	Job insecurity
Elderly	Reduced hearing	Tension from isolated feelings	Retirement

stressors. These stressors are classified by the developmental continuum and the dimensions of man.

The nurse begins by identifying what she believes to be actual or potential stressors, but there needs to be extremely clear communication between client and nurse because what might be considered an overwhelming and destructive stressor to the nurse may not be viewed so by the client, who might see it more as a challenge. In order to do this, you ask questions which give you some idea of the client's and family's perception of the problem. Sample questions to ask include

1. What stressors are the individual and his family actually experiencing? The answer to this question will give you an idea of how the client perceives his situation. Asking this question is critical because all too often nurses assume that everything is a stressor; this assumption may lead to nursing care which is inappropriate.
2. What effect does this individual and/or his family believe this stressor will have on their life style? You must consider the client's and family's perception of the duration, type, and number of stressors they are experiencing at the present time; then you can determine if they feel these would be taken in stride or if these stressors would cause a major disruption in their living style.
3. Does the individual and his family believe they have the capacity and energy to meet the challenges of stressors? This question will help you to determine which support systems the client utilizes. For instance, he may lean very heavily on other family members for support in his illness, therefore, you must act as a support to the family.
4. Does the individual need help? After asking the above questions, you should be able to determine whether or not the individual needs further help. Actually, all four questions will tell you what the client and his family are going through at the present time and will help you plan your nursing interventions.

Table 6–5 should also assist you in assessing the client's perception of the stressor and its impact by presenting a model relating this perception to health, habits, personal relationships, and current events. The emphasis in this model is on perceptions, the change aspect of stress, and areas of man's response. The situation used to demonstrate this model is that of an individual who has been threatened with a job layoff and has now developed a peptic ulcer. If the person perceives a recent diagnosis of peptic ulcer as a danger, he will be activated to help himself, complain, or use some other means of expression. There is always the possibility he is denying the threat even though he has been told the diagnosis. Through careful questioning this area can be explored selectively to determine strengths to build on and weaknesses to work with. Using this model and moving to the right along the change perception category, one can identify a number of changes which may be perceived as stressful. For example, in the perception of change row, the nurse

TABLE 6-5
Model of perceptions of client with relationship to change, limitations, and resources

	STATE OF HEALTH	PERSONAL HABITS	PERSONAL RELATIONSHIPS	CURRENT PERSONAL EVENTS
Perception of Changes	Recent ulcer	Dietary changes	New food preparation to fit in with family meals	Threat of job layoff
Perception of Limitations	Recent hospitalization	Reduced responsibility	Reduced family provider role	Period of waiting
Perception of Resources	Health provider support	Received health instruction re: relaxation	Open discussion with family members	Determine alternate means for finances

may think "Does he perceive dietary changes as stressful?" and follow with relevant questions.

Strategies for Stress Reduction

Now that you have a basis for measuring the stress state in man, you proceed by analyzing this information and developing a plan of care. Keep in mind that the goal of nursing is to assist the individual and his family to obtain and maintain the optimal level of health by

1. Recognizing where the client is on the health-illness continuum.
2. Determining the effectiveness of coping mechanisms.
3. Intervening appropriately to promote adaptation.

All these steps must be carried out in collaboration with the client because without his interest and input your care plan will not be effective. Interventions are planned according to where the patient falls in reference to the type of care he will require. We will consider each of these levels separately.

Primary Level. At this level, you and the client determine what stressors existed in his life and his perceptions of them. Then you and he develop a protection plan. This plan is a means of attempting to balance work and play, and it is composed of a list of things which will help the client cope with stressors before they become major problems. For instance, a busy executive who must cope with many stresses during the day would find life more tolerable if he could engage in vigorous exercise. You might suggest that he jog for ten minutes a day. Other hints for what might be appropriate in a protection plan might include provisions for rest, exercise, an activity the client really enjoys, organizing time, altering the environment, verbalization, and diversion.

Secondary Level. On this level, this patient is ill and is hospitalized. The nurse modifies, reduces, or removes stressors in order to get the client through the crisis. This is done by establishing a climate of trust and effective communication and by supporting adaptive processes. Such measures may include administering antibiotics, providing emotional support, or modifying the patient's environment.

Tertiary Level. This is the rehabilitation level. The client's lines of defense are broken but are in a state of repair. At this stage it is also appropriate to formulate a protection plan. This plan will assist the client to actually get back on his feet. Some techniques that are effective at this level include yoga, meditation, knowing your own limitations, diversional activities, and relaxation techniques. How would you go about determining the techniques that would be effective for Jenny? For example, yoga might be more effective for Jenny at her young age than for an elderly client.

SUMMARY

This chapter introduces the reader to stress adaptation theory by first defining and explaining the concepts of stress and stressors. The relationships are further explored by a discussion of both the nature of stressors and the classification of stressors. Against this background the reader is introduced to how man adapts to stress-producing stimuli. Man's adaptation is strongly influenced by the fact that he is an open system. Stress theory is then related to systems theory. The chapter concludes by applying stress theory to nursing, particularly in the areas of assessment and planning. Key points to remember are

1. The characteristics of stress and stressors define and differentiate these two concepts.
2. There is no one right way to classify stressors; however, classification systems are helpful in organizing the information concerning stressors for each client.
3. All theories related to man overlap as demonstrated by the relationship between systems and stress theory.
4. Each man responds as a unique individual utilizing all dimensions when encountering stressors. The goal of his response is adaptation.
5. Identification of the stress state involves application of stress theory to the assessment and planning process.
6. Though numerous techniques can produce stress reduction, these techniques must be individualized when applied to clients.

REFERENCES

Bailey, J. "Stress and Stress Management: An Overview." *Journal of Nursing Education* 19 (6) [1980]: 5–7.

Bailey, J., Streffer, S., and Grout, J. "The Stress Audit: Identifying the Stressors of ICU Nursing." *Journal of Nursing Education* 19 (6) [1980]: 15–25.

Benson, H. "Your Innate Asset for Combating Stress." *Nursing Digest* 3 (3) [1975]: 38–41.

Burdis, C. "Biofeedback—Does It Work? *The Canadian Nurse* 76 (2) [1980]: 44–46.

Byrne, M., and Thompson, L. *Key Concepts for the Study and Practice of Nursing.* St. Louis: The C. V. Mosby Co., 1978.

Calkin, J. D. "Assessing Small Children: Are Hospitalized Toddlers Adapting to the Experience as Well as We Think?" *The American Journal of MCN* 4 (1979): 18–23.

Coddington, R. D. The Significance of Life Events as Etiological Factors in Disease of Children. *Journal of Psychosomatic Research* 16 (1972): 7.

Coelho, G., Hamburg, D., and Adams, J., eds. *Coping and Adapting.* New York: Basic Books, Inc., 1974.

Coleman, J. C. Life Stress and Maladaptive Behavior. *The American Journal of Occupation Therapy* 27 (4) [1973]: 169–173.

Dubos, R. *Man Adapting.* New Haven: Yale University Press, 1965.

Frazier, C. "The Anxious Mind and Disease." *Nursing Care* 19 (1) [1977]: 16–19, 34.

Goodwin, S. "Curbing the Caveman in Us." *Nursing Mirror* 150 (20) [1980]: 22–24.

Havighurst, R. *Developmental Tasks and Education.* New York: Longmans, Green, 1952.

Holmes, T., and Rahe, R. N. "The Social Readjustment Rating Scale." *Journal of Psychosomatic Research* 11 (2) [1967]: 213–218.

Janis, J. "Stages in the Decision Making Process." In *Theories of Cognitive Consistency: A Sourcebook*, edited by R. Abelson, et al. Chicago: Rand McNally and Co., 1968.

Jones, P. "An Adaptation Model for Nursing Research." *American Journal of Nursing* 78 (1978): 1900–1906.

Lawrence, S., and Lawrence, R. "A Model of Adaptation to the Stress of Chronic Illness." *Nursing Forum* 18 (1) [1979]: 33–42.

Lyness, A. "Interview Observations Between Mothers and Nurses at Selected Child Health Conferences." Unpublished Master's Thesis, University of Pittsburgh, Graduate School of Public Health, 1971.

MacFarlane, P. "The Stress Test." *The Canadian Nurse* 76 (4) [1980]: 39–40.

Mason, J. W. "A Historical View of the Stress Field, Part I." *Journal of Human Stress* 1 (1) [1975]: 6–12.

Mason, J. W. "A Historical View of the Stress Field, Part II." *Journal of Human Stress* 1 (2) [1975]: 22–36.

Murray, R., and Zentner, J. *Nursing Concepts for Health Promotion.* Englewood Cliffs, NJ: Prentice-Hall, Inc., 1979.

Pender, N. *Health Promotion in Nursing Practice.* Norwalk, CT: Appleton-Century-Crofts, 1982.

Pollitt, J. "Symptoms of Stress, Part I." *Nursing Mirror* 144 (24) [1977]: 13–14.

Pollitt, J. "Symptoms of Stress, Part II." *Nursing Mirror* 144 (25) [1977]: 24–26.

Rahe, R., and Ransom, A. "Life Studies: Past History and Future Directions." *Journal of Human Stress* 4 (1) [1978]: 3–15.

Reich, C. *The Greening of America.* New York: Random House, Inc., 1970.

Richter, J., and Sloan, R. "Stress, a Relaxation Technique." *American Journal of Nursing* 79 [1979]: 1960–1964.

Robinson, A. "Stress Can Make You or Break You." *RN* 38 (1975): 73–76.

Saxton, D., and Hyland, P. *Planning and Implementing Nursing Intervention.* St. Louis: The C. V. Mosby Co., 1979.

Scully, R. "Stress in the Nurse." *American Journal of Nursing* 80 (1980): 912–915.

Selye, H. "A Code for Coping with Stress." *AORN Journal* 25 (1) [1977]: 35–42.

Selye, H. "The Stress of Life." *Nursing Forum* 4 (1) [1965]: 28–38.

Selye, H. *The Stress of Life.* New York: McGraw Hill Co., 1956.

Sloboda, S. "Understanding Patient Behavior." *Nursing 77* 7 (9) [1977]: 74–77.

Tierney, M., and Strom, L. "Stress: Type A Behavior in the Nurse." *American Journal of Nursing* 80 (5) [1980]: 915–918.

Wallace, J. "Living with Stress." *Nursing Times* 74 (11) [1978]: 457–458.

7

Learning theory

DEFINITION OF TERMS

Accommodation The process whereby the child modifies or changes his thinking process in order to adapt to reality.

Assimilation The process by which the child takes in information.

Bit A single unit of information.

Classical Conditioning A theory of learning which explains changes in behavior or responses as a result of pairing the conditioned stimulus with the unconditioned stimulus.

Emitted Behavior Behavior that is originated initially without any identifiable stimuli.

Interference A process whereby the previous learning interferes with new learning or new information interferes with previous learning.

Law of Effect When a modifiable connection between a situation and a response is made and is accompanied or followed by a satisfying state of affairs, then that connection's strength is increased. When the connection is made and accompanied or followed by an annoying state of affairs, its strength is decreased.

Memory Information that is retained within a human learning system.

Short-Term Memory (STM) Information that is currently in the focus of attention and is retained through a conscious, active process.

Long-Term Memory (LTM) Information that has high utility and has been stored for permanent retention.

Percept An impression of an object obtained solely by use of the senses.

Perception A two-step process in an open system by which data are taken in and then interpreted as information.

Reinforcement The process whereby an event occurs after a behavior and increases the probability that the behavior will recur.

Remembering The process of retaining information within a learning system.

Respondent Behavior Behavior that results from an identifiable stimulus.
Response Specific measurable behavior or output.
  Conditioned Output or behavior which occurs as a result of a conditioned stimulus.
  Unconditioned Output or behavior which occurs without previous learning and as a result of an unconditioned stimulus.
Stimulus A specific measurable input which will produce a response.
  Unconditioned Stimulus Specific input which will produce a measurable response without previous learning.
  Conditioned Stimulus Specific input which has been paired with an unconditioned stimulus so that it will produce the same measurable response as the unconditioned stimulus.
Structuring The organization of data taken into the human system in a way in which it can be recognized, interpreted, or understood as information.
Stimulus-Response Unit An event in which a specific measurable input results in a specific measurable output. The input is referred to as the stimulus or the S and the output is referred to as the response or the R.

Nurses work in such a variety of settings with such different clients that there are very few tasks which all nurses must do. One exception is teaching. Nearly all nurses are required to teach at some time and it can be your most rewarding or most frustrating experience. Let's eavesdrop on a few nurses and see just how they discuss this experience.

Nurse 1: I explain to every woman who comes in this office as a client how to do breast-self exams, but I don't know why I bother. Those who are interested already know how and do them every month. Most of the other women tolerate my explaining but I know they will never follow up.

Nurse 2: Yes, I know just what you mean, yet the other side of that coin is what happened to me today. I asked one of the clients why she never takes her children's temps when they are sick. She has two preschoolers and a new baby. No one has ever shown her how to take a rectal temp. She was so happy to learn this was something she could do, and I feel so much better knowing all three of those kids are safer because their mother is better able to care for them.

Nurse 3: Well, I had a situation today which was the same as and different from both of yours. My client was interested but still didn't learn. Mrs. S. is to take her husband home in two days. He is in a body cast and needs help even with turning over. Mrs. S. really wants to take good care of him but she is so nervous and tries so hard that everything I showed her she did wrong. I just don't understand.

The task each of these nurses is discussing is teaching, yet unless one understands learning, effective teaching can be nothing more than trial and error.

Man as an open system lives in an ever changing, ever demanding world. His successes as well as his failures in life are directly related to his skills in adapting to ever changing demands. Man, more than any other system, is dependent on his ability to learn as his means of developing his adaptive skills. But what is known and what can be explained about this process is far from complete. No one theory of learning exists but what we have is a variety of interrelated, overlapping, and, at times, conflicting theories.

It is beyond the purposes of this book to review each of the various theories of learning. However, since there is a great deal of overlap and interrelation, the major theories can be classified into three approaches to learning. These approaches are the behavioral, the information processing, and the developmental. Although each approach influences the definitions of learning, teaching, and the teaching-learning process, an operational definition of each term will be given. How learning theory relates to nursing practice will then be explored. Principles of learning which should guide the nurse will be given. The relationship between learning and the nursing process will be examined.

At the completion of the chapter, the reader will be able to

1. Define and explain three major approaches to learning theories.
2. Define teaching, learning, and the teaching-learning process utilizing concepts and terms basic to learning theory.
3. Identify principles of learning.
4. Give examples of how learning principles influence the teaching process.
5. Relate nursing process to the teaching-learning process.

BEHAVIORAL APPROACH

Modern learning theories began to evolve around the turn of the twentieth century when it became clear that the scientific method of inquiry was very successful for understanding the physical sciences. The physical sciences had demonstrated that all kinds of substances are made up of the simplest chemical elements. It was anticipated that complex learning (i.e., problem solving) was also made up of simple elements. Therefore, the beginning efforts to understanding learning were an attempt to reduce learning to the simple elements involved. For this reason, the behavioral approach is sometimes referred to as the *reductionist* approach (Travers, 1977).

While the reductionist approach is aimed at breaking learning into its constituent parts, this is done within the framework of the scientific method. From the beginning these theories were developed from experimentation conducted in controlled laboratory conditions with rigor and objectivity. This is the main reason why animals as opposed to humans have been utilized in much of the research.

Four of the most commonly recognized and influential learning theorists of the reductionist approach are Pavlov, Thorndike, Hull, and Skinner (Snelbecker, 1974). Although each of these theorists presented different theories of learning, each theory utilized as the basic element of learning, the **stimulus-response** (S-R) **unit.** This unit attempts to explain behavior in terms of an observable input, the stimulus (or S) and a measurable output, the response (or R) (Biggs, 1971).

The first of these four theorists is Ivan Pavlov who evolved the theory of **classical conditioning** (Snelbecker, 1974). He theorized that food without previous learning will produce salivation. Therefore, he considered the food an **unconditioned stimulus** and the salivation an **unconditioned response.** An unconditioned stimulus or response is one that occurs without previous learning. If an additional stimulus, for example a bell, was presented at the same time as the unconditioned stimulus, the two stimuli would become paired. After the pairing of the two stimuli either stimulus could produce the response. The new stimulus in this case, a bell, which had become paired with the unconditioned stimulus, would now function as a **conditioned stimulus** (see Figure 7-1).

The response which occurs before learning or conditioning is termed the **unconditioned response.** After learning, when the response is produced by the conditioned stimulus alone, it is referred to as a **conditioned response.** A child who has had a series of negative experiences with people in white uniforms may show a negative response to anyone in a white uniform no matter what the situation. Such a child may have paired the unconditioned stimulus (the negative experience) with the conditioned stimulus (the white uniform).

Shortly after Pavlov began developing his theory of classical conditioning, Edward Thorndike began his research, which approached the learning process as a series of laws or principles which explained the S-R unit. The main conclusion of his research has been called the **law of effect** (Snelbecker, 1974).

Thorndike noticed that an animal in a new situation will demonstrate a variety of behaviors. If any of these behaviors happened to produce positive

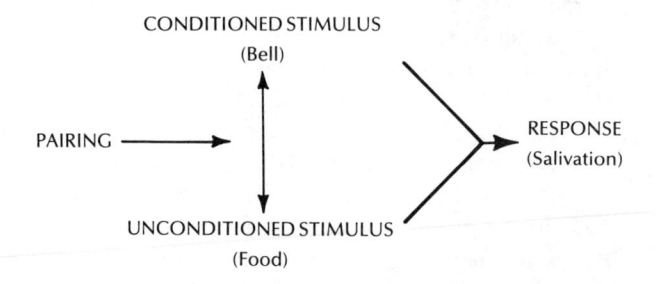

Figure 7-1 Pavlov's Classical Conditioning. If a bell is rung when food is presented, the food and the sound of the bell will become paired so either the sound or the food will result in salivation.

results (like food), the behavior was likely to be repeated. If a behavior produced negative results (like pain), the behavior was not likely to be repeated (see Figure 7-2). In other words, in a given environment we learn to perform those behaviors which produce pleasurable or positive results and avoid the behaviors which produce unpleasant or negative results. In Thorndike's words

> When a modifiable connection between a situation and a response is made and is accompanied or followed by a satisfying state of affairs; that connection's strength is increased. When made and accompanied or followed by an annoying state of affairs its strength is decreased. (Thorndike, 1913, p. 4)

Thorndike's theory of learning has been referred to as connectionism because it identified a connection between the stimulus and the response. In nursing, many behaviors exist that can be explained by this connection. If an individual who is being treated with medication for an illness feels better when he takes the medication, he is more likely to continue. If, on the other hand, the medication has side effects which make him feel worse, he is more likely to stop. There are many times when the client who is experiencing side effects should continue his medication. In this case, the nurse who explains this and points out the positive results of the medication may prevent the client from stopping needed medication.

Clark Hull, who was influenced by Pavlov and Thorndike, believed that behavior was adapted to maximize the likelihood that needs would be satisfied. Therefore, if a particular stimulus evoked a response which satisfied a need of an organism, then for that organism the connection between the stimulus and response would be strengthened. These strengthened connections increased the possibility that the behavior would occur again when the need (drive) recurred. Hull believed that need reduction or need satisfaction

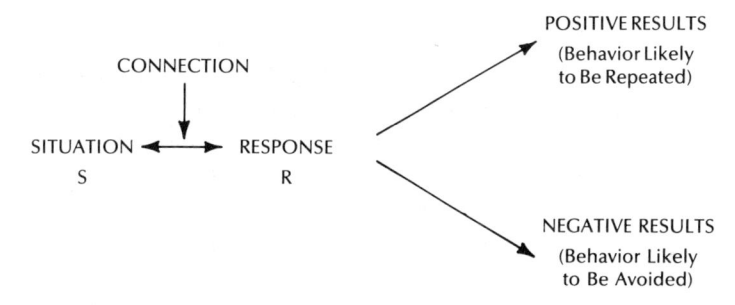

Figure 7-2 Thorndike's Law of Effect. The law of effect states that when a modifiable connection between a situation and a response is made and is accompanied or followed by a satisfying state of affairs, that connection's strength is increased. When made and accompanied or followed by an annoying state of affairs, its strength is decreased.

reinforced the behavior. In fact, his theory has been called the "true reinforcement theory of learning" (Snelbecker, 1974).

The final major theorist to represent the behaviorist position is B. F. Skinner. Skinner's writing represented a major break with the traditional explanation of the S-R unit. Pavlov, Thorndike, and Hull had all described learning as a matter of building connections between the stimulus and the response. Skinner considered this true for only some behavior, which he classified as **respondent behavior.** By respondent behavior, Skinner was referring to behavior that results from an identifiable stimulus. However, for a large number of behaviors, there is no identifiable stimulus. These Skinner classified as **emitted behaviors** (Travers, 1971; Snelbecker, 1974).

Skinner believed that one way the learning process began was with an organism which emitted a large amount of random behavior. For example, an infant will produce or emit a large amount of random vocal behavior. Through a complex learning process these behaviors come under the control of various stimuli. For example, the stimulus "thank you" will frequently produce the response "you're welcome."

Today, much of what is termed behavior modification therapy is based on principles and ideas Skinner developed. However, behavior modification therapy is only one of the influences the behaviorist approach has produced. Another influence this approach has had is on the definition of learning. One of the definitions most commonly used represents the behavioral approach and considers learning as a relatively permanent change in behavior. Travers describes this by saying "that learning involves a relatively permanent change in a response (R) as a result to a stimulus (S)" (Travers, 1977, p. 7).

This definition that considers learning in terms of what can be observed can be useful if the nurse is functioning in the role of educator. The nurse plans by developing behavioral objectives which clearly state what changes are to occur in behavior. The effectiveness of the learning experience is then evaluated by the presence or absence of these behaviors.

The method by which the change in behavior is produced for the behaviorist is usually through use of reinforcement. However, for many, reinforcement or the S-R unit fails to explain the wide variety of learning of which man is capable. As a result, a new group of theories began to develop around mid century. These theories are aimed not at finding the basic element, but at understanding the overall process. They are less concerned with animal learning, but rather, focus on the complex learning patterns of humans. These are the information processing theories.

INFORMATION PROCESSING APPROACH

Information processing theories are a comprehensive look at complex learning. Because it is such a comprehensive look at a very complex process the individual theorists are not the homogeneous group that the behaviorists are. For example, the research which has been done on how an individual perceives has considered one part of learning. The research itself is important in understanding the whole picture. Therefore, information processing theory is presented here using the concepts of input, throughput, and output rather than the individual theorist's work, as was done with the behaviorists.

Input considers how information that is being learned is perceived and moved into the system. Throughput considers how the information is both utilized and stored (or not utilized or stored) within the individual system. Output looks at the behavior which demonstrates that the learning has occurred.

Input

Human systems take information in through a process termed perception. **Perception** refers to the ability to take information from the environment. This can be conceptualized as a two-step boundary function. First, the data from the environment are transported to the system via the sense organs (see Table 7-1). However, the data do not become information within the system until they are interpreted by the system. For example, if you would look at a page written in a foreign alphabet, you could see the color, character, and shape of the letters. But you would not perceive the content of the information on the page. Therefore, perception involves interpretation of the sensory experience and is always limited by the ability of the system to interpret the data.

Studies of the perception process have identified a number of factors which influence both the accuracy and the completeness of the information taken into the system. The first factors one should consider are the presence of each of the sense organs and the degree to which each is intact. Though each sense organ should be assessed, remember that the individual rarely uses one

TABLE 7-1
Sense organs and related senses in the human neurological system

Sense Organs	Sense
Ear: utricle, saccule, and semicircular canal	Acceleration
Ear: organ of corti	Hearing
Eye: rods and cones	Vision
Nose: olfactory neurons	Smell
Tongue: taste buds	Taste
Muscle Spindles, Golgi Tendon Organ, Skin: nerve endings	Touch and Position

sense organ alone. At any point in time, he will be collecting data via each organ in concert. It is the total data on which he will base his interpretation.

A second factor affecting accuracy and completeness of information is the preference of the individual for the use of specific sense organs. A dramatic example of this can be seen in those individuals who have been blind since birth and gain their sight as adults. These individuals do not automatically begin using their eyes. In fact, some continue to live as if they were blind (Von Senden, 1961). Several common examples can also demonstrate these same preferences. Some people prefer to *hear* new information, as in a lecture; others prefer to *read* new information, as in a textbook.

Both of these factors concerning sense organs, intactness and preference, have a variety of implications for nurses who are teaching. First, one needs to assess the client for physical limitations which directly or indirectly affect the sense organs. For example, it is not unknown for a diabetic client to try to learn how to pull up the correct amount of insulin into a syringe when he cannot see the numbers on the syringe. Needless to say, if the client is to learn self-care, a different arrangement is necessary.

A second implication is the need for the nurse to assess not only for the intactness of the organs, but also for the preferences. These are not always identifiable. Many individuals are not aware of or cannot verbalize their own preferences. There are also no simple standard tests for this. However, there are usually clues to the individual preferences of clients. If an individual rarely reads, it is unlikely that reading is his preferred mode of information intake. The nurse who does a complete assessment will have some ideas of preferences; however, she can never be sure she has a complete picture. Therefore, it is wise to use a variety of modes in presenting information. The wider the variety of ways that information is presented, the more likely it will be taken in.

Man's senses of sight and sound, followed by touch, are of main interest in health education. The amount of information available to these systems is large, in fact, larger than the system can possibly process. As a result, man filters entering information at his boundary. For example, while reading this page you have not been aware of sounds in the background or even the type of print used on this page. Without the ability to filter, an individual cannot function. Overload of information produces disorganization.

In teaching, when too much information is provided too quickly, the boundaries are bombarded and the learner is unable to utilize an effective filtering system. The learner will try to slow down the process and bring in one piece of information at a time. When the system is bombarded the point of the information is missed. Students verbalize this experience when they say, "I don't understand, but I don't know enough to ask a question." Patients verbalize this same experience when they say, "Yes, someone told me about my operation, but I can't really tell you what they said."

The process of overload at the boundary occurs much quicker if the information is new to the individual. This is because perception is a two-step process. The data the sense organs have taken into the system must be interpreted. New information which does not fit into an existing, interpreting structure must first be structured. Notice the natural tendency to slow down and think through each sentence when reading new and complex information.

In this context, the term **structuring** means the organization of data in a way in which it can be recognized. The process of structuring has several implications for the nurse when teaching. First, new information should be presented slowly to allow for structuring. It should be organized and presented in a method which encourages the development of percepts. A **percept** is an impression of an object obtained solely by use of the senses (American Heritage Dictionary of the English Language, 1973). In the situation at the beginning of this chapter, Nurse 2 was teaching a mother how to take a temperature. To encourage the development of a percept, the nurse starts with an enlarged picture of the thermometer which emphasizes the numbers used for reading.

As a result of all the factors which influence perception, the nurse must constantly validate what data are being received and how those data are being interpreted. However, the nurse cannot validate one part of the learning process unless she understands the complete process. Once the data are taken into the system, they will be processed within the system. These are the throughput functions.

Throughput

Once information is taken into the system a variety of throughput functions are possible. In other words, the information taken in can be utilized in a variety of ways. If information is going to be utilized within the system, it must first be retained. The process of retaining information within the system is a boundary function termed *remembering*. The information that is retained is termed *memory*. While the concepts of *short-term memory* (STM) and *long-term memory* (LTM) do have general acceptance, a review of the literature reveals controversy concerning the number of memory systems represented. At this point it is not clear whether STM and LTM are two different memory systems or represent aspects of one memory system. At any rate, incoming information goes first to STM.

Short-term memory is information that is the focus of attention and is retained by a conscious active process. The STM is what we use when we look up a phone number and remember it long enough to dial. It is the type of memory most likely in use as you read this page. Each sentence that you read is considered in terms of the content of the previous sentences. The content of the previous sentences at this point is in short-term memory. In other words, STM processes that incoming information with which you are currently dealing (Bower, 1975).

The STM has several basic characteristics. First, because the information is at the focus of attention, there is fast access to the items in STM. This may be why many students find that "cramming" just before a test usually improves their scores. However, this would lead one to anticipate that these students would tend to experience poor long-term retention of this information. The information would be mainly in the STM, and, therefore, it would fade.

Cramming may be more difficult to do if the exam is comprehensive. This is because a second characteristic is that STM has a severely limited capacity. Somewhere between four and seven bits of information can be retained. A **bit** is a single unit of information. What constitutes a bit of information varies from individual to individual. For example, the word **memory** may be one bit of information for one individual and seven bits of information for another. As can be seen from this example, chunks or units of information can vary greatly in size. This is why concept learning is so important. It provides for large chunks of information.

A final characteristic of short-term memory is the tendency to preserve the temporal order in which the information is given. This is demonstrated when someone is asked to repeat back a string of items. The tendency is to repeat the information in the order it was presented. As a result of this characteristic, it might be anticipated that cramming would be more effective with tests which require direct recall. It might also be anticipated that cramming would be less effective with tests which require interpretation or application.

As opposed to STM, which deals with the focus of attention, LTM is reserved for the permanent storage of information that has high utility. For example, one's knowledge of basic math or language is information that has high utility and can be recalled over a lifetime.

Like STM it has a set of basic characteristics. First, although LTM is relatively permanent it does not rule out forgetting or the loss of information. With STM, loss was inevitable and occurred by fading. In LTM, loss occurs through **interference**.

Interference occurs when previous learning interferes with new learning or when new information interferes with previous learning. In a profession such as nursing where learning is a continuous lifelong process, the loss of information from LTM is of special concern. The continuing education which the nurse plans for herself or for others must try to counteract interference. The nurse must constantly be alert that previous learning does not interfere with new learning ("That's the way we always did it"). She must also be alert that new learning does not result in a loss of previously learned material. In a field with a continuous parade of new developments, this implies that there must be plans for review of previous learning.

A second characteristic which differentiates LTM from STM is in the area of capacity. The STM has a limited capacity, but the LTM appears to have a very large capacity. If one were to write out every piece of information one is able to remember, it would obviously be a great deal of information. But just how large the capacity of LTM is is a matter of controversy (Travers, 1977). Common experience would indicate there is a great deal of individual difference in how much can be remembered.

There may also be individual differences in the third characteristic of LTM. This is how one categorizes or stores the information in long-term memory (Hunt, 1975). Individuals may also have more than one organizational system. Tulving (1972) suggested that LTM is organized in two major ways—episodic and semantic. With episodic memory, information is organized in terms of time. Many events in our personal lives are recorded this way. It would be this system of memory which would be tapped when doing a nursing history. Semantic memory is organized in the ways that knowledge is organized. In other words, it would be hierarchically arranged with specific ideas categorized under more general ideas. Much of the theory studied in nursing would be remembered in this system.

Because LTM contains a large amount of information which is organized in a variety of ways, retrieval requires time. As a result, access to information tends to be slower, which is the final characteristic of LTM. How many times have you said, "Give me a second to remember."? In other words, let me search back through my data bank of information to see if I can retrieve this fact.

There are five factors or characteristics which distinguish short-term memory from long-term memory (see Table 7-2). In nursing these factors are important to us because health education, if it is to be utilized, must be remembered. It must first enter STM and then be transferred to LTM. How to effectively encourage this transfer becomes the next issue.

Several factors influence transfer of information. Good teaching takes advantage of these factors. First of all, information which is learned over time as opposed to one concentrated effort shows better long-term retention. If the nurse would spend fifteen minutes over four days teaching a client, she or he should see more long-term retention than if she spent one hour on one day covering the same information.

TABLE 7-2
Factors and characteristics that distinguish STM and LTM

LTM	STM
1. Loss of information by interference	Loss of information by fading
2. Slower access to information	Quick access to information
3. Information stored in a variety of ways	Storage is usually in temporal order
4. Retention tends to be permanent	Loss is inevitable
5. Large capacity	Limited capacity

Along with an increase in retention, the total amount of time spent on learning will increase the transference of information to LTM. In other words, if in the example above, the time periods were twenty minutes in place of fifteen, there would be even more retention of information.

A third factor that will influence transfer of information from STM to LTM is the intention to retain the information. This is called intentional learning. This is as basic as explaining to a client the importance of what is to be learned. "When your baby is sick and you call your doctor, he will want to know the baby's temperature. Therefore, I am going to show you how to take the temperature." Many times nurses and other health personnel forget to describe the intent of the teaching. In this situation, it would be obvious to the nurse that a mother would need to know how to take a baby's temperature. But it may not be obvious to the mother. It may never have occurred to her to anticipate the possibility of illness with an infant.

One of the techniques used in intentional learning is a fourth factor which influences transfer of information to LTM. This technique is called planned rehearsal or reviewing of material. It is what you use when you "memorize" your notes. You look at the material, then look away and repeat it in your mind; then you look back at your notes to check if you have it. It is a technique which is well learned by the time you reach college. However, it is a learned technique; not every client has learned this technique. The nurse, when teaching, needs to determine if the client has learned this technique and, if not, assist the client in learning to review. Even if the client is well versed in rehearsing or reviewing the material, it can be impossible for the client if the material is presented too fast. Therefore, when teaching a client, give the information slowly and encourage the client to repeat information back to you.

The fifth and final factor which encourages transfer of information from STM to LTM is inherent in all the others given. If they are followed, the fifth factor comes automatically. This is the overlearning of information. The more the information is overlearned, the better the long-term retention. One of the oldest techniques in teaching is based on this fact—the drill. Although there are a number of factors which influence transfer of information from STM to LTM, these five are among the most commonly recognized and utilized. They are summarized in Table 7-3.

Memory is only one aspect of the throughput learning processes. Obviously the processes of thinking and learning are very complex. Other aspects of this process will be further discussed in the developmental approach.

Output

The only way that the nurse who functions as a health teacher can determine if the client perceived the correct information and transferred it from STM to LTM so it is now ready for use is to measure the resulting behavior. The resulting behavior is the output of the learning system.

TABLE 7-3
Summary of factors influencing transfer of information from short-term memory to long-term memory

Factors
1. Distributing the learning over time.
2. Planning to retain the information.
3. Rehearsal or reviewing the material.
4. Increasing the time spent on learning.
5. Overlearning.

Effective measurement of changes in behavior is a very difficult process. The first step in dealing with this is to classify the behavior. Traditionally, behavior has been classified into three types

1. Cognitive behaviors are those which demonstrate intellectual skills. If you as a student would take a written test on the content within this chapter, your responses on that test would be cognitive behavior or cognitive output of your learning.
2. Affective behaviors are those which demonstrate attitudes. If you as a nurse made a medication error of which no one was aware and decided to report this error, your behavior would demonstrate your attitude. This would be an affective behavior or output.
3. Psychomotor behaviors are those which demonstrate motor skills. If you as a nurse give an injection, you would be demonstrating psychomotor skill or output.

Looking at the type of behavior helps the nurse decide which method of measurement may be most effective. For example, if the desired behavior from a learning experience is of the psychomotor type, then the most effective method for testing would be a demonstration by the learner. For each type of behavior, there are certain methods of measurement which tend to be more effective than others. The study of testing and measurement has become an extensive field of study in itself.

DEVELOPMENTAL APPROACH

In the previous section on information processing, the only throughput process considered was memory. Yet it should be obvious this is not the only learning process. Information is not only remembered but it is also rearranged and utilized in a cognitive process called thinking. In thinking, we utilize the knowledge we have to make decisions in order to adapt our behavior to the world in which we live.

Although the cognitive process of thinking is a throughput process, it is presented in this book under the major heading of developmental approach. The reason for this is that much of the research related to these cognitive processes demonstrates that they change as the organism grows and develops. This is especially true with the human learner, who is our main concern. In other words, the thinking that is done by a two-year-old child is very different from what is seen when the child becomes a person of twenty years.

Developmental learning theories tend to be divided into two types: child and adult. In the child developmental learning theories, the name Piaget stands out (Travers, 1977). In his theory, cognition is explained as a set of irreversible stages each building upon the previous stage. The emphasis is on the common elements of development seen in rational human beings. In adult developmental learning theories, which are as a group less well established than child developmental learning theories, a variety of theorists have been identified (Knefelkamp, 1980). The adult theories, like the child theories, recognize or identify stages of development. However, the adult theories differ in that they place an emphasis on the individual differences or styles of learning. This may be because individual differences are more obvious in the adult learner.

At any rate, for the purpose of discussing the cognitive process of thinking, a brief summary of Piaget's theory will represent child developmental learning theories. A summary of Kolb's theory, which was built on Piaget's, will represent the adult learning theories.

Child Developmental Learning Theories

According to Piaget's theory, child development is divided into four basic stages. These stages extend from birth through adolescence. Essential to each of the four stages are the twin processes of assimilation and accommodation. **Assimilation** is the process by which the child takes in information. **Accommodation** is the process whereby the child modifies or changes his thinking process in order to adapt to reality (Almy, 1972). What information is taken in and how it is utilized varies depending on which of the four stages the child is currently in.

The first stage, the sensory motor stage, exists from birth until about two years of age (Jennings, 1975). The infant at this stage makes two great discoveries. First, he discovers his ability to take information in through his senses. He sees, hears, feels, and tastes his world. His second discovery is his ability to manipulate this world through his muscles. With these two discoveries he now has the basis for the development of internal representation of the world. He can see in his "mind's eye" objects and events which exist in time and space. This is the beginning of language and of thinking.

The infant at this stage is totally dependent on his care givers. They may recognize his physical and even his emotional independence, but it is also important that they recognize his intellectual dependence. He is dependent on his care givers for an environment which maximizes the safe use of all his senses and of his beginning muscular coordination for his intellectual development.

The second stage in Piaget's theory spans a time period from about eighteen months to seven years. This stage, with its three main characteristics, is termed preoperational. First, there is extensive growth in the ability to see and remember objects and events in the "mind's eye." This growth in the internal representation and memory of objects and events is growth both in terms of numbers and complexity. As one would anticipate, language development is extensive during this time period. The second main characteristic of the preoperational stage builds upon the first. With an increase in the number and complexity of images, the child develops the ability to classify and arrange objects. During this development, things such as finding all the blue objects on a page or all the square objects in a room can be great fun. At the beginning of this stage, the child can classify with only one dimension the blue blocks, for example. However, by the end of the stage, the child has great ease in handling a variety of dimensions, for example, all the large, blue squares.

The ability to classify is limited by the third main characteristic of the preoperational stage. The child's decisions are based on what he actually sees. The same amount of liquid in a tall slender container or a short fat container is seen as two different amounts. Any mother who has pulled out a variety of glasses in order to give lemonade to her child and friends has seen a clear example of this. The mother will look for unbreakable glasses, regardless of shape; however, if the glasses are different shapes, the children are all sure they received different amounts.

The children are fussing, the mother may try to show them the drinks are equal in amount. She pours the lemonade into a ½-cup measure and then into each of their glasses. However, the children will still be convinced they have received unequal amounts. They lack the ability to reverse or cancel. Even though they see the liquid being measured, when it is poured into different shaped containers, it is seen as different amounts. The child at the preoperational stage is able to label objects but is unable to relate or compare the properties of the objects.

The third of Piaget's stages occurs between the ages of seven and eleven. This stage is termed concrete operations. A child at this stage is able to manipulate numbers, space, and time and can reverse his thinking. As a result, he is able to solve problems using trial and error and to give an explanation. However, his explanations are in terms of the concrete data (Almy, 1972).

If the child is given several objects and asked which will sink and which will float he will test this out with trial and error. He may arrive at the conclusion that heavy objects sink and light objects float. He may even note there is a relationship between the size of the object and whether it will float. But a child at this stage cannot conceptualize the displacement of the water dependent on the size and weight of the object. He cannot yet think in abstract symbols.

The ability to think propositionally, using abstract symbols, occurs in the fourth stage, formal operations. This stage develops in adolescents and is for Piaget the final stage since it represents the thinking abilities that occur in the adult. With the use of formal operations, the individual is able to devise theories in his mind, verbalize them, and then test them (Almy, 1972). For example, in the problem above, the individual would be able to note that objects of the same size can have different weights and that objects of the same weight can have different sizes. He would be able to generalize his observations so that he would be able to conceptualize and state the theory of specific gravity. With the ability to theorize, the stages of human learning are complete for Piaget. But for a whole group of learning theorists (the adult learning theorists) this was just the beginning.

Adult Learning Theory

Although Piaget believed that the fourth stage of his theory explained the adult learner, others who have focused their studies on the adult have been impressed by the individual differences that exist (Almy, 1972). These differences are usually grouped under various cognitive or thinking styles. One of the more comprehensive theories of adult learning which deals with these individual differences is Kolb's experiential learning theory (Fry & Kolb, 1979). Kolb, in the development of his theory, was greatly influenced by Piaget. This influence can be seen in the close relationship between the four stages of both theories.

Kolb's learning theory can be conceptualized as two interacting continuums (see Figure 7-3). From these two continuums a four-stage learning cycle has been identified (see Figure 7-4). According to Kolb, learning begins

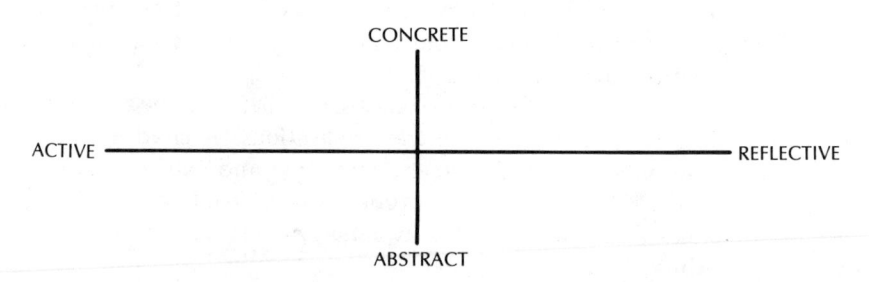

Figure 7-3 Experiential Learning Model Continuums. (From: Kolb, D. "Learning Styles and Disciplinary Differences." In *The Modern American College*. Edited by A. Chickering, et al. San Francisco: Jossey-Bass Publishers, 1981, p. 235.)

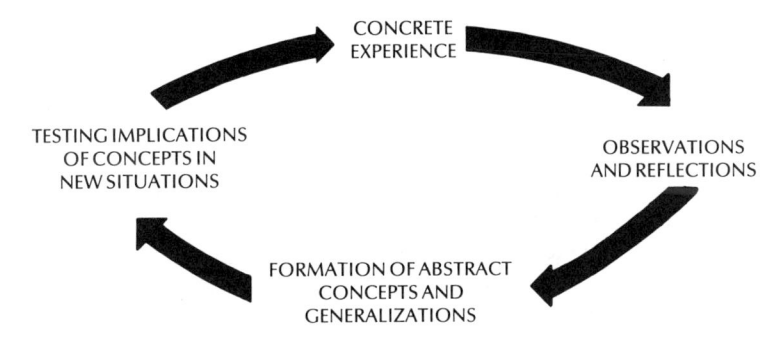

Figure 7-4 The Experiential Learning Model. (From: Kolb, D. "Learning Styles and Disciplinary Differences." In *The Modern American College.* Edited by A. Chickering, et al. San Francisco: Jossey-Bass Publishers, 1981, p. 241.)

with a concrete experience and moves in a clockwise fashion around the cycle.

The first stage, the concrete experience, is the stage where experience forms the basis of learning. For example, in tasting a new food, you experience the taste; or in hearing a new piece of music, you experience the music. You move from this concrete experience to observing and reflecting on what has taken place—the watching stage. It should be noted that the processes in these first two stages are very similar to perception. Information is first taken in through the senses, then interpreted. In abstract conceptualization, the concepts which have been created are integrated into logically sound theory. This is called the thinking stage. It is similar to Piaget's fourth stage. Once the theories are formulated, they are used to make decisions. This process of decision making based on theory is termed active experimentation or the doing stage (Kolb, 1976).

The adult learner will, to some degree, utilize elements from each of the four stages, but each adult learner has his own combination. This unique combination, which is reflected in what stages are emphasized, makes up the learning style of the individual. For example, learners who emphasize reflective observation and/or active conceptualization tend to prefer learning situations such as lecture. On the other hand, individuals who emphasize concrete experience and/or active experimentation benefit more from discovery, discussion type learning (Kolb, 1976).

APPLICATION TO NURSING PRACTICE

We have been discussing learning as a very abstract process, but the rest of the chapter will focus on how to utilize this information in concrete situations. When a person experiences an abundance of health, there can be feelings of zest and vigor, yet also a measure of contentment. How often have you felt that way? Every part of you operates effectively and you may have only a general awareness of your body. But just bump your toe. What happens? Suddenly you zero in on that toe and give it concentrated thought. You want to fix it and to prevent bumping it again. You become motivated to help yourself because something has happened to you.

What if you had not bumped your toe? Consider this situation. You are feeling fine and generally satisfied. You happen to see a booklet on home safety and while scanning through it you notice a section on preventing obstacles in walkways. Hmmm, interesting. The information is well presented and makes sense. You appreciate the booklet a few moments, put it down, and turn to other business of the day. However, the client who just bumped his toe on a toy left in the walkway responds differently. He is more attentive to the booklet.

The clients that you work with are in a variety of responding states. Sometimes they may feel like learning new material. Other times they may not. It is through your assessment that you can tailor a plan to help clients promote, maintain, and restore well-being.

Not only are clients responding to health situations at hand, but they have also developed ways of thinking and acting over a lifetime. No one has all the answers as to how one develops response patterns but the ability to learn is universal and can be tapped for bringing about a healthier state. However, before you as the nurse can tap this universal ability to learn, we need to examine some terms that can be confusing. These terms are *health education, patient education, learning,* and *teaching.*

Definitions

School health programs, industrial safety campaigns, and well-baby promotions are all examples of health education. Health education is a dynamic process directed toward increasing the health of people. It is broad in scope, involving formal classes as well as informal learning experiences. Patient education, on the other hand, tends to be viewed as a narrower term. Patient education refers to a teaching-learning process that occurs when a patient, usually in a hospital or clinic, requires information for a health condition, i.e., enters the health care system for maintaining or restoring health when an illness, accident, or disability occurs. You may see the term *client education* used similarly; however, the word *client* often connotes more of a wellness orientation.

Learning is an actual change that takes place within a person and is reflected in areas such as knowledge, attitudes, and skills. Learning may result from incidental events or from planned teaching. Teaching means interaction and communication designed to promote learning. Can the teacher learn it for the person? Only the learner can do the learning, but the teacher can be a facilitator and can provide a climate for learning. The nurse who communicates in such a way to change a person's health behavior is teaching—health teaching. When you study about teaching you will see ways in which information and activities are put in motion to increase the likelihood of learning.

Principles for Guidance

Learning theory has resulted in a number of guiding statements or principles that may serve as a frame of reference. The following list is a condensation of a number of teaching and learning principles you will see in the literature (Redman, 1984; DuGas, 1972; Fleming & Levie, 1978). A solid foundation with these principles will help you in the clinical setting.

1. *The client's perception of what is to be learned influences the extent of his learning.*

    Perception involves taking in and interpreting stimuli from the environment. Such special senses as vision and hearing are used during perception, and the brain begins cognition trying to make sense out of the new input. A client takes in only a select amount of stimuli, usually the numbers he can handle and in the forms recognized from prior experience. The client's overall feeling of well-being will affect his perception. If he feels well he may take in greater amounts of external stimuli. If he is aching or in pain, his perceptions to external stimuli will diminish.

    Consider the patient with a heart condition who is going to have a heart examination called a cardiac catheterization. Patients often feel stressed when learning the procedure is indicated. The invasion into the body and concerns about what the results of the procedure will show are fear producing and stress producing. The nurse informs and instructs the patient so he can handle the experience more easily and is better prepared. It would not be unusual for a patient in this situation to miss some of the information. He is seeing and listening but also concentrating on interpreting the effects on his survival. Only so much input can be handled at a time.

2. *Meaningfulness assists learning.*

    If the patient cannot relate the instruction to himself, he may block it out. On the operative day of orthopedic surgery, the patient will probably be interested in instruction that leads to comfort. He will not receive content on an exercise program in the same way because it will not be as meaningful at that point. Only later when the patient is more comfortable will he be ready to hear about exercising. This relates to what was said about perception. Meaningful stimuli are perceived according to an individual's own priority.

    Meaningfulness also implies that what is taught is comprehended by the client. Material should be taught in language the client can understand, not technical jargon. To save time, the nurse may find it very easy to slip into using abbreviations. Anyone who has interacted with computers knows this. Numerous words are coded into a short form, but the computer has been programmed to recognize the codes.

Clients are not programmed similarly. They have developed their own abilities to decode words from diverse backgrounds. You may instruct a patient whose primary language is not English and who may miss important meanings. Verifying the client's understanding periodically is recommended. The evaluation stage of the nursing process will help you know where learning has occurred according to the objectives of your teaching plan.

3. *Taking in new material through more than one modality can facilitate learning.*

Here is where audiovisuals often come into use. Adding an illustration that shows injection sites could help the diabetic patient understand more of your explanation on rotating sites. Giving a patient the opportunity to hold and manipulate an ace bandage in addition to explaining about it will improve his later ability to wrap it effectively. Adding slides to a discussion with a preoperative patient could fill out concrete details of the anticipated experience and assist him to raise questions in areas of concern. Audiovisuals can also be overdone or used inappropriately. Selection of media requires an analysis of the learning situation, including criteria related to the learner, the setting, and the content to be taught.

If you want to show walking with a cane then a dynamic presentation that moves, such as a videocassette, will be more informational. If you want to differentiate types of infant cries to a mother, an audiocassette will be useful. What is it you are trying to get across? Do you have a clear objective or goal in mind? If you want to change an attitude or increase motivation a dramatic presentation may be best. The picture, words, and music all come together to work on feelings. The various audiovisuals have attributes which make them more effective in certain cases.

4. *Concept learning is enhanced through the use of examples.*

Concepts are general ideas that reflect a category of similar specific items. The word *patient* may stand for patient X, inpatient, outpatient, and home care patient. Some concepts are broader and include more specific categories. Broad concepts include health, education, teaching, and learning. In order to make broad abstract ideas clear it is necessary to add concrete examples. Otherwise the learner may think of a mistaken example of his own in an effort to find relevance in what you have said.

When a nurse uses general terms, such as health care delivery system or preventive health care, with clients during instruction, what examples might be thought of? Can you recall times when a teacher's examples clarified a point for you? Memorable examples have been found to be important to comprehension and to the retention of learning.

5. *Emotional appeals have the potential to change attitudes and behaviors.*

Knowing does not assure change. To change habits a durable, emotional response must be integrated with the knowledge. One area where this has been observed has been in the antismoking campaigns. Are you a smoker or do you know a smoker who has tried to stop smoking? It has been reported over and over that smoking is a very difficult habit to stop. Intelligent individuals with substantial knowledge have continued to smoke in the face of evidence linking cigarette smoking to serious diseases such as cancer and emphysema. Even people with chronic coughs or a family history of cancer have continued to smoke. This problem becomes compounded in the individual who is already debilitated and is trying to maintain as much health as possible to begin the road to recovery.

Antismoking campaigns have introduced affective aspects such as humor, scare tactics, testimonials, authoritative statistics, and social supports. Still the habit remains. One can only conclude that the satisfaction from smoking is outweighing the effects of emotional appeals in people who still smoke. The unfortunate part is that cognition may change rather than the behavior, i.e., the evidence is faulty, cancer and emphysema won't get me, I must be on the right track since I feel good, I feel relaxed when I smoke and that is better for me, smoking prevents obesity which is worse. These forms of cognition are compatible with continued smoking.

Some emotion-directed appeals have worked. We know that many people have been persuaded away from smoking in recent years. There has been progress related to improved health habits in other areas, such as early disease detection, hypertension, and cancer. Often these appeals contain warnings as to the consequences of delaying treatment. No one can predict with certainty how an emotionally focused message will be received, but timing and appropriateness are important in increasing effectiveness of the teaching.

6. *Participation and practice augment the retention of learning.*

When a client participates during instruction it assists in keeping him more attentive and involved. The active person takes in and deliberates on small portions of the material to be learned. Suppose you are working with a patient who is recovering from surgery and who has recently decided to become a vegetarian. Involving him in menu selection will assist him in learning to eat a balanced meal. Questions and answers periodically throughout will also assist. You might find a fun way such as a game or puzzle to give additional support to his activity.

7. *Learning takes place intentionally and unintentionally.*

The parents of a high-risk infant listen to the nurse's instruction about washing and gowning before reaching into the isolette to touch their baby. As they follow the procedure correctly they demonstrate intentional learning. There will be many other areas of learning intended by staff and indicated as such to the parents. There will also be areas of learning that will occur on an incidental basis. The parents might not even be aware of this learning at the time. Incidental learning can occur daily and includes vital changes of thought, attitudes, and behaviors even though it was not planned or mentioned. The parents who initiate contact with an infant by shaking a certain toy in front of him while they stroke his shoulders and arms and begin softly voiced words may not recall that this was the manner by which a nurse initiated contact in their presence.

These seven principles will serve as a frame of reference to you as you begin to develop plans of care and teaching. As you gain in experience you will probably use some principles more than others. You will also generate additional principles which you will add to the list. For example, what principles of learning can you generate from the section of this chapter from the behavioral approach to learning?

Use of the Nursing Process

Many of the same steps used in the nursing process can be applied to teaching and learning. Table 7-4 relates these two processes and Table 7-5 provides a

140 SELECTED THEORIES UTILIZED IN NURSING

TABLE 7-4
Use of the nursing process in health teaching

Nursing Process	Health Teaching
ASSESSMENT	
Data Collection	
Sources—e.g., patient, family, other professionals	What does the patient want to know?
Methods—e.g., examination, observation, interview	What questions are being raised? What elements should assist patient learning? What interferences exist?
Data Analysis	
Note gaps	Is there an aspect important to the patient's condition that has not been explored?
Apply standards	
Note relationships	
Identify norms	
Nursing Diagnosis	Learning Diagnosis
Draw conclusions based on analysis	Identification of specific learning need(s)
PLANNING	
State goal(s) e.g., the patient will	A teaching objective has these parts— who, what task, to what extent, under what conditions
	Domains—cognitive, affective, psychomotor
Identify criteria for evaluation	Identify criteria for evaluation
State approach	Identify teaching method(s)
Plan jointly	Plan jointly
IMPLEMENTATION	
Plan is carried out	Provide a climate for learning
Verbal report	Carry out teaching plan
Written documentation	Document activities
EVALUATION	
Use of criteria	Evaluate if patient has achieved the learning objective(s)
Judgment—was goal achieved?	
Analysis	Evaluate use of teaching method selected
Recycle to assessment if needed	
	Evaluate learning environment

TABLE 7-5
Client example

Assessment Situation
The mother, a twenty-year-old breastfeeding primipara (first child) at two-days post delivery, has asked many questions about breastfeeding in relationship to her breasts, ability to nurse, the infant's ability to suck, and nutritional questions related to both mother and infant.
Specific questions raised by the mother include
How long should I nurse him?
How frequently should he be fed?
How will I know when he has had enough?
Sometimes he's sleepy. How can I help him to start sucking?

TABLE 7-5 (*Cont.*)

Elements assisting the client to learn are
    Nurse observes mother's high motivation to breastfeed.
    Mother and newborn are both healthy.
    The mother was first introduced to breastfeeding information in prenatal classes and is now reviewing and learning new details about breastfeeding.
    Bonding between mother and infant is occurring effectively.
    The father is in favor of breastfeeding.
    The nurses and physicians are supportive of breastfeeding.
    When the mother goes home, she will have assistance from her mother for a month. The client has said she is glad for the help.

Interferences to learning are
    The infant has lost 50 grams since birth. The mother is concerned she won't be able to provide for his nutritional needs adequately.
    The mother's right nipple is not as prominent as the left and the infant does not latch on as easily. The mother expressed that she viewed this as a problem.

Aspects not explored:
    The mother's comfort in breastfeeding in the presence of others.

Nursing Diagnosis: Knowledge deficit: Anxious about breastfeeding related to lack of information

INSTRUCTIONAL PLANNING

Goals: When asked, the mother will correctly describe infant behaviors that indicate an effective breastfeeding situation. (Cognitive)

    When feeding her infant, the mother will effectively assist the infant in latching on. (Psychomotor)

    The mother will appear relaxed while breastfeeding and in discussions about breastfeeding. (Affective)

Criteria for Evaluation: For the cognitive objective—
    Describes infant behaviors and changes:
    1. Infant sucks with consistency, beginning with several minutes on one side at a feeding and eventually building to ten minutes on each breast at a feeding.
    2. Hunger cry diminishes with the feeding.
    3. Sleeps between feedings.
    4. Wets 6 or more diapers/day.

Criteria for Evaluation: For the psychomotor objective—
    1. Mother rolls her nipples, especially the nonprominent nipple, between her thumb and forefinger.
    2. Positions herself seated comfortably or lying on her side.
    3. Positions the infant so that his body is turned toward the breast and his mouth is close to the nipple.
    4. Inserts the nipple and as much of the areola as possible directly into the infant's mouth.

Criteria for Evaluation: For the affective objective—
    1. Mother shows relaxed posture and facial expressions when feeding and discussing breastfeeding.
    2. Rests or sleeps between a number of feedings.

Teaching Methods:
    Small group patient teaching session with 4 to 6 postpartum mothers. Include discussion of feeding in the presence of others.
    Individual teaching follow-up session.
    Use of breast model
        —breastfeeding posters
        —videotape on breastfeeding

client example. When the nurse conducts an assessment, learning needs are identified. Think about questions you would ask. You will ask about health-related habits of the client and his family and you will try to determine if behaviors and circumstances have placed the client at risk. You will want to assess the client's readiness to learn.

For learning to occur there must be a stimulating factor which increases the energy level or provides the motivation to learn. A person must want to learn. The client will be motivated if he believes the learning will help meet needs and/or lead to a future desired state. However, the learner will not automatically believe this just because the teacher does. Many times in health teaching we make this mistake. We have such a strong belief in the importance of the material to be learned it does not occur to us that the client does not have the same belief. For example, we may be teaching a teenager about birth control when that teenager has no interest in avoiding pregnancy.

A stimulating force is necessary for client motivation, but if the client and the person doing the health teaching agree on what is to be learned, it is not necessary that they always have the same stimulating force or motive. A good example of this is brushing teeth. The great majority of people brush their teeth to avoid bad breath, not cavities. But the end result is that they brush their teeth.

Although a motive can stimulate the learner, this is only the beginning of the process. Once the desire to learn is initiated, it will not automatically be maintained. The learner must believe his learning will result in a desired future state and/or a satisfied need. For example, the mother of a child with cystic fibrosis may desire no further chest infections. This desire could motivate her to learn chest physiotherapy. However, if in learning the chest physiotherapy she decides this behavior will not help her child in preventing infections, she would not continue the learning. The learner must be able to see and believe in the relationship between the specific learning and the motive for his learning.

The learner must also believe he as an individual is capable of the learning. The learner may have a clear realization of his motive or desired future state. He may also believe this specific learning will result in achieving this desired state. Yet he may not attempt to learn because he does not believe he is capable of learning this specific material. Clients who say, "I could never give myself a shot; I could never care for my mother at home; or I could never stay with my wife in delivery" are saying, "I am not capable."

Once you have assessed the client and identified his specific learning needs, the planning process begins. Planning starts with writing a clear, precise statement of the desired learning outcome or long-term goal (LTG). Because long-term goals are the final outcome intended, they usually involve weeks or months to achieve. Objectives or short-term goals (STG) are the stepping stones to achievement of LTG's and can usually be achieved in a few hours or days. Since LTG's tend to be written in more general terms, they need to be supported with a list of specific behavioral objectives or short-term goals.

A well-written objective (STG) has four components. The first component is the actual task or behavior to be accomplished. The task or behavior component consists of two parts: verb and noun. The actual task is a noun. The "to be accomplished" part of the objective is a verb, frequently referred to as an action verb. The verb determines the actual domain of the objective. For example, if the task or behavior to be accomplished is planning a nutritious menu, the objective reflects the cognitive or knowledge domain. If the task to be accomplished is to verbalize a willingness to follow a diet, the objective reflects the affective or feeling domain. If on the other hand, the task is to prepare the meal, then the objective reflects the psychomotor domain.

Note that the verbs in these examples demonstrate observable behaviors. The measurability of an objective is directly related to the observability of the verb in the objective. If the verb in an objective is reflective of an internal state and not clearly observable, it is difficult to measure. For example, "to really understand" or "to appreciate" are verbs that reflect an internal state and are difficult to measure.

The second component of a behavioral objective is who will demonstrate the task that is to be accomplished. Objectives should be stated in terms of the learner, not the teacher. The learner, however, may be the individual, family, or community.

The third component of a behavioral objective is the time frame, i.e., when will the objective be achieved. The time limit tells you when to measure achievement of the objective. Examples of the time component are such statements as, "within two weeks" or "by the end of this session."

The final component of a properly written objective deals with the condition under which the behavior will occur. The condition usually indicates the setting and the supports the client can utilize in demonstrating the behaviors. For example, condition statements generally include words such as, "during a clinic visit," "when selecting menu items," and "with the support of a teaching pamphlet."

When the objectives have been decided, you will want to develop certain criteria for checking the achievement of the objectives. Did the learner do what was intended? How can you determine the outcome of learning? A written test is a way that you are familiar with, but what other ways would help you know if the client had learned and completed activities successfully? Cognitive objectives are often tested by quizzing. There are a variety of ways to make quizzes. The attainment of affective objectives may be observed through role playing, feedback in discussion, or through selected observations put on anecdotal notes. Psychomotor objectives are often evaluated by having the client return a demonstration.

After you have developed the objectives and criteria for attainment you will be selecting methods that assist learning. Some of this you may already have thought through when considering how you would evaluate. There are many teaching methods. Some are traditional, such as lecture and discussion, demonstration, and audiovisuals, and others are innovative, such as games and simulations. However, most of all you want the client to learn and so you need to consider his time and energy levels.

During the implementation stage you will carry out the teaching plan. The method must be capable of bringing out the desired content and activities to achieve the objectives. The environment should be conducive to learning and place the client in as much physical and psychological comfort as possible. There needs to be a relaxed and unhurried climate. Ground rules could include the client being able to stop at any time and the nurse leaving if needed.

The evaluation looks at whether or not the client achieved the objectives. It also looks at the process involved in the teaching and learning situation. What things were effective, what were not and why? Was the poster not big enough for everyone to see? Was the session too long? Was the environment conducive to learning?

SUMMARY

The first part of the chapter reviewed a variety of learning theories as a basis for understanding how man as an open system adapts to his ever-changing environment through learning. These theories have been divided into three approaches: behavioral approach, information processing approach, and developmental approach. Although these approaches interact, overlap, and, at times, conflict, each of the theories brings to nursing an understanding of man and how the nurse may help him maximize his potential. The second part of this chapter focused on how the nurse utilizes learning theory in health teaching. Key definitions were given and guiding principles identified. Finally, application of learning theory is described utilizing the nursing process.

Key points are

1. A variety of learning theories help to explain the learning process.
2. The process by which we learn is as individualized as any other aspect of our being.
3. Health teaching involves teaching and learning in an interactive process.
4. Principles for guiding the teaching-learning process are derived from learning theories.
5. The nursing process provides the framework by which the nurse utilizes the teaching-learning process.

REFERENCES

Almy, M. "Wishful Thinking about Children's Thinking." In *The Psychology of the Elementary School Child*, edited by A. R. Binter and S. H. Frey. Chicago: Rand McNally and Co., 1972.

American Heritage Dictionary of the English Language. New York: American Heritage Publishing Co., 1973.

Biggs, J. B. *Information and Human Learning.* Glenview, IL: Scott, Foresman and Co., 1971.

Bower, G. Cognitive Psychology: An Introduction. In *Handbook of Learning and Cognitive Processes: Introduction to Concepts and Issues*, edited by W. K. Estes. New York: John Wiley and Sons, 1975.

Claxton, C., and Ralston, Y. "Learning Styles: Their Impact on Teaching and Administration." *AAHE-ERIC/Higher Education Research Reports*, no. 10, 1978.

DuGas, B. *Introduction to Patient Care.* Philadelphia: W. B. Saunders, 1972.

Estes, W. K., ed. *Handbook of Learning and Cognitive Processes: Introduction to Concepts and Issues.* New York: John Wiley and Sons, 1975.

Fleming, M., and Levie, W. H. *Instructional Message Design.* Englewood Cliffs, NJ: Educational Technology Publication, 1978.

Fry, R., and Kolb, D. "Experiential Learning Theory and Learning Experiences in Liberal Arts Education." *New Directions for Experiential Learning* 6 (1979): 79–92.

Ganong, W. F. *Review of Medical Physiology.* Los Altos, CA: Lange Medical Publications, 1983.

Hunt, E., and Lansman, M. "Cognitive Theory Applied to Individual Differences." In *Handbook of Learning and Cognitive Processes: Introduction to Concepts and Issues*, edited by W. K. Estes. New York: John Wiley and Sons, 1975.

Jennings, F. G. "Jean Piaget: Notes on Learning." In *Issues and Advances in Educational Psychology*, edited by P. Torrance and W. White. Itasca, Ill.: F. E. Peacock Publishers, Inc., 1975.

Kolb, D. "Learning Styles and Disciplinary Differences. In *The Modern American College*, edited by A. Chickering et al. San Francisco: Jossey-Bass Publishers, 1981.

Kolb, D. *Learning Style Inventory: Self-Scoring Test and Interpretation Booklet.* Boston: McBer and Co., 1976.

Knefelkamp, L. "Faculty and Students Development in the 80's: Renewing the Community of Scholars." In *Current Issues of Higher Education: Integrating Adult Development Theory with Higher Education Practice*, no. 5. Washington, DC: American Association for Higher Education, 1980.

Pohl, M. L. *The Teaching Functions of the Nursing Practitioner.* Dubuque, IA: Wm. C. Brown, 1981.

Redman, B. *The Process of Patient Teaching in Nursing.* St. Louis: The C. V. Mosby Co., 1984.

Snelbecker, G. *Learning Theory, Instructional Theory and Psychoeducational Design.* New York: McGraw-Hill Co., 1974.

Thorndike, E. *Educational Psychology, the Psychology of Learning.* New York: Teachers College, Columbia University, 1913.

Travers, R. *Essentials of Learning.* New York: Macmillan Publishing Co., 1977.

Tulving, E. "Episodic and Semantic Memory." In *Organization and Memory*, edited by E. Tulving and W. Donaldson. New York: Academic Press, 1972.

Von Senden, M. *Space and Sight.* Translated by Peter Heath. Glencoe, IL: Free Press, 1961.

8

Communication theory

DEFINITION OF TERMS

Channel A means through which communication can be detected by the special senses.
Communication The process and structure of sending and receiving messages by a variety of means.
Feedback A portion of receiver output that is returned to the source of the communication.
Interaction Mutual exchange between two or more systems revealing influence.
Message Verbal or nonverbal expressed content of communication.
Receiver The system that inputs the sent message.
Referent The event that motivates or triggers the communication.
Sender A source of communication.
Source An initiator of communication.

In man's existence, communication is considered a universal element. All of us are continually in the process of communicating with the world around us. At times, this communicating is effective, and we find the whole process beneficial. At other times, communication is not so effective and life is not so pleasant. Nurses, if they are to assist a client to optimal well-being, cannot depend on chance. They need specialized knowledge about communication theory and its use. Let's look at two situations to ascertain the outcomes of various types of communication.

SITUATION 1

A nurse, Mrs. Joseph, meets Mrs. Kappa for whom she has previously provided nursing care while the woman was in the recovery room. The woman is now a patient on the unit where the nurse currently works. The conversation is as follows:

Mrs. Joseph: (Smiling) "Hello. I remember you. You were a patient of mine when you had your surgery."
Mrs. Kappa: (Smiling) "Oh, really."
Mrs. Joseph: (Still smiling) "Yes, you carried on and cried like a baby."
Mrs. Kappa: (Looking serious and eyes down) "Oh, I'm a regular baby when it comes to pain." (voice apologetic)
Mrs. Joseph: (Still smiling) "Oh, that's OK. When I had my surgery I carried on, too. Don't worry about it. But my surgery was just terrible."
Mrs. Kappa: (Silent, nods head, face downcast)
Mrs. Joseph: (Walking away, smiling) "Well, I'll be seeing you. Nice to see you again."

SITUATION 2

Three months later the nurse meets this patient again while she is undergoing follow-up treatment for cancer. The conversation is as follows:

Mrs. Joseph: (Smiling) "Hello, Mrs. Kappa. I'm Mrs. Joseph, one of the nurses who cared for you on Unit 85. How have you been lately?"
Mrs. Kappa: (Looking serious) "Oh, I'm so glad some of the same nurses are still here. Oh, I'm OK ... almost OK."
Mrs. Joseph: (A little more serious) "What does almost OK mean?"
Mrs. Kappa: (Silent at first, then) "I thought I was doing OK ... then the doctor told me I have to come back for more treatment."
Mrs. Joseph: "Why don't we walk back to your room where we can both sit down and talk about this?"

They both start back to the patient's room.

From these two situations one might assume that the nurse in the first instance was less caring, concerned, or interested in the patient. In reality she was simply less effective in communicating her interest and concerns. Her change in effectiveness came about because of an increased knowledge base in communication. The second situation demonstrated how she used her knowledge to assist Mrs. Kappa. This chapter focuses on presenting an overview of the communication process. Key terms are defined and components of the communication process identified. The communication process is analyzed to determine factors that influence communication, methods of achieving effective communication, and some of the barriers to effective communication. At the completion of this chapter, the reader will be able to

1. Define communication.
2. List purposes for communicating.
3. Describe common components of the communication process.
4. Identify factors that influence communication.
5. Recognize barriers and facilitators to effective communication.

DEFINING COMMUNICATION

Many definitions for the term *communication* exist. For example, if you look in any dictionary for the word communication you will not find just one definition. Webster gives numerous definitions for communication

1. An act or instance of transmitting a verbal or written message.
2. A process by which information is exchanged between individuals.
3. Personal support.
4. Technique for expressing ideas effectively.
5. Technology of transmitting information. (Webster, 1981, p. 225)

The complexity of the concept and the focus of the definer add to these numerous definitions. For our purpose, we will use one broad definition that can be applied in many situations. Communication is the process and structure of sending and receiving messages by a variety of means. Key in this communication process is the idea that communication is a cyclic and continuous process. If the circle is broken, then communication stops or becomes ineffective. Simply sending a **message** does not guarantee that the message is received or understood. For effective communication to take place, the message must be received and understood by the **receiver.** How does one know if this has occurred? In fact, you don't know unless you receive **feedback** about the message, thus completing the circle. For example, how many times have you said something and, when the receiver did not respond, you commented, "Am I talking to the walls?" This definition also implies that communication is dynamic in that it is a process. Being dynamic requires the systems, both the **sender** and the **receiver,** to use energy when communicating.

The many different features to communication help us recognize that it is communication. When one first thinks about the communication process, language or the spoken word usually comes to mind; however, messages can be sent through several means. One of the ways by which communication is analyzed then is through a classification system: form. Form is transmission of the message, either verbal or nonverbal. Verbal communication is the use of spoken words to convey the message. Nonverbal communication includes all other forms of sending messages such as symbols, physical movements (kinetics), and melodies. Most messages contain both verbal and nonverbal forms. Both forms can assist man in expressing himself fully; in presenting himself as a unique individual. Verbal forms allow for cognitive and emotional outputs while nonverbal forms mainly involve expression of emotion, feeling, or affect. Handily, nonverbal forms cross populations whose spoken languages are different. For the most part a smile is welcomed universally. It makes a statement that is broadly understood.

While these two forms can provide unlimited ability for expression, many times they are misinterpreted or incongruent. Incongruency occurs when the verbal message is different from the nonverbal message. For example, as a nurse you may interview a patient who is scheduled for surgery. The patient may verbalize no concerns or fears, but nonverbally he may ring his hands and pace the floor. In this case, you would identify the incongruency between the verbal and nonverbal message and explore this with the patient. Misinterpretation results, however, when the receiver inaccurately interprets the message being sent. Although the sender may have congruence between verbal and nonverbal forms, the receiver simply reads the message the wrong way.

REASONS FOR COMMUNICATING

Now that communication has been defined, we need to examine why people communicate, i.e., what purposes communication serves. All communication has a purpose. The effectiveness of communication is determined by the extent to which the communication achieved its purpose. Pluckhan (1978) identifies three major purposes for communicating: to influence or persuade, to receive pleasure, and to survive.

All systems spend time and energy trying to impress others; to influence or persuade them to our way of thinking, acting, or supporting. Part of the way we in nursing influence or persuade others is through the teaching process. During the teaching process we try to motivate the client to respond in a new way; to change his behavior; or to acquire new knowledge that will change his way of thinking or acting. We provide the client with information so that he can make educated or informed decisions about his health care. In addition, we as nurses band together to communicate our concerns to our leaders, politicians, and administrators in an attempt to influence health care policies.

Although much of our communication is directed toward influencing others, we also communicate for the pleasure we derive from interacting with others. Man is a social being and as such receives pleasure from communicating with others. Communication provides an opportunity for man to express his thoughts and feelings, to share and develop relationships. This process of obtaining pleasure from communicating helps man to develop his "self," to understand who he is. In addition, communication serves to entertain man, to help man escape from silence. Although everyone has a need for periods of silence, man also has a need for noise. Total silence for an extended period of time results in man making sounds just to make sounds.

All critical processes which are needed for a system to function require communication. When we lose control over our environments, our very existence is threatened. Survival communication deals with our ability to inquire about meeting our needs, to request information, to clarify misunderstandings that can threaten our existence, and to request aid or help in obtaining what is necessary for survival.

COMPONENTS OF A COMMUNICATION MODEL

Communication models help the nurse develop a way of handling this complex process. Models provide the communicator with a frame for analyzing and, in turn, improving their communication skills. A variety of communication models have been developed. These models range from simple to complex, from one person models to mass communication models. These models often present a structure composed of parts and a process revealing relationships. Although various model developers describe the structure and the relationships in a variety of ways they share a common orientation. This common orientation was utilized in the basic communication model presented here.

First, there is usually a prompt or trigger, which is frequently called the **referent** (Hein, 1980). This referent causes the **interaction** to occur (see Figure 8-1). The referent energizes the communication networks of man's systems. It motivates and mobilizes the system to activate in relationship to another system, and establishes a climate of meaning for the communication. Inherent in the triggering event is the reason for the communication. Many possible reasons for communication exist. Table 8-1 demonstrates one possible way of classifying referents.

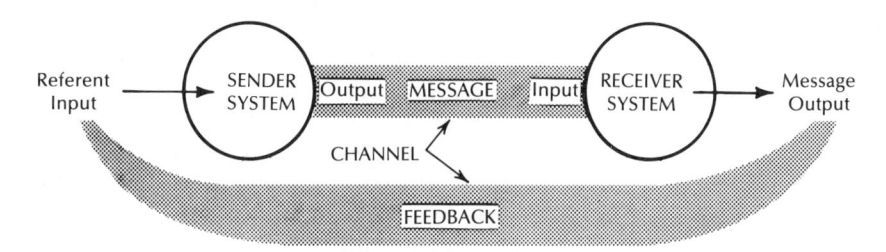

Figure 8-1 Basic Communication Model.

TABLE 8-1
Communication referents of man

Man	Referent
Physiological dimension	- ask for or offer assistance designed to meet physical and safety needs - cough, sneeze, or make other sound producing body activities that assist the body and carry a message at the same time
Psychological dimension	- express feelings - express unconscious ideas - release sexual desires - conceal or make evident problems - express creative thinking
Sociocultural dimension	- transcend generations - appreciate human differences in world - establish territories - bridge nations and/or distinct populations
Developmental continuum	- make new sounds and words - reflect abilities and/or limitations associated with age level

Although dimensions overlap, referents reflecting a physiological dimension primarily deal with physical self and safety. The psychological referents set in motion communication of inner thoughts and feelings, some of which are unpleasant. Referents that can be categorized as sociocultural in orientation tend to involve distances between people in time and space. The developmental referents involve expectancies and pronouncements related to age or period of life.

Several examples of a referent that you may have experienced are the need for more money from home, the need for a delay in taking an exam, or the need to tell someone how you feel about him. Another example of a referent can be seen with a breast-feeding mother and her baby at feeding time. A fullness occurs in the mother's breasts as she realizes it's almost time for her baby to be fed. The expectancy to feed and the realization of appropriateness about the timing and the situation set the tone for the communication that will follow.

The second part of the structure comprises the **source**, that is, the sender of the communication. The source is the system that begins the communication. Each source develops his own personal style of initiating communication. Personal style is reflective of the culture in which man's system exists. This personal style in communicating is a learned form of behavior that is passed down from generation to generation. The mother, well aware that it is approaching the time for her baby to be fed, nears the crib. If she is a verbal mother she may begin by calling out endearments to her infant. The manner by which the mother slips her arms around the infant to pick him up, all the while smiling and chatting, represents her own personal style embedded against a larger cultural framework. Here she is the source of communication.

A third structural part often included in communication models is the message. The message is the information being transmitted. It reflects what is to be transmitted and how this information is to be transmitted. The content of the message reflects that it is time to be held and fed. The pleasantries and endearments uttered by the mother to her infant make up the verbal part of her message. The tender movements of her hand on his head provide a nonverbal message. The how of the transmission, then, refers to the next structural part of the communication model—the **channel.** The channel addresses how the message is transported. The channel, or channels as the case may be, include hearing, touch, smell, and taste. Verbal and nonverbal events work through these channels. In this instance, the mother spoke sounds that could be detected by the infant's auditory channel, the ear. Moving toward the crib within the infant's visual field permitted his channel of vision to detect the event. Stroking his head evoked his sense of being touched.

The fifth main structural part of communication models is often the receiver, the system making contact with the new communication. The input has to be understood by the receiving system for communication to have occurred. As the mother rubbed the infant's head, he stirred. He felt his mother's touch and was activated. At first he had random movements but as sleep faded, and he became more alert, his attention increased. He could see and hear his mother. He made a sound between a coo and a cry. He felt an internal sensation of hunger and began to cry louder. The infant received the mother's messages and was able to respond.

The last major structural component of communication models is feedback. In feedback a part of the output returns to the system as input. Feedback in communications tells the source system that the message was or was not received. When the infant stirred immediately subsequent to the mother's touch, this was feedback to her that the infant had received the nonverbal stimulus, her output, emanating from her hand.

If one looks at the above example in a summary manner, the following exemplify the structural communication parts: (1) anticipation of feeding—referent; (2) mother—sender (source); (3) utterances and hand and arm movements of mother—message; (4) hearing and touch—channels; (5) infant—receiver; and (6) infant's cry and stirring—feedback.

Although this short example is easy to understand, it is simplistic. It is imperative when working with clients that the nurse is cognizant that human communication is never simple. There are models to provide a base for examining this complex process.

LEVELS OF COMMUNICATION

Besides the communication model, one can also facilitate an understanding of the communication process by examining levels of communicating. These levels are intrapersonal, interpersonal, and extrapersonal. Intrapersonal communication focuses on the communication that takes place within man. This is the communication that takes place between the subsystems within the system of man. When man is stimulated by a referent, a code composed of symbol clusters is channeled into his system.

To deal with the symbol clusters the system must first give these data attention. Once the data are given attention, they are channeled through the memory bank to establish meaning. If a coded message is logical when aligned with stored past referents, the system can recognize and understand the message. The system then responds. If the message is incongruent with what is stored, it is recycled through memory in an attempt to align it logically and meaningfully to other comparable coded messages. If not possible, the message remains meaningless to the system and therefore is lost to response, even to posing a question. Figure 8-2 depicts this process. Two common examples of this type of communication are talking to yourself or thinking through a solution to a problem.

The interpersonal communication level refers to two or more people communicating with each other. This communication serves to establish a common purpose between or among these individuals. Communications tend to be task oriented or support oriented. Task oriented communications assist in doing the jobs that have to be done by these individuals while support communications cushion the feelings and handle the human needs of these individuals. A balance has to be achieved between task and support communications.

Analysis of interpersonal communication tends to focus on the depth of personal relationships that are established by the personal communication. A common example of this is the revealment model developed by Powell (1972). This model contains five deepening levels of revealment (see Figure 8-3).

The first level is termed *surface communication*. People exchange brief surface communications daily. These communications are simply designed to acknowledge awareness so that if desired, further, more involved interpersonal communication may follow. If not, the communicators terminate the exchange, going their separate ways. Surface communications contain often repeated phrases, such as "Hi," "How are you," and "Fine." They use less energy since they are used within a range of fairly predictable circumstances.

Communications which are one level more involved than surface communications are "reports others" communications. These statements give facts and stories about others and very little is revealed about the source system. Attention is deflected away from the source while still attracting other

Communication Theory 155

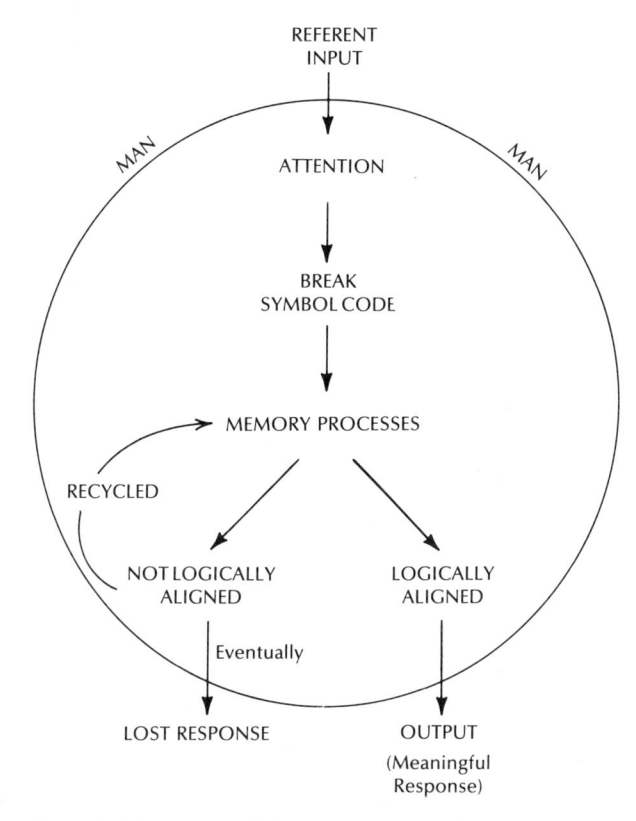

Figure 8-2 Intrapersonal Communication Level.

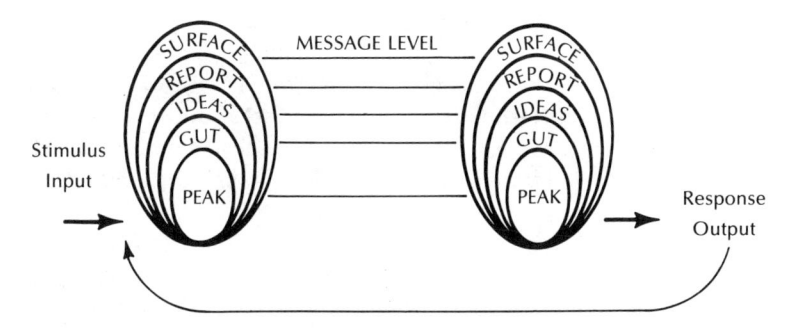

Figure 8-3 Levels of Revealment Communication Model. (From: "Interpersonal Encounter and the Five Levels of Communication." In *Bridges Not Walls*. Edited by J. Steward. Menlo Park, CA: Addison-Wesley Publishing Co., 1972.)

systems to maintain interpersonal communications. This level avoids loneliness without risking self-exposure.

The third level of revealment is one of "my ideas." In this level, the system does risk self-exposure through the giving of own ideas and conclusions. However, the feelings that lie beneath the ideas are not revealed and the overall communication is still fairly easy to terminate or protect.

The fourth level is the "gut" level of communication. Here the feelings that lie beneath one's ideas are shared and explored. There are some formalities and some guardedness continued in this level but they have been noticeably diminished. In all probability, the receiving system has tuned in well to the trust involved for the source to reach this point. Gut communication occurs when understanding is highly desired. One often sees this operating in the family, among close friends, and between a trusted provider and consumer of health care. For example, a client who discussed with a nurse problems related to sexual dysfunction is usually communicating on this level.

The fifth level of communication is referred to as "peak" communication. At this level both communicating systems are completely open. Boundaries function to accord each system with free transfer between them. There is extensive understanding and enhancement of feelings that takes place within a short time span. A pouring of energy is released from the system during peak communication. There is intense concentration of attention given to the communication with feedbacks operating effectively. Peak communication is an extreme condition and happens in rare instances between individuals. This type of communication is most likely to occur between individuals with a long-standing, close, personal relationship. You may have an opportunity to observe this communication in the delivery room. Couples frequently communicate at this level during the birth of their child.

Interpersonal communication has also been analyzed in terms of proximity. Hall (1966) used four levels in describing interpersonal distance zones. The intimate zone is the area closest to the person, generally considered within arms length, 6 inches to 18 inches. The personal zone ranges from 1 ½ feet to 4 feet. The social zone is from 4 feet to 12 feet, and the public zone is the most distant from 12 feet to 25 feet. Zones can be seen in this illustration. As the expectant mother drove up to the hospital to attend prenatal classes she was guided into the parking lot by a parking attendant who was in the center of the traffic flow (public zone). Upon arriving at the classroom, she was greeted by the nurse instructor (social zone). During the class she talked with some of the other women as they sat in their seats (personal zone). At one point the instructor showed restful positions for sleeping during the last few weeks of pregnancy. She assisted the mother, who at this time was lying on a mat to demonstrate the position, by placing a pillow to take the pressure off the abdomen (intimate zone). The distances themselves send a message understood within a cultural setting.

Extrapersonal communication level refers to that communication which has the capacity to reach thousands, perhaps millions of people. Another more common term used to refer to this level of communication is *mass communication.* Mass communication comes to individual man from a network of systems much larger than his own or that of his family. Broad sweeping communications such as television fall into this category.

Mass communication can be classified as electronic and nonelectronic (see Figure 8-4). Electronic media has enormous influences on man and particularly in recent years has made substantial attempts to influence man's health. Although health content can also be carried by means of radio, television is probably the single most influential means of communication ever invented. The potential to influence man's health through television is limited only by the imagination. Researchers in the various helping professions have sought ways to learn the effects of television. This area remains to be more fully studied and analyzed in terms of man's health. Television offers information to the public. Some of the information is visibly identified as health related, in fact, an entire program may have a health label for its title. It may be a nutrition program or an exercise program. Indirectly a program may also state health information that has been incorporated into a plot primarily designed for entertainment purposes. News shows are somewhere in between. Sharing of information about new drugs or treatments on the market is a typical information giving service by network news. Often times there are brief interviews with experts, including nurses, who provide additional pertinent information.

```
                    MASS COMMUNICATION
                            |
            ┌───────────────┴───────────────┐
        ELECTRONIC                      NONELECTRONIC
            |                               |
            |                       ┌───────┴───────┐
            |                     PRINT          NONPRINT
            |                       |               |
       • Television            • Books         • Photographs
       • Radio                 • Newspapers    • Artwork
       • Movies                • Magazines     • Artifacts
```

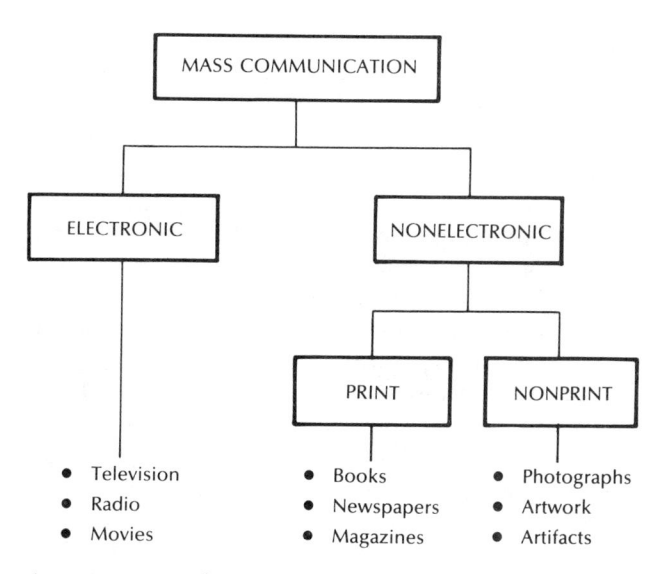

Figure 8-4 Types of Mass Communication.

There is a vast segment of mass communication that is not electronic. Newspapers, magazines, books, and other forms of print are circulated to millions of people on a daily basis. What is different is that print communication can be examined at the pace of the person and details can be included to enhance understanding. In addition, its highly portable quality allows the communication to be put into the system when convenient for the system. Because words in print remain, the person can return to them again and again to study thoroughly as needed. The effectiveness of print material is limited to the reading level of the reader.

Nonprint communications include such things as photographs, art work, artifacts, and realia of all types. Nonprint material can be combined with print material to enhance the reader's understanding. For example, several children's museums communicate information by letting the children play with models of the heart, crutches, wheelchairs, and other similar materials.

In this section of the chapter we have been discussing levels of communication: intrapersonal, interpersonal, and extrapersonal. These levels assist you in analyzing the communication process. In each of these levels a number of factors influence the process. The remaining sections of this chapter will focus on influences on communication as well as facilitators and inhibitors to effective communication.

INFLUENCES ON COMMUNICATION

If you were to sit and list each factor that could influence communication, the list would become overwhelming. This problem can be avoided by organizing the influences in terms of the sender and receiver, the message and channel, and the environment. In the communication model we identified the people who are communicating as senders and receivers. Since communication is cyclic, these roles are continuously being reversed. The receiver becomes the sender and the sender becomes the receiver. As a result, messages which are being sent and received are influenced by the unique characteristic of the sender and the receiver. Influences which originate from the source can be classified by the dimensions of man.

The physiological dimension provides the physical means to talk or to make physical gestures. It also provides the physical means by which we receive and comprehend a message. Certainly, if one has lost the ability to talk or to hear, communication is influenced. It is also influenced if one has lost the physical ability for nonverbal communication. A client who has lost the ability to move the muscles of the face is often described as without affect. Such a client may have deep feelings of frustration but his/her face will be unexpressive.

Communication is also influenced by the cognitive and emotional or affective aspects of the psychological dimension. The cognitive aspects include the overall knowledge base of the individual as well as his individual thinking pattern. For example, a client who has experienced a previous hospitalization will have a knowledge base which influences his communication with hospital personnel. How he uses this information will be determined by his individual thinking pattern or approach to problems. One person may ask questions of all staff in order to gather information from a variety of people. Another person may identify an "expert" and ask his questions of only that person. For example, he may decide his physician is the only one who can answer his questions.

The affective aspect of the client tends to be reflected in the personality. Personality includes such things as personal feelings, attitudes, biases, and values. If a client values health, he may be interested in learning about preventative measures and in turn his interest will be reflected in his communication.

The sociocultural influences on communication are broad and sometimes subtle. Factors such as attitudes, values, and norms from the culture have a persuasive influence. For example, the culture of the health care system includes a variety of roles and many norms related to how individuals in these roles communicate with each other. How the nurse informs the physician of a patient's condition is different from how she explains the same information to the patient. How the nurse communicates with a young person is different from how she communicates with an older person. Some of these differences are the result of cultural norms about communication between different age groups.

The dimensions of man are helpful in identifying influences on communication. All characteristics of the sender and receiver do not easily fit in this classification system. For example, the overall health of a client will have a direct influence on his communication. If he feels well he may have more energy to use in communicating. On the other hand, if he is weak and tired, he may have very little interest in talking or relating to another person.

Although the relationship between a sender and receiver influences communication, the message also plays a role in influencing the communication process. For example, if we receive a message that we interpret as pleasant or pleasing, we frequently are stimulated to continue the interaction. If on the other hand, we interpret the message as negative, we may react in one of two possible ways. First, we may be motivated to stop the interaction and terminate the negative experience. Or secondly, we may be motivated to continue the interaction in order to counteract the negative message. Many times as nurses we need to communicate information which is unpleasant for the client. The content of these messages greatly influences how the communication process progresses.

The final set of influences are those related to environment. Think about how you would relate to a friend you meet at a carnival as opposed to meeting the same friend in a church. Clients communicate differently in the hospital setting from the way they do in their own homes. In the hospital setting, the client is in the nurse's territory and plays the role of the patient. In his home, the nurse is in the client's territory and includes in her role the role of guest. In other words, the setting influences the communication process by altering roles and priorities.

The result of the numerous influences on communication is a dynamic process. Communication happens and effects happenings. Sometimes the influences facilitate the communication and the results are positive. Other times, they can act as barriers and the results are negative. In most situations, a combination is occurring. However, the nurse, in order to have some control over these influences, needs to know what can facilitate and what can inhibit communication.

FACILITATORS AND INHIBITORS TO COMMUNICATING

A review of the literature demonstrates numerous techniques that are effective in encouraging or blocking communications. Those techniques which encourage effective communication are termed *facilitators*, while those techniques which block communication are termed *inhibitors*. In most situations the nurse selects and develops those techniques that she can use with comfort. Hopefully, the nurse's repertoire of techniques leads to clear effective communications. In this section of the chapter, we will use the communication model presented earlier to analyze why facilitators encourage effective communication and inhibitors act to block communication. Though all of these facilitators and inhibitors will not be discussed in this chapter, examples of some of them will be presented in our analysis.

Referent

The referent serves to facilitate communication by providing the sender and receiver with a common bond or purpose. The referent can also serve to motivate those involved to want to communicate effectively, to spend the energy necessary for effective communications. If a nurse's purpose for communicating is to teach the client specific information and the client wants to learn this information, then the stage is set for effective communicating. If, on the other hand, the client wants to socialize, then communication problems will emerge. Both the sender and receiver must be headed in the same direction for effective communication.

Differences in referent or reasons for communicating may interfere with the effectiveness by heading the sender and receiver in different or noncompatible directions. The time spent in communicating is then diluted by each person trying to meet his individual needs or purpose. Each person brings the conversation back to his referent, and the interaction is terminated with a feeling of frustration and nonaccomplishment. One of the rationales for careful assessment and planning with clients before intervention is related to identifying a common purpose. Many times the nurse establishes the referent or purpose for communicating at the beginning of the interaction. An agreed upon purpose and direction, which was negotiated at the beginning of the interaction, serves to set the stage for effective communications because both parties are headed in the same direction and are committed to the interaction through the negotiation process.

Sender and Receiver

Facilitators and inhibitors related to the sender and receiver include (1) knowledge and use of appropriate verbal communication techniques, (2) observation and perception skills, (3) listening habits, (4) planning, and (5) emotions, values, and beliefs. The ability of the sender to know and use techniques with comfort influences the interaction. Some of these common techniques are described in Table 8-2. At this point in your education you

TABLE 8-2
Communication techniques: facilitators

Facilitators	Examples
1. Using silence	
2. Accepting	Yes.
	I follow what you said.
3. Giving recognition	Good morning, Mr. S.
	I notice that you have combed your hair.
4. Offering self	I'll sit with you a while.
	I'm interested in your comfort.
5. Giving broad openings	Is there something you'd like to talk about?
	What are you thinking about?
6. Offering general leads	Go on.
	And then?
	Tell me about it.
7. Placing the event in time or in sequence	What seemed to lead up to . . . ?
	Was this before or after . . . ?
	When did this happen?
8. Making observations	You appear tense.
	Are you uncomfortable when you . . . ?
9. Encouraging description of perceptions	Tell me when you feel anxious.
	What is happening?
10. Encouraging comparison	Was this something like . . . ?
	Have you had similar experiences?

(Continued)

TABLE 8-2 (*Cont.*)

Facilitators	Examples
11. Restating	*Patient:* I can't sleep. I stay awake all night. *Nurse:* You have difficulty sleeping?
12. Reflecting	*Patient:* Do you think I should tell the doctor . . . ? *Nurse:* Do you think you should?
13. Focusing	This point seems worth looking at more closely.
14. Exploring	Tell me more about that. Would you describe it more fully?
15. Giving information	My purpose in being here is . . . . I'm taking you to the . . . .
16. Seeking clarification	I'm not sure that I follow. What would you say is the main point of what you said?
17. Presenting reality	Your mother isn't here; I'm a nurse.
18. Voicing doubt	Isn't that unusual? Really?
19. Seeking consensual validation	Tell me whether my understanding of it agrees with yours.
20. Verbalizing the implied	*Patient:* I can't talk to you or to anyone. It's a waste of time. *Nurse:* Is it your feeling that no one understands?
21. Encouraging evaluation	What are your feelings in regard to . . . ? Does this contribute to your discomfort?
22. Attempting to translate into feelings	*Patient:* I'm dead. *Nurse:* Are you suggesting that you feel lifeless? *or* Is it that life seems without meaning?
23. Suggesting collaboration	Perhaps you and I can discuss and discover what produces your anxiety.
24. Summarizing	You've said that . . . . During the past hour you and I have discussed . . . .
25. Encouraging formulation of a plan of action	What could you do to let your anger out harmlessly?

Adapted with permission of Macmillan Publishing Co. from Hayes, J. and Larson, K. H. *Interacting with Patients.* New York: The Macmillan Company, 1963.

will be learning these techniques but are not yet skillful in using them. Frequently during this learning process, learners feel awkward and stilted when using these various techniques. You will be experimenting with difficult combinations of these techniques and trying them out in different situations to develop a repertoire that works for you. You will also be analyzing why they worked or didn't work for you. Table 8-3 shows one process by which you might begin to analyze your communications. In learning communication

TABLE 8-3
Analysis of communication

SITUATION 1:	
INTERACTION	ANALYSIS
Mrs. Joseph: Hello. I remember you. You were a patient of mine when you had your surgery.	Recognizing.
Mrs. Kappa: Oh, really.	Recognizing.
Mrs. Joseph: Yes, you carried on and cried like a baby.	Rejecting.
Mrs. Kappa: Oh, I'm a regular baby when it comes to pain.	Patient attempts to gain acceptance by agreeing.
Mrs. Joseph: Oh, that's OK. When I had my surgery I carried on, too. Don't worry about it. But my surgery was terrible.	Approval. Introducing an unrelated topic (the nurse's surgery). Disparaging.

SITUATION 2:	
INTERACTION	ANALYSIS
Mrs. Joseph: Hello, Mrs. Kappa. I'm Mrs. Joseph, one of the nurses who cared for you on Unit 85. How have you been lately?	Recognizing. Broad openings.
Mrs. Kappa: Oh, I'm so glad some of the same nurses are still here. Oh, I'm OK . . . almost OK.	Recognizing and informing. Patient is testing to determine if nurse will respond if problem is introduced.
Mrs. Joseph: What does "almost OK" mean?	Exploring.
Mrs. Kappa: I thought I was doing OK, then the doctor told me I have to come back for more treatment.	Informing.
Mrs. Joseph: Why don't we walk back to your room where we can both sit down and talk about this?	Nurse is providing an environment physically and psychologically (suggesting collaboration) for communication.

techniques you will discover that some of the accepted facilitators work better for you, as an individual, than others do.

Anxiety during this process is common and tends to block effective communication. The sender is so busy trying to remember what to say next that little time is spent observing and listening to the receiver. Sometimes the anxiety causes us to say things that tend to represent our wishful thinking, to be nice. For example, a client has just been told he has cancer. You may feel an urge to reassure him that everything will be all right. If you tell him everything will be OK, you have provided him with false reassurance. He will soon realize that everything is not all right and he has, in fact, many problems with which he must deal. He may now feel uncomfortable sharing these problems with you since you have told him you believe everything will work out. Knowing when and how to reassure or provide support for the client takes time and practice. Table 8–4 summarizes some of the common errors or

TABLE 8–4
Communication techniques: inhibitors

Inhibitors	Examples
1. Reassuring	I wouldn't worry about.... Everything will be all right.
2. Giving approval	That's good. I'm glad that you....
3. Rejecting	Let's not discuss.... I don't want to hear about....
4. Agreeing	That's right. I agree.
5. Disagreeing	That's wrong. I don't believe that.
6. Advising	I think you should.... Why don't you...?
7. Probing	Now, tell me about.... Tell me your life history.
8. Challenging	If you're dead, why is your heart beating?
9. Testing	What day is this? Do you know what kind of a hospital this is?
10. Defending	This hospital has a fine reputation. No one here would lie to you.
11. Requesting an explanation	Why do you think that? Why did you do that?
12. Indicating the existence of an external source	What makes you say that? What made you do that?
13. Belittling feelings expressed	*Patient:* I have nothing to live for.... I wish I were dead. *Nurse:* Everybody gets down in the dumps.
14. Making stereotype comments	I'm fine, and how are you? Just listen to your doctor and take part in activities—you'll be home in no time.
15. Giving literal responses	*Patient:* I'm an Easter egg. *Nurse:* What shade? *or* You don't look like one.
16. Using denial	*Patient:* I'm nothing. *Nurse:* Of course you're something. Everybody is somebody.
17. Interpreting	What you mean is.... Unconsciously, you're saying....
18. Introducing an unrelated topic	*Patient:* I'd like to die. *Nurse:* Did you have visitors this weekend?

Adapted with permission of Macmillan Publishing Co. from Hayes, J. and Larson, K. H. *Interacting with Patients.* New York: The Macmillan Co., 1963.

inhibitors to therapeutic communications. Everyone at some point uses these inhibitors especially when feeling uncomfortable. As you gain skill in sending messages you will also become more skillful in receiving them.

Observation and perception skills are significant facilitators of communication if used appropriately. Through observation, facts and events are taken into the system, i.e., noted and recorded. This can be done through any of the senses but one most often thinks of vision and hearing as the major collecting instruments. Observation is not usually confined to a single channel but combines all the responding senses. Once an observation is made, then the system analyzes and gives meaning to the data. This act of analysis or giving personal interpretations to the data is referred to as perception. No two systems have identical perceptions. Once an analysis to an observation is made, verification for accuracy and completeness is made with the client. Without verification, an error in conclusions could result.

As an illustration of observational and perceptual skills note the following: The nurse observes that a patient has left her breakfast untouched. She analyzes this observation. The food looks and smells fresh, the patient seems content otherwise, and the overall situation in the semiprivate room is unremarkable. One conclusion is that the patient is not hungry or the food is bad. She asks, "I noticed that you didn't touch your breakfast. What seems to be the difficulty?" "Oh, there's no difficulty," the patient replies, "I'm going home early today and I took a couple of pieces of fruit from my fruit basket, so I didn't think I needed anything more right now." The nurse responded, "Oh, yes, I see," and was glad she had verified her tentative conclusion that something might have been wrong with the food or the patient's ability to eat the breakfast. Many times, however, the nurse does not stop to verify what she believes the client is trying to say or communicate. She assumes her observation and perception to be correct and proceeds in that direction, thereby inhibiting communication.

The third area related to the sender and receiver is listening. Listening is more than just hearing. It is a highly perceptive process where the listener is purposely attentive to the speaker (sender). In therapeutic listening the full message is received by focusing on both the sender and the message. Time is utilized to collect data about the sender while hearing the message. A problem can arise if the receiver is listening faster than the sender is speaking. During this gap, receivers many times let their minds wander or mentally complete the sentence for the sender.

To develop good listening habits one must develop the concurrent techniques of silence. Silence can function as a facilitator or inhibitor. If the silence is comfortable, then time is provided to organize thoughts, plan how the message will be sent, support the sender, and provide reassurance. If the silence is uncomfortable, then pressure is exerted on both the sender and receiver to verbalize, to fill the void created by the silence. Uncomfortable silence can be converted to comfortable silence by providing permission for the silence. For example, the nurse may say to the client, "Just take your time and think about what you want to say."

Proper planning on the part of the sender, the fourth area, can facilitate effective communication by appropriate timing of the message and by creation of an environment conducive to privacy, comfort, and attentiveness. Timing of the message refers to assessment of the receiver's readiness for the message. A number of factors may interfere with the receiver's readiness for the message. He may be overloaded with new information from others. He may need time to assimilate what has been communicated to him recently. He may be tired, in pain, or distracted by other problems. An effective sender would consider all these factors and negotiate with the client for a time he may be more receptive to an interaction. Sometimes when this is not possible, acknowledging your understanding and concern of these difficulties will help make the receiver more receptive to the message.

Proper planning also includes consideration of the environment in which the interaction is to occur. The environment includes all that surrounds the interaction, i.e., privacy, comfortable furniture, room size, emotional tone, and temperature. Creating a comfortable nonthreatening environment facilitates the communication process. To illustrate this point, consider the following situation. A nurse is assigned to complete an admission interview with a young patient with a pelvic infection. The nurse takes the patient to the lounge, closes the door, and conducts the interview. She is paying attention to environmental influences on the communication process. Contrast this with the nurse who enters the patient's room, stands at the bedside, and proceeds to conduct the interview while the roommate is behind the curtain with her visitors. Can you anticipate which situation will probably result in a more effective interview, in a better level of interaction?

The last facilitator or inhibitor that relates to the sender and receiver is emotions, values, and beliefs. For example, if the sender is very anxious she may not hear the message sent. You have this experience when you mean to say one thing but actually say another. This same thing occurs with the receiver. High anxiety blocks the ability to receive information.

Values and beliefs function much like the environment. If there is a commonality of values and beliefs between the sender and the receiver, communication is supported. If there is not a commonality, communication can be inhibited. For example, if a client believes that illness is the result of fate alone he will not receive and understand information related to primary prevention; or if a nurse believes that people from a certain ethnic background are poor parents, the nurse may provide little or no information on parenting to individuals from that ethnic background. On the other hand, if the nurse and the client value medical care, the nurse may recommend and the client may follow the suggestion that the client present medical problems to a physician.

Message

So far we have been focusing on facilitators and inhibitors related to the referent and sender and receiver. We will now focus on facilitators and inhibitors related to the message. The message refers to what is communicated; that information conveyed that is both planned and unplanned. Unplanned messages relate to what we inadvertently convey; planned messages refer to what we want to say. For example, we may say to a client, "I'm going to teach you how to arrange your diet," but if the nurse is standing throughout the communication while the client is sitting, we are also sending a message about who is in charge. Facilitators frequently show congruence between planned and unplanned messages. Inhibitors, on the other hand, frequently demonstrate incongruence between planned and unplanned messages, i.e., double messages.

In order for a message to be conveyed the sender must decide on its content, code it, and transmit it. Decisions related to content involve how much and what is to be in the message. When the sender selects the appropriate amount and nature of the content, communication is facilitated. On the other hand, when the sender includes too much information or includes the wrong information, the communication can be inhibited. How does one make these decisions? A few rules of thumb might help. First, be aware of the attention span and health status of the receiver. Short, more frequent messages are better when giving information. Longer, less frequent interactions are better when the intent is to promote self-understanding and time for reflection. Generally, receivers in discomfort and in distracting environments have short attention spans. Before sending the message, the nurse should provide comfort for the client and a quiet, unhurried environment. Second, be aware of the needs of the client. What clues has the receiver given you regarding his readiness to receive your message or your support? Use these clues to determine what information to transmit and provide hints of additional information that you, in your professional judgment, feel is needed.

The next component related to message is coding it. Language, i.e., words, is most often thought of when discussing coding messages. The words that a nurse selects in explaining a procedure to a client become crucial in facilitating the client's understanding and acceptance of the procedure. For example, in teaching a diabetic person how to give his insulin the nurse may refer to the injection as a shot or hypo. The term *shot* may carry a negative emotional message. The term *hypo* may not be understood by the client. The nurse must work with the client to clarify information, to use words understood by the client, and not to use medical jargon or abbreviations. Terms that are carefully defined and understood are key facilitators. Selecting words based on the client's educational level and using several different words to convey the same message aids in facilitating an understandable message. The nurse needs to set a climate whereby the client feels free to ask for words to be defined. Prefacing the message with a statement, "Sometimes we use words that clients don't understand. If I do this, please let me know so I can define the words. Your understanding this information is critical," can set the climate conducive to open communication.

While language is most frequently thought of when discussing coding messages, symbols are another form of coding. The use of symbols facilitates flexibility among ideas to be communicated. Symbol manipulation can suggest a relationship, association, convention, or resemblance (Webster, 1981). When the symbol system is understood, a clear message can be sent and perceived. Symbols can be pictures, people, color, inanimate objects, animals, and probably any other item that can be discretely identified so that it can stand for another item. A surgical mask for sterile field, green fabric for operating room dress, green "Mr. Yuk" stickers for poison, a banded white cap to designate nurse, and stethoscope to depict a technical skill are all symbols that can move a communication along readily within a particular context. Nurses need to be aware that how they manipulate symbols can influence the message either negatively or positively. Walking into a room with a clipboard may convey to the client that although you want to see how he is doing, you have no intention of providing nursing care. His response to you will reflect his interpretation of this message. The nurse facilitates communication by relying on her observational and perceptual skills to assist in identifying how the client reacts to her use of language and symbols. The nurse also validates these perceptions with the client.

The last facilitator and inhibitor related to message is transmission or treatment of the message. How will the message be conveyed? What channel will be used? What nonverbal techniques will be used to enhance the verbal transmission? Verbal techniques to facilitate conveying the message were discussed with sender and receiver. Two additional facilitators related to message transmission are presented here.

The first facilitator related to message transmission is skillful use of space and movement. Skillful use of space and movement can be as difficult to learn as those of language and symbols. Learning when and how to touch the client to provide for feelings of comfort is especially difficult in our non-touching society. For example, imagine a situation where a family has returned to the hospital because their family member has become seriously ill. As they approach the nurses' station, the nurse comes around from behind the desk, places her hand on the shoulder of the closest family member and states, "I'm sorry we had to call you back like this." She briefly explains the changing condition and walks back to the room with them. She makes sure there is room and chairs for all the family members. A short time later she returns, briefly examines the patient, and sits down with the family to explore whether they have any questions. Note in this situation how much of the message was sent not with language but via touch and body movement. While learning when and how to touch a client to convey your concern and caring, the best rule of thumb to follow is to touch judiciously. Some people do not like being touched by others; other people do. Once you have touched the client during an interaction, you need to observe how he responds. If the response is positive, then the nurse could use this technique during communications with this client. If, on the other hand, the reaction is less than positive, this communication facilitator could be an inhibitor for this client.

The second facilitator related to message transmission is selection of the appropriate channel. What is the best way to communicate this message? Some messages need to be conveyed both verbally and nonverbally. Some messages need to be reinforced in writing. Think about how many channels your teachers are using to teach you information related to communication. How was related class content presented? Were there lectures, slides, overheads, and movies? As a general rule the more channels in use the more likely the message will be received.

SUMMARY

This chapter has described communication theory and related this theory to the practice of nursing. A broad definition of communication was presented, followed by the purposes for communicating. Components of the communication process were presented through use of a communication model. These components are referent, sender, message, channel, receiver, and feedback. This model then provided a method for analysis of the influences and identification of the facilitators and barriers to effective communication.

The key points to remember related to communication are

1. Communication is a cyclic process involving alternating sender and receiver roles.
2. Communication models can serve to assist you in dealing with the complex nature of this process.
3. Any factor that influences man in his environment can be a factor in influencing communication.
4. Although many communication techniques have been identified, effective utilization of these techniques involves an understanding of why and how they influence the process of communicating.
5. Effective communication skills can be learned, but they require time and energy to develop.

REFERENCES

Caldwell, E., and Hegner, B. *Foundation for Medical Communication.* Reston, VA: Reston Publishing Co., 1978.

Cohen, A. R. "Some Implications of Self-Esteem for Social Influences." In *Personality and Persuasibility*, edited by I. L. Janis, et al. New Haven: Yale University Press, 1959.

Curtis, D. B., and Kline, J. A. *Effects of Message Organization on Attitude Change.* Paper presented at the annual meeting of the Western State Communications Association. Albuquerque, New Mexico: November 1973, ERIC No. ED 090596.

Davies, E. "Say It with Symbols." *Nursing Times* 75 (44) [1979]: 1900–1901.

Dembroski, T., and Pennebaker, J. W. *The Effect of Guilt-Shame Arousing Communications on Attitude and Behavior.* U.S. Department of H.E.W., Office of Education, April 1972. ERIC No. ED 072361.

Evans, R. I., et al. "Fear Arousal, Persuasion and Actual Versus Implied Behavioral Change." *Journal of Personality and Social Psychology* 16 (1970): 220–227.

Festinger, L. "Cognitive Dissonance." *Scientific American* 207 (1962): 92–102.

Hall, E. *The Hidden Dimension.* New York: Doubleday and Co., 1966.

Hart, G. "The Earliest Medical Use of the Caduceus." *Canadian Medical Association Journal* 107 (1972): 1107–1110.

Hays, J., and Larson, K. H. *Interacting with Patients.* New York: Macmillan Co., 1963.

Hein, E. *Communication in Nursing Practice.* Boston: Little, Brown and Co., 1980.

Hovland, C. I., and Weiss, W. "The Influence of Source Credibility on Communication Effectiveness." *Public Opinion Quarterly* 15 (1951): 635–650.

Janis, I. L., and Feshbach, S. "Effects of Fear-Arousing Communications." *Journal of Abnormal Social Psychology* 48 (1953): 78–93.

Karlins, M., and Abelson, H. *Persuasion.* New York: Springer Publishing Co., 1970.

Kelly, A. D. "A Crash of Symbols." *Canadian Medical Association Journal* 109 (1973): 515–518.

Murray, R. B., and Zentner, J. P. *Nursing Concepts for Health Promotion.* Englewood Cliffs, NJ: Prentice-Hall, Inc., 1979.

O'Brien, M. *Communications and Relationships in Nursing.* St. Louis: The C. V. Mosby Co., 1978.

Pluckhan, M. *Human Communication.* New York: McGraw-Hill Co., 1978.

Powell, J. "Interpersonal Encounter and the Five Levels of Communication." In *Bridges not Walls*, J. Steward, ed. Menlo Park, CA: Addison-Wesley Co., 1972.

Raia, J. R., and Osipow, S. H. "Creative Thinking Ability and Susceptibility to Persuasion." *Journal of Social Psychology* 82 (1970): 181–186.

Robertson, L. S., et al. "A Controlled Study of the Effect of Television Messages on Safety Belt Use." *American Journal of Public Health* 64 (1974): 1071–1080.

Shannon, C., and Weaver, W. *The Mathematical Theory of Communication.* Urbana, IL: University of Illinois Press, 1949.

Steiner, M. J., and Rothberg, S. "Teaching Home Health Care with Videotapes." *Nurse Educator* 5 (4) [1980]: 5–7.

Thayer, L. Communication Systems. In *The Relevance of General Systems Theory*, edited by E. Laszlo. New York: George Braziller, 1972.

Webster's New Collegiate Dictionary. Springfield, MA: G & C Merriam Co., 1981.

Wiedenbach, E., and Falls, C. *Communication: Key to Effective Nursing.* New York: Tiresias Press, 1978.

9

Change theory

DEFINITION OF TERMS

Change   Alternation of the present state, to be different.
Change Agent   An individual or group of individuals who attempt to control a direct change.
Change Model   A plan depicting the various steps or phases to be utilized when planning, implementing, and evaluating change.
Change Theory   That body of knowledge which exists to describe the phenomena of change.

At the beginning of each of the chapters in this unit on theories a situation is presented. Each situation was chosen to focus the learner on a specific theory. Yet, if you look back at these situations you will note that each one deals with change. This is because each of us is in the process of changing as we go about living in a changing world. We are constantly experiencing change and producing change. Therefore, we need to know what change is, how people react to change, and how to produce change. This is done by application of change theory.

For example, let us look at a situation involving change. Sophomore nursing students at Wakefield University have been studying primary prevention in Nursing 001. Today's discussion focused on the hazards of smoking. After class a group of these students decided to go to the student lounge for a break. They noticed that the lounge was smokier than ever. This stimulated a discussion of the fact that there was not a no-smoking area or lounge. Why should they let themselves be exposed to all this harmful smoke? No one, however, was willing to ask the smokers to stop smoking. Everyone felt it would only produce an embarrassing scene. Surely there was some logical, systematic way to change this situation. What could they do? How could they get a no-smoking area or lounge? Once obtained how could they get the smokers to observe the no-smoking areas or lounge?

The purpose of this chapter is to present relevant concepts related to change theory that can be used not only by those who hope to produce change but also by those who are experiencing change. At the completion of this chapter, the reader will be able to

1. Define change and change theory.
2. Explain how people react to change.
3. Identify the information needed to plan for change.
4. Describe principles that can be applied in planning for change.
5. Identify strategies that can be used in implementing change.

CHANGE DEFINED

According to the American Heritage Dictionary, **change** is "to cause to be different; alter" (Morris, 1973, p. 224). Change is a phenomenon that occurs all around us, but with varying degrees. In other words, it may be seen on a continuum from minor changes, e.g., a hair cut, to crisis type changes, e.g., loss of family in an accident (see Figure 9–1). Where change is placed on this continuum is determined by the amount of alteration required in the system's structure and function. The greater the degree of alteration, the closer one moves to the crisis end of the continuum.

Although change can be seen on a continuum reflecting degree of change experienced, it can also be considered on a related continuum reflecting the degree of control of that change. This continuum moves from an end point of little or no control over the change to an end point of major control over the change (see Figure 9–2). For instance, a client is placed on a new diet. A nurse has limited control over an individual's diet when he leaves the hospital but has more control while he is in the hospital. Examples of the no or little control end of the continuum would include inflation, organizational structure, weather, pollution, height, eye color, and sex. Examples of the major control end of the continuum would include buying habits, size of car you drive, weight, and eating habits. Changes where you feel you have little or no control are more likely to be crisis situations. People who experience a sudden

MINOR CHANGE ——————————————————— CRISIS CHANGE

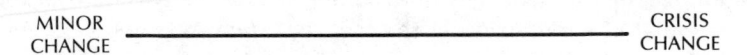

Figure 9–1 Degree Change Continuum.

```
LITTLE OR                                              MAJOR
NO CONTROL    ─────────────────────────────           CONTROL
OVER CHANGE                                         OVER CHANGE
```

Figure 9-2 Control Change Continuum.

major change in their health status frequently feel they have little control over that change.

No discussion of change would be complete without addressing types of change. Types of change can be classified according to who is changed, what is changed, and the process of change. Who is changed refers to the target system changed. This can be an individual, a family, a group, an institution, or a community. Knowledge of who is to be changed facilitates selection of change strategies, prediction of scope or magnitude of change, and resources needed to implement the change.

What is changed refers to the aspect of the system to be changed. Are you changing structure, function, or purpose or some combination of these? Because the system functions as a whole, change usually affects each of these aspects. For example, if the nurse wanted to facilitate changing the health practices of a high-risk coronary artery disease client, the nurse might help this client by first promoting exercise to increase the efficiency of the heart muscle and circulation. This is mainly a structural change. Next, you might convince the client to adjust his dietary habits and stress patterns. These are mainly functional changes. Finally, you might also facilitate the client valuing good health so that he spends his time and energy in health-related activities. These changes represent changes in purpose or goals. As you can see, change is more successful if it addresses as many aspects of the system as possible.

Considering the process of change is the most common way of looking at change (see Figure 9-3). Process of change refers to how change occurs. Change occurs by nonplanning or planning. Nonplanned change refers to change which occurs by drift. Planned change is change which occurs either by planning *with* the client system, commonly referred to as collaborative change, or by planning *for* the client system, commonly referred to as traditional change (Brooten, Hayman, & Naylor, 1978).

Change by drift (nonplanned change) includes that change which occurs without our awareness. This type of change generally involves small subtle changes in the system which eventually results in large major changes that hit all at once. It is with this type of change that you wonder how it happened. Examples of drifting change might be the gradual weight increase a person experiences over the winter months or the aging process.

Planned change involves a change agent. A change agent is either an individual or a group of individuals who attempt to control a direct change. For

```
                        ┌──────────┐
                        │  CHANGE  │
                        └────┬─────┘
              ┌──────────────┴──────────────┐
   ┌──────────────────┐            ┌────────────────┐
   │ NONPLANNED CHANGE│            │ PLANNED CHANGE │
   │        OR        │            │                │
   │      DRIFT       │            │                │
   └──────────────────┘            └────────┬───────┘
                            ┌───────────────┴───────────────┐
                  ┌──────────────────┐            ┌──────────────────────┐
                  │PLANNED FOR CHANGE│            │ PLANNED WITH CHANGE  │
                  │        OR        │            │         OR           │
                  │TRADITIONAL CHANGE│            │ COLLABORATIVE CHANGE │
                  └──────────────────┘            └──────────────────────┘
```

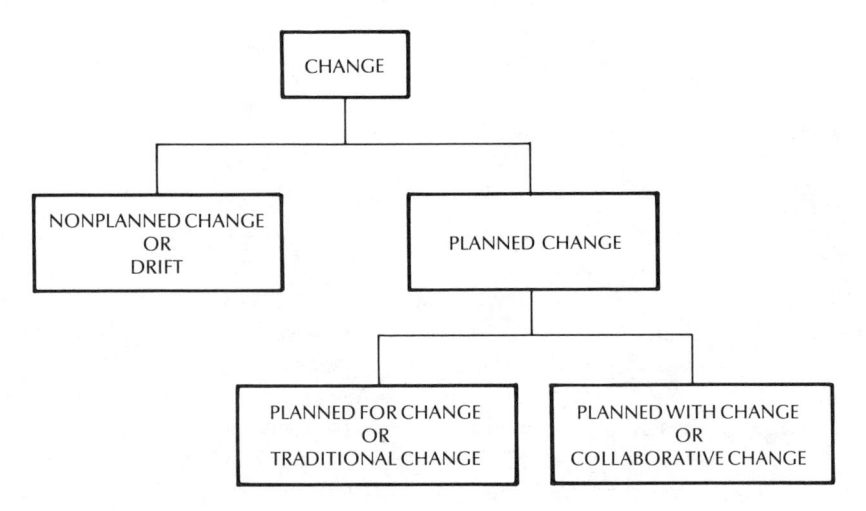

Figure 9-3 Process of Change.

example, a nurse who encourages a client to change his diet is functioning as a change agent. So, too, is the nurse who works with legislators to help enact a law requiring car seats for children. In each case the type of planned change is determined by the amount of direct client involvement in goal setting.

Traditional change (planned for change) involves that change which occurs through the use of three basic strategies—education, emotional appeal, and coercion. Examples of these basic strategies include providing facts and statistics to the system, appealing to emotions, and developing rules and regulations which enforce this change. These examples can be seen in society's attitude about cigarette smoking. While individuals continue to smoke, the nonsmoking public has demanded their rights to non-smoke-filled places. After much education of the public related to the hazards of smoking; emotional appeals made by children, cancer victims, and various organizations; and laws regulating places for smoking and nonsmoking, society's attitude toward the nonsmokers' rights is gradually changing.

Collaborative change (planned with change) involves a change agent who works with a client system defining and working toward specific change related to mutually established goals. Collaborative change has the most potential for helping the nurse function as an effective change agent. An example of this type of change might be a nurse who works with a client and establishes a goal that the client will lose fifty pounds in eight months. They then will select appropriate strategies for achieving this goal.

Having defined change, the question now becomes what is change theory? **Change theory** means that body of knowledge which exists to describe the phenomenon of change. As a relatively new theory, change theory is not as well developed as some of the other theories we have discussed. This chapter will present those aspects of the theory that will be useful to the nurse as she functions in her role as a change agent.

CHANGE MODELS

The term *model* refers to a plan or object representing some aspect of reality. A **change model** is a plan depicting the various steps or phases to be utilized when planning, implementing, and evaluating change. Many change models exist; each has its advantages and disadvantages. Each seems to focus on slightly different aspects of the system, steps in the change process, and strategies for changing the system. Each situation you are involved in is slightly different and may require some changes or adaptations of a model; however, these models can serve as a useful guide to facilitate the process by reminding you of important aspects of change. These models should help keep you pointed in the right direction when you are involved with change.

Chin (1961) has identified three types of models. These three types of models are systems, developmental, and changing. A systems model is based on systems theory and focuses on maintaining stability of the system. Stresses, strains, and tensions are the presenting symptoms; and adjustment and adaptation are the goals of intervention (Rodgers, 1973, p. 162). In other words change occurs in this model as a result of structural tensions when incompatible and conflicting parts emerge. For example, a current change that can be analyzed using this model is occurring with the financing of health care in this country. Dissatisfaction with the high cost of health care is the presenting symptom. The development of diagnostic related categories (DRG's) is an adjustment to financing with the goal of reducing cost, therefore making the system more stable. The change process in this model involves an external change agent and structural alterations.

The developmental model focuses on maintaining system existence. Concern is with phases and stages of change which are not planned but occur with time. In other words change is natural and occurs when there is a gap between what is actually present and what is potentially available. A change that can be analyzed using this model is the change that occurs as a student moves over time to the role of professional nurse. The faculty of the school constantly work assisting the student to develop into a future professional nurse. This change model also requires an external change agent who focuses on removing the gaps through tending, cultivating, and guiding the system.

The last model, the changing model, focuses on variable goals and is deliberate and planned. It includes aspects of both the above models and is the one most commonly used today. Change in this model occurs as a result of the system and change agent perceiving a need to change. The change process requires a participant change agent who facilitates identifying the need for change and then helps see that the desired change occurs.

The most frequently discussed changing model is the one developed by Lewin (1947). Lewin's model consisted of three phases—unfreezing, moving, and refreezing. During the unfreezing phase the change agent focuses on dissolving old behaviors and creating an imbalance between facilitators and barriers. In other words there must be more facilitators than barriers for the change to move in the desired direction. In the moving phase the change agent helps shift system behaviors to the desired behaviors by using motivating forces. Examples of motivating forces are status, money, praise, fear of job loss, and peer pressure. This is the phase frequently referred to as implementing the planned change. The refreezing phase involves maintaining the new behaviors by reinforcing and rewarding them. This phase continues until the new behaviors become a permanent part of the system's behaviors.

Most of the other changing models are adaptations and expansions of this model (Reinkemeyer, 1970; Havelock, 1973; Capelle, 1979; Spradley, 1980). These models generally expand the phases from three to five or seven. All these models in one way or another include diagnosing the need to change, selecting strategies or solutions, implementing the change, evaluating the change, and then stabilizing the change. Most of these models present a problem-solving approach to dealing with change. Regardless of which model you select to use when functioning as a change agent, a key point to remember is to select a model which fits your style and the situation. Then, use this model as a guide during the change process. Doing this will help facilitate the change process.

ASSESSMENT OF THE NEED TO CHANGE

Before a change agent can begin to change any system, he must be able to diagnose, that is, to develop a clear statement of the problem. Any diagnostic process begins by collecting data. A change agent collects two types of data. The first type of data collected deals with the basic problem or need. While collecting this, data which will help him select appropriate strategies and plan appropriate solutions are also collected. In other words, he looks at both the system and its environment.

Lewin's (1976) diagnostic process begins by assessing facilitators and barriers (supporting and opposing forces) and then creating imbalances in the proper direction. Capelle (1979) has provided a more specific guide for assessing a system for change. In using this guide the data are usually collected from the systems level through to the client consultant relationship (see Table 9-1). By system level, Capelle is referring to the individual, family, group, community, or organization. Systems analysis includes information on input into the system, throughput, output from the system, feedback, boundary, and environment. Developmental stage refers to the system's age and appropriateness of age and behavior. Information on objectives, structure, roles,

TABLE 9-1
Capelle's consultants' human systems assessment model

1. Systems Level
2. Systems Analysis
   a. Input
   b. Throughput
   c. Output
   d. Feedback
   e. Boundary
   f. Environment
3. Developmental Stage
4. General Factors
   a. Objectives
   b. Structure
   c. Roles
   d. Communication
   e. Reward System
   f. Power
   g. Time
   h. Space
5. Client System-Change Agent Relationship

From: Capelle, Ronald G. *Changing Human Systems.* Toronto: International Human Systems Institute, 1979. P. 32. Used with permission.

communication, reward system, power, time, and space is included under the heading of general factors. The last information the change agent collects would be on the change agent and system relationship. Table 9-2 demonstrates sample questions and data you would collect using this assessment guide.

TABLE 9-2
Change assessment of the individual

Area to be Assessed	Specific Content	Sample Questions
1. Systems level	Individual	— —
2. Systems analysis		
Input	Matter Energy Information	What is this system taking in?
Throughput	Cognitive processes Psychological processes	How does this individual feel? What are his defenses? How does he perceive the situation?
Output	Matter Energy Information	Does this individual work? What are his contributions to society? Are his outputs appropriate for the situation?

(Continued)

TABLE 9–2 (Cont.)

Area to be Assessed	Specific Content	Sample Questions
Feedback	Physiological Psychological Sociocultural	Are the feedbacks received appropriate?
Boundary	Defined boundary	How open or closed is this individual's boundary?
Environment	Physical space People	What is this individual's environment? Describe it. Who are this individual's significant others? Describe them.
3. Developmental state	Stages of development	Is this individual's age and developmental level appropriate?
4. General factors		
Objectives	Present Future	Does this individual have objectives? If so, are they realistic, obtainable? List them.
Structure	Generally refers to groups and not included with individual system.	
Roles	Specific ones Numbers Conflict Enactment	What roles does this individual occupy? How many are there? Are they compatible? How does the individual perceive himself in these roles?
Communication	Patterns and ability Effectiveness	How does this individual communicate? How articulate is he? Does he speak English? Does he read?
Reward system	Motivators	What motivates this individual?
Power	Assertiveness Self-control	Does the individual have the power to obtain objectives?
Time	Client history Present state	Any factors from past which will influence or affect present and future? What is individual's present state?
Space	Territoriality	How does the individual feel about distances?
5. Client system—change agent	Interrelationship	How well do the change agent and client get along? Is there respect for the change agent? Is the change agent seen as a professional?

IDENTIFICATION OF CHANGE REACTIONS

Information about change reactions will help the nurse whether she is a change agent or an individual encountering and experiencing change. As a change agent, you can use this information as a basis for planning possible strategies which deal with reactions to change. As an individual experiencing change, this information provides a basis for analyzing and evaluating the change, not just reacting to it. Havelock (1973) has classified reactions to change into three types—do nothing, reflex, and problem solving. Do nothing is the most primitive reaction to change. "If you do nothing it will go away" is a frequent response heard in the health field. This means you do not change your behavior, you continue the way you were before the change was begun. For example, the hospital you work in is changing the sign-in and sign-out procedure. In the do nothing reaction you would continue to sign in and out following the same procedure you did before the change. The second reaction, simple reflex, is responding to the change by utilizing the least amount of energy. Continuing with the example above, you would respond to the changed signing in and out procedure by complying with it. Third, the problem solving reaction is responding to a change by active involvement in the proposed change from the planning stage through the implementation phase. Using the same example from above, the nurse when learning about the proposed change in the signing in and out procedure would become involved in the revision of the procedure as well as in educating the other staff to the new procedure.

The most common universal reaction to change is resistance. Resistance is one change reaction to which a change agent must always be alert. Other common reactions to change include negativism, anger, hostility, denial, depression, frustration, indifference, and acceptance.

How and why do people react to change as they do? How do you assess and anticipate these reactions? Generally, people respond to change as they do when they believe their basic needs are being challenged. Brill and Kilts (1980) state that reactions to change result when our basic needs for self-esteem, safety, and security are being threatened. It becomes important then for the change agent to be aware of how these needs are being challenged and to plan strategies for reducing these threats.

Asprec (1975) has identified several factors which need to be assessed in order to anticipate and deal with these reactions. Since any change will have behavioral, psychological, and social effects on the system and since systems are largely comprised of individuals, predicting the reactions to change becomes one of predicting key individual's responses to the change. These factors which need to be assessed are feelings of insecurity, trust, historical events, apprehensions and expectations, cultural beliefs and norms, manner of change, and predisposed feelings. Some of this information can be ob-

TABLE 9-3
Change reaction identification

Area to be Assessed	Sample Questions
1. Feelings of insecurity	How will this change affect this individual's job security? Self-esteem?
2. Trust	How much does the individual trust you?
3. Historical events	How did the individual handle past changes? What was the result of past changes? What were the individual's experiences with past change agents?
4. Apprehensions and expectations	Can the individual develop the skills needed for the new job? How will responsibility be affected with this change?
5. Beliefs and norms	Does the individual hold any values which will influence the change process? What norms exist that will influence the change?
6. Change manner	To what method(s) of change has this individual been exposed? How did he react to the various methods? How much time will the individual need to assimilate the change?
7. Predisposed feelings and attitudes	What feelings can the individual describe related to change from the past? How does the individual generally feel about change?

tained by using the change assessment guide presented earlier; however, it might be wise to add an additional section on change reactions (see Table 9-3). This would help the change agent to remember and anticipate the system's possible reactions when planning strategies and selecting solutions.

Feelings of insecurity result when one is concerned with job security and financial future. Looking at all the changes occurring as a result of the energy crisis demonstrates how these feelings of insecurity are hindering energy conservation. Many people's jobs are tied closely with their confidence and self-worth. Changes which affect their jobs result in feelings of insecurity. As a change agent you must ask yourself, how will these changes affect job security, self-esteem, and financial status of these individuals involved in the change?

Another factor to consider which influences people's reactions to change is trust. How well does this individual or group of individuals trust the change agent and others involved in the change? If an individual trusts you, he is more apt to feel that you will look after his best interests regardless of this change. If little trust exists, then negative change behaviors will develop. Developing trust then becomes an important part of the change strategy.

Awareness of historical events can have a profound effect on how people will react to the current change. As a change agent you need to collect information about past changes in terms of how the change was handled, outcomes of past changes, and trustworthiness of change agents. This information helps you anticipate and prevent undesirable reactions. For example, knowing that the system has experienced a change where the change agent said one thing but did another helps you anticipate difficulty in the system-change agent relationship. You would then need to work on developing a working relationship before and during the current change.

Apprehensions and expectations an individual holds related to this particular change need also to be determined. Factors in this area include what will be required of one after the change. Does the system have the skills for this new assignment? Does the system have the ability to learn the new things which will be required? Will this mean increased recognition, responsibility, status, etc.? These are all questions which need to be answered in anticipating reactions in the area of apprehension and expectations. As the individual's apprehensions increase, so too do the negative change reactions.

Beliefs and norms held by systems lead to conflict if the change is not consistent with these beliefs and norms. The change agent needs to be aware of what these beliefs and norms are and whether the change is consistent with them. If the change creates conflicts then the change agent must first work to change the beliefs before tackling the change. For example, if the cultural belief is anticontraceptives and you are trying to reduce overpopulation in that culture through use of contraceptives, you must first change the cultural belief before you can begin to educate the populace in the proper use of contraceptives.

The "how" of a change becomes just as important as the actual change in generating positive or negative reactions. When speaking about the manner of change, such things as timing, strategies, and type of information dispensed are included. In other words the change process itself will help determine reactions to the change. For example, a nurse wants to change the method of scheduling staff. The nursing director decides to bring an outside consultant in to do time-work studies. A recommendation and plans for implementation are made. The staff nurse becomes hostile to this change even though she wanted this change. She resents the way the change occurred because she is not accustomed to direct orders without her input. Another important aspect of the change manner is the timing. Most systems need time to assimilate the change and adjust themselves to it.

Predisposed feelings about change and attitude determinants are the last factors that need to be assessed in anticipating and reducing negative change reactions. Predisposed feelings about change refers to those vague, unpleasant feelings systems have when confronting change. Some of these feelings developed in childhood and remain through adulthood. The nurse cited above reacts to change with suspicion and distrust and must be helped to see the rewards generated by the change. Attitude determinants, on the other hand, generally refer to the resistant feelings generated by change and need to be dealt with similarly to predisposed feelings.

Assessing the above factors will place the change agent in a better position to proceed with the planned change. This data will facilitate selecting strategies to reduce possible negative reactions. Giving careful consideration to this information will make the change process more effective and satisfying instead of frustrating.

CHANGE PRINCIPLES

Regardless of what model one chooses to follow for changing, there are several general principles which the change agent can find helpful in planning for change. Paying attention to these rules can reduce frustration, anger, and hostility during the change process.

General Principles

1. Effective change is usually a slow process. Keeping this in mind is important to reduce frustration. Since systems did not develop overnight, the change agent cannot expect them to change quickly.
2. Multiple simultaneous changes are more difficult to handle than step-by-step changes. In other words, change is easier to accept if many elements of the system are held constant and time is permitted to assimilate each change. Since change is a stressor too many simultaneous changes can overwhelm the system.
3. Since systems have a tendency to maintain a steady state, resistance to change is natural. People tend to prefer the status quo because they know what to expect, how to react, etc.
4. The change agent can minimize resistance to change if the agent involves the people affected by the change in the planning for the change.

Principles Related to Structure

1. Since systems exist in an environment, changing behaviors in some part of the system requires you to make relevant changes in the existing environment. If these additional changes are not made, it may result in failure of permanent change. For example, changing the eating patterns of a child will not result in permanent change unless the family environment is also changed. The mother who continues to serve high calorie desserts will not facilitate changing the eating patterns of a diabetic child.
2. Since systems exist in a hierarchy, change must occur from above and below the system which is to be changed. When assessing the system, you must also pay attention to how the subsystem and suprasystem will be affected and what aspects of those systems will also need to be changed.

Principles Related to Process

1. Change in any part of a system affects the whole system. Keep in mind that in order to effectively change a system you must also consider changing relevant aspects of the system's components.

2. Change is more effective and easier if you maintain an individual's self-esteem. Remember that resistance to change and other negative reactions will increase in proportion to the degree of perceived threat to the individual's basic needs.
3. Begin change where some stress already exists in the system. This stress can serve as motivation to facilitate the change. Remember, though, that you do not want to begin change at those points already overloaded with too much stress.
4. Change behaviors need to be reinforced if they are to continue. Making a change and then not reinforcing the new behavior will result in a return to the old behavior.

STRATEGIES FOR IMPLEMENTING CHANGE

Chin and Benne (1976) have identified three basic types of change strategies. The types are empirical-rationale, norm-reeducative, and power-coercive. No one strategy will work all the time and generally you need a combination of these three types of strategies. Which strategies are actually used and how they are implemented is determined by the degree and type of collaboration that has been established in planning for this change. Using the situation at the beginning of the chapter, let us now identify how these three strategies might be utilized.

Empirical-Rationale

This strategy implies that you believe human beings are rational and will follow you if you convey your rationality. Specific strategies that fall into this category are basic research and dissemination of knowledge, personnel selection and replacement, use of systems analysts, utopian thinking (develop image of future), etc. Since man is guided by reason, the change agent only needs to provide expertise, i.e., change lies with experts. Using this strategy, the group of students might hang posters showing statistics that demonstrate the relationship between smoking and a variety of health problems. They might also plan a seminar in which the keynote speaker is a clinical specialist in respiratory nursing. She as an expert could educate the students on the kinds of health problems they might expect to experience if they continue on as smokers. This presentation could be dramatized through the use of case studies and slides. While these two techniques might encourage change, used alone they would produce little or no change.

Normative-Reeducative

This strategy works on the assumption that human beings are guided by internal meanings and are committed to the norms of the culture in which they reside. Specific techniques utilized in this category are improving problem solving capacity of the system, promoting growth in persons, encouraging peer pressure, and using group process. Using this strategy, the students might organize a self-help group aimed at helping fellow students to quit smoking. While this technique might strengthen the students' change program, they may also need the support of the power structure.

Power-Coercive

This strategy works on the assumption that knowledgeable people are in political and economic power. These people will exert change through legitimate law-making activities. Specific techniques utilized in this category include using nonviolent techniques, using political institutions (law-making bodies), and changing or manipulating the power elites. Using this strategy the students might petition the administration for the establishment of a no-smoking area or lounge.

Using these strategies requires a variety of skills. These skills include the establishment of professional relationships, the ability to communicate effectively, the ability to negotiate, coordinate, and collaborate, and a knowledge of the system. As one can see these are not skills which are developed easily or quickly. It takes much time and practice at becoming a skilled change agent. To develop these skills one needs both a knowledge base and an opportunity to practice.

SUMMARY

While change has existed from the beginning of time, research that describes and analyzes the change phenomenon is relatively new. This chapter defined change and classified types of change. Three change models were introduced. Guides for assessing need for change and change reactions were discussed. Principles that can be used in planning for change were identified, and several change strategies presented.

The nurse experiences change from two perspectives—as the initiator of change and as a system experiencing change. Since change is a constant, the nurse must learn to deal effectively with it. Knowledge of change will assist the nurse to better understand and promote effective change.

Some key points to remember as you use change theory in nursing are

1. Change is a constant phenomenon that individuals produce as well as experience.
2. While there are a variety of change models, no model is inherently better in and of itself than any other.
3. Effective change is usually based on a problem-solving approach.
4. Effective change usually involves a variety of different strategies and techniques.
5. Collaborative change has the most potential for helping the nurse function as an effective change agent.

REFERENCES

Asprec, E. "The Process of Change." *Supervisor Nurse* 6 (1975): 15–16, 18–24.

Bennis, W., Benne, K., Chin, R., and Corey, K. *The Planning of Change.* New York: Holt, Rinehart, and Winston, 1976.

Bennis, W., Benne, K., and Chin, R., eds. *The Planning of Change: Readings in the Applied Behavioral Sciences.* New York: Holt, Rinehart, and Winston, 1961.

Bennett, T. *The Leader and the Process of Planned Change.* New York: Association Press, 1962.

Brill, E., and Kilts, D. *Foundations for Nursing.* New York: Appleton-Century-Crofts, 1980.

Brooten, D., Hayman, L., and Naylor, M. *Leadership for Change: A Guide for the Frustrated Nurse.* Philadelphia: J. B. Lippincott Co., 1978.

Capelle, R. *Changing Human Systems.* Toronto: International Human Systems Institute, 1979.

Chin, R. "The Utility of Systems Models and Development Models for Practitioners." In *The Planning of Change: Readings in the Applied Behavioral Sciences*, edited by W. Bennis, K. Benne, and R. Chin. New York: Holt, Rinehart, and Winston, 1961.

Chin, R., and Benne, K. "General Strategies for Effecting Changes in Human Systems." In *The Planning of Change*, edited by W. Bennis, K. Benne, R. Chin, and K. Corey. New York: Holt, Rinehart, and Winston, 1976.

"Change, Conflict, Continuing Education, Competency." *Supervisor Nurse* 10 (1979): 26–27, 30–32, 34.

Clark, C. C., and Shea, C. A. *Management in Nursing, A Vital Link in the Health Care System.* New York: McGraw-Hill Co., 1979.

Copp, L. A. "Inservice Education Copes with Resistance to Change." *Journal of Continuing Education in Nursing* 6 (1975): 19–27.

Havelock, R. G. *The Change Agent's Guide to Innovation in Education.* Englewood Cliffs, NJ: Educational Technology Publications, 1973.

Lancaster, J., and Lancaster, W. *Concepts for Advanced Nursing Practice: The Nurse as a Change Agent.* St. Louis: The C. V. Mosby Co., 1982.

Lewin, K. "Group Decision and Social Change." In *Readings in Social Psychology*, edited by T. M. Newcomb and E. Hartley. New York: Holt, Rinehart, and Winston, 1947.

Lewin, K. "Quasi-Stationary Social Equilibria and the Problem of Permanent Change." In *The Planning of Change*, edited by W. Bennis, K. Benne, R. Chin, and K. Corey. New York: Holt, Rinehart, and Winston, 1976.

Lindquist, J. *Strategies for Change.* Berkeley, CA: Pacific Soundings Press, 1978.

Lippitt, R., Watson, J., and Westley, B. *The Dynamics of Planned Change.* New York: Harcourt, Brace, and World, Inc., 1958.

Mauksch, I. G., and Miller, M. M. *Implementing Change in Nursing.* St. Louis: The C. V. Mosby Co., 1981.

Morris, W., ed. *The American Heritage Dictionary of the English Language.* Boston: American Heritage Publishing Company, and Houghton-Mifflin Co., 1973.

Olson, E. M. "Strategies and Techniques for the Nurse Change Agent." *Nursing Clinics of North America* 14 (1979): 323–336.

Reinkemeyer, A. "Nursing's Needs: Commitment to an Ideology of Change." *Nursing Forum* 9 (4) [1970]: 340–355.

Rodgers, J. A. "Theoretical Considerations Involved in the Process of Change." *Nursing Forum* 12 (2) [1973]: 160–174.

Saunders, L. "Permanence and Change." *American Journal of Nursing* 58 (1958): 969–972.

Schaller, L. E. *The Change Agent.* Nashville, TN: Abingdon Press, 1972.

Spradley, B. W. "Managing Change Creatively." *Journal of Nursing Administration* 10 (5) [1980]: 32–37.

Welch, L. B. "Planned Change in Nursing: The Theory." *Nursing Clinics of North America* 14 (1979): 307–321.

10

Role theory

DEFINITION OF TERMS

Position   Location in a social system.

Role   Acts or behaviors expected of one who occupies a given social position.

Role Enactment   Observable social conduct.

Role Expectations   "... rights and privileges, the duties and obligations, of any occupant of a social position in relation to persons occupying other positions in the social structure" (Sarbin & Allen, 1968, p. 497).

Role Learning   The process involved in locating yourself accurately in the social structure.

Role Socialization   The process of acquiring specific roles.

Role Stress   Felt difficulty the role enacter experiences when trying to meet role obligations.

Role Structure   Way of viewing and examining the components of role.

Role Theory   "... a collection of concepts and ... hypothetical formulations that predict how actors will perform in a given role or under what circumstances certain types of behaviors can be expected" (Hardy & Conway, 1978, p. 17).

Mrs. Smith is a thirty-year-old woman who comes to you because she does not know where to turn. She feels overwhelmed. Mrs. Smith is married, has a twelve-month-old son, maintains the house, works full-time as a professional nurse, and goes to school part-time to obtain a BSN degree. She is basically healthy and prides herself in her organizational ability. She believed everything was under control and she could handle all these demands. After all she chose to be a wife, mother, nurse, and student; her friends can do it and she enjoys being active. Lately she finds herself daydreaming, sleeping and eating more, being irritable, and doing repetitive nonessential tasks.

Where would you begin to help Mrs. Smith in this situation? While knowledge of systems and stress-adaptation theories would provide you with a starting point, knowledge of role theory would provide you with an increased understanding of a particular type of stressor—role.

Roles are an integral part of our lives and are essential when people live together. Roles serve the purpose of dividing tasks which need to be done. In addition to dividing the tasks, roles give guidance for developing relationships and for transmitting knowledge from one generation to the next. Generally little thought is given to the idea of roles until some problem arises with individuals. Role theory then provides a perspective for viewing these existing or potential problems at an organizational, familial, or individual level. Knowledge of role theory assists the nurse to help man function.

At the completion of this chapter the reader will be able to

1. Define role and related terms.
2. Identify the common elements inherent in three role-theory perspectives.
3. Explain the components of role.
4. Describe the process of role socialization.
5. Identify and describe types of role stress.

ROLE DEFINED

Although roles have existed from the beginning of time, the current use of the term *role* had its origin in the 1920s (Biddle & Thomas, 1966). Today there exist many related definitions for "role," reflecting a variety of disciplines and their specific interest in the concept of role. Kramer defined role as ". . . a set of expectations about how a person in a given position in a particular social system should act" (Kramer, 1974, p. 52). Oeser and Harary take a slightly different approach to defining role. Role is defined as " . . . positions within a structural system that includes persons, positions and tasks" (Oeser & Harary, 1962, p. 92). Inherent in these two definitions are three common elements—people, tasks or behaviors, and positions— in social systems. **Roles** then are acts or behaviors expected of one who occupies a given social position.

Role is distinguished from the term *position* by many role theorists; however, many writers use these two terms interchangeably. Many dictionaries use one term to define the other. When the terms *role* and *position* are not used interchangeably, **position** is defined as a location in a social system. Position is the social identity assigned to a person by others in that system. Positions are static in that certain rights and obligations are expected of the person who occupies that position. Sarbin and Allen (1968) define rights, as what is expected of another, and obligations, as behaviors directed toward others. Patients have certain expectations of nurses, for example, competent care, respect, and confidentiality. These examples represent patients' rights. In turn, nurses are obligated to perform competently, respect the patient, and maintain confidentiality. Generally the rights of one person are the obligations of the person in the complementary position.

So far we have defined position. How then is role defined when a distinction is made between role and position? Roles are the acts or behaviors expected of one who holds a particular position. The concept of position is subsumed in the definition of role. These acts or behaviors include both the rights and obligations expected of a person who holds that position. In other words, roles include the specific acts and behaviors of one in a position, while position alone locates that person in the social system.

Positions then are locations in social systems such as staff nurse, public health nurse, doctor, or teacher. Each position has a complementary position: doctor-patient, nurse-patient, teacher-student, mother-child, etc. These positions contain specific rights and obligations. People who occupy these positions collectively share certain common characteristics or behaviors. These specific behaviors with these positions constitute the roles. Therefore, roles like positions have a counterpart termed *counterrole*. Examples of counterroles include leader-follower, researcher-subject, and care-giver-care receiver.

Just as there are many different definitions and uses of the terms role and position, there are many ways they can be classified. One of the simplest ways to classify positions is to consider positions as ascribed and achieved. Ascribed positions are those which the individual has little or no control over. There is no decision making involved. These positions are assigned to you without concern for your abilities or preferences. One example of this type of position is family relationships. Ascribed positions are generally assigned to you at birth. At birth you are assigned an age, sex, and family location, depending on whether you are a son or daughter, youngest or oldest sibling, etc. Although you have little or no choice about these position assignments, the specific behaviors (roles) enacted in these positions generally vary from individual to individual within a range for that position in that system. To further clarify this point, let's use the example of sex. You and your sister are assigned your sex at conception. Both of you are females. Your sister remains at home to take care of her family and home. You go to work as a nurse and hire a babysitter and housekeeper. Both behaviors—going to work and staying home—are considered within the range of acceptable behaviors in today's society for a person occupying the position of female.

Achieved positions are those positions over which you exert some degree of control. You make a decision to participate in these positions. You obtain them through personal effort. Examples of this type of position include occupation, marital status, and social status. Let's use marital status as an example to elaborate on this type of position. You graduate from nursing school and obtain a position as a staff nurse with the public health department. While dating you meet someone with whom you might like to spend the rest of your life. You two decide to be married. You had control over this decision and will now spend time enhancing your marriage.

It is important for the nurse to be alert to this position classification or some other way of classifying positions. The way a position is assigned could have an impact on how one feels about the position and then how one enacts the role. For instance, let's take the ascribed position of gender again. How individuals feel about their sex will influence their relationships with others, their career choices, their outlook on life, and, ultimately, their role enactment.

ROLE THEORY DEFINED

There exist many concepts and hypotheses concerning particular segments of role theory; however, there is as yet no one integrated theory of role. **Role theory** is a "... collection of concepts and ... hypothetical formulations that predict how actors will perform in a given role or under what circumstances certain types of behaviors can be expected" (Hardy & Conway, 1978, p. 17). Generally when one refers to role theory, the basic components are similar but the specific focus is different. There are three main perspectives for studying role theory (Hardy & Conway, 1978; Biddle & Thomas, 1966).

The first approach to studying role theory is that of the structuralist. This approach analyzes roles in terms of their structural elements and function within the system. In this approach the focus is on the system. Structural elements are viewed as the organization of positions in that system. Specific information you would collect using this approach would emphasize the division of labor, role prescriptions, and position identification. An analysis would then be undertaken to determine the function that each position plays in the total system. The focus in this approach is on the system not the individual. Positions and roles exist to serve the system. For example, using this approach the role theorist would look at the organizational chart of a hospital and identify all the positions, job descriptions, and rules and regulations affecting the positions. The role theorist would then determine the function of each position as it relates to the total hospital. Individuals are only considered as a function of the position. Another example of this approach would be analysis of a family. The structure of the family would be identified, i.e., positions, role prescriptions and norms, values, and beliefs affecting role behaviors. Then the function of each position and its relationship to the total working of the family would be analyzed. No attempt would be made to evaluate the effectiveness of each individual in implementing the role.

A second approach to studying role and role theory is that of the social psychologist. In this approach the focus is on the interaction between the individual occupying the positions and the system. Some of the issues of concern in this approach are questions like: How does one learn to enact a role? What role does language play in role development? How do counterroles interrelate? In other words, this approach focuses on concepts such as role, self, language, and role taking. To further explain this approach we will go back to the previous hospital example. The role theorist using the interactional approach would interview and observe the individuals who occupy the positions identified by the structuralist. Data which would be of concern to this theorist would be how the individual perceives the role, how he enacts the role, and how he was socialized into the role.

The last role theory approach is that of the psychiatrist. This perspective focuses on the individual as opposed to the system or the individual within the system (Sullivan, 1953). Key concepts of this approach are the self, communication, and interpersonal behavior. The role theorist utilizing this perspective would collect information about the individual, the communication patterns, and the interpersonal behaviors, as they relate to role implementation. The environment is only considered as it influences the individual and his role implementation. For example, in analyzing the individual in the role of patient, you would collect information about the number of roles the individual occupies, the importance or priority of each role, the interference with other roles, the way he acts out the patient role, his communication patterns with counterroles, and his perceptions about the patient role. You would collect information about hospital structure, role learning positions, etc., but only as it influences this individual's role.

While these three approaches to the study of role theory focus on different aspects of roles, they present many common elements. It is these common elements which will be the concern of the remainder of the chapter.

ROLE STRUCTURE

Role structure refers to the components of role. These components, as were identified in the definition of role, are individuals or persons, acts or behaviors, and positions or status. The following section describes these components.

Persons

There are many terms used to describe the person. Some of these terms are ego, self, actor, and referrent (Biddle & Thomas, 1966). The term one uses to describe the person being studied or the person enacting the role will be determined by the role theory approach taken by the examiner. This approach taken will also determine the extent or focus given the person. Regardless, positions are filled by persons. This means that someone occupies the position. This person has a set of attributes. The structuralist will stop here, as the specific attributes are defined only by the description of the position tasks. The interactionalist will describe the set of attributes as they relate to role enactment, persons perception of role, and the interaction of roles. The psychiatrist will describe the person in terms of personal attribute, i.e., personality as it relates to role enactment.

Acts or Behaviors

Acts or behaviors are generally described in terms of the actions taken by the role enactor. These acts or actions are influenced by norms and sanctions. Acts and behaviors are learned. In many cases these acts and behaviors are goal directed and voluntary. A term frequently used when describing acts and behaviors is *prescription*. Prescriptions refer to what ought to or should be done by persons in a certain position. Prescriptions imply norms and sanctions. Prescriptions may be positive, if they sanction a behavior, or negative, if they forbid it. Prescriptions are associated with home, church, school, leisure, and work. Some examples of prescriptions include: you must not commit adultery, honor thy mother and father, work before play, and honesty above all.

To further elaborate on acts or behaviors let's discuss the care-giver role of a person in the position of staff nurse in an acute care hospital. Specific behaviors required of the staff nurse in the care giver role could include: conducts complete assessment on all patients assigned; plans care, based on data collected and analyzed; implements care, which is individualized; evaluates and revises care; and competently implements all technical skills. These specific behaviors are influenced by peer group, supervisors, and the rewards system of that hospital.

Positions

Positions are socially defined in terms of age, sex, and education. In other words, you may hold specific positions based on your age, sex, or education. Positions generally require specific skills, intelligence, and/or temperament. People occupying specific positions should have the ability to do the tasks required of the person in that position. Positions also imply that people occupying them are identified by titles like nurse, teacher, or doctor. People in those positions are exchangeable but positions are not.

ROLE SOCIALIZATION

Role socialization is the process of acquiring specific roles. Role socialization includes role expectations, role learning, and role enactment. These three components may be viewed in terms of input into the system, throughput processes, and output.

Role Expectations

Role expectations are what you expect to happen because of "... rights and privileges, the duties and obligations, of any occupant of a social position in relation to persons occupying other positions in the social structure" (Sarbin & Allen, 1968, p. 497). In other words role expectations are those beliefs which are held by others regarding the specific behaviors inherent in specific positions. Regardless of who occupies the position, the obligations are the same. Role expectations help integrate the individual into the system and are communicated by direct instruction, expression of approval or disapproval, and suggestions made by peers and significant others.

Generally role expectations can be viewed via several dimensions (Sarbin & Allen, 1968). The first dimension is whether the expectations are general or specific. General expectations permit more latitude in implementing roles. The expectation that nurses should be kind and gentle is general. Specific ways of meeting that expectation could include vocalizing concern, therapeutic touching, and paying attention to small details of care. A nurse demonstrating any of these behaviors could be considered kind and gentle.

Another dimension of role expectation is the scope or extensiveness of the behavior. Some expectations are extensive in scope, such as those dealing with sex and age. Regardless of your position, certain things will be expected of you if you are female and thirty. These expectations will transcend all of your roles. On the other hand, some expectations are very narrow in scope and apply in only a few positions. The expectation that a nurse will accurately interpret an electrocardiogram applies in very limited positions within the hospital.

The third dimension of role expectations is clarity. Some expectations are very clear, i.e., as a nurse you will perform psychomotor skills competently. Some expectations are not so clear and are generally those with which there is some degree of disagreement. An example of this is the expectation that as a nurse you are responsible to the institution which employs you. The question then becomes, Who is your first line of responsibility—the institution, the doctor, or the patient?

The last dimension related to role expectations is the degree of formality. Degree of formality varies from informal to formal. Some expectations are formal; these are many times written and communicated in the form of codes of ethics, behavioral objectives, and descriptions of norms. Informal expectations are those which are usually not written and are communicated indirectly, many times, after the fact. For example, a patient is expected to wear pajamas when he is admitted to the hospital; however, in most cases this expectation does not appear in writing. If a nurse sees a patient in regular clothes, he is told to put on his pajamas.

Role Learning

Role learning is the process involved in locating yourself accurately in the social structure. It is generally agreed that role learning begins in infancy and young childhood. This role learning prepares the child to assume adult positions. It continues as the person moves through the life cycle (Hardy & Conway, 1978).

Role learning requires development of some basic skills. These basic skills are language, role taking ability, development of self, interpersonal competence, motivation, and moral values (Hardy & Conway, 1978). These skills, regardless of age or role, require learning. Language skills are basic for the facilitating of the other skills necessary for role learning. Without language the role learner would be unable to develop the additional skills needed to learn roles, i.e., to socialize.

Role taking is the ability of the role learner to act out his perception of how he and others would behave in that position. The role learner anticipates the response of others in that position. Role taking ability is influenced by the individual's social experience, timing of social experiences, and attention to that experience (Hardy & Conway, 1978). When you see children "playing house" what you are witnessing are children learning role taking—the ability to behave as mother and father. Providing role learners the opportunity to practice role taking is important in facilitating the role-learning process. This applies to all age levels and is an important point to keep in mind as you work with people who are learning new roles. For example, many clients have had little or no opportunity to learn the role of patient before they become patients. Some health professionals are now providing some limited opportunities for selected types of patients to try on their roles before elective or preplanned hospitalizations. Some of the more common examples occur in pediatrics where children are given the opportunity to act out their future surgery as well as in maternity settings where opportunity is provided to simulate the labor and delivery experience.

Development of self involves identifying who you are. This is done by interacting with others and through play activities. Important in this skill is the ability to define self and to internalize attitudes of significant others.

Interpersonal competence, motivation, and moral values all relate to the ability to interact with others effectively. It helps the role learner to decide what behaviors to present in which situations and to develop the behaviors acceptable to the significant others. In other words, the role learner internalizes the attitudes, beliefs, and morals of the significant others in the social system.

Although role learning involves play, coaching of some form, and observations of others in those roles, there are some differences in role learning between children and adults. Hardy and Conway (1978) have identified these differences as (1) the influence of previous experiences on the ability to role learn, (2) differences in specific information that needs to be learned, and (3) differences in relationships between adults and among children and adults or other children.

Role Enactment

Role enactment focuses attention to overt or observable social conduct. It refers to what we do. Sarbin and Allen (1968) have identified three components inherent in understanding role enactment. These components consist of the number of positions you hold, the intensity or involvement in these positions, and the preemptiveness of the positions.

The number of positions any person holds at any point in time will influence his role enactment. No person occupies only one position; each person occupies multiple positions. Sometimes it is these multiple positions which cause conflict and difficulty in role enactment. Note, for example, Mrs. Smith at the beginning of this chapter.

As a wife, mother, student, and professional, she may have difficulty due to amount of time needed to effectively implement each position. A person may also get caught between conflicting role expectations. For example, as a professional you are expected to commit yourself to lifelong learning, which requires time outside your normal working hours. At this same time you are to be available to your children when they need you.

Another component to role enactment is intensity of involvement. Intensity of involvement is the degree of effort exerted in enacting a role. The effort can range from noninvolvement such as being a card-carrying member of an organization, to total engrossing involvement such as being president of an active organization which requires extensive time, thought, and energy. Some roles require intense involvement while others require less involvement. The difficulty arises when a person becomes involved in many roles, all of which require intense enactment.

The last component to role enactment is preemptiveness. Preemptiveness is the amount of time a person spends in one role relative to the other roles the person occupies. Generally this component is applicable only to achieved positions. A person occupies ascribed positions most of the time, i.e., normally you are a male or female all your life. Some roles a person occupies may require a large amount of time. Difficulty arises when the person occupies multiple roles, all of which require a large amount of time.

Role socialization therefore involves role expectations, role learning, and role enactment. Role expectations may be viewed as input into the system, role learning as throughput in the system, and role enactment as output (see Figure 10-1).

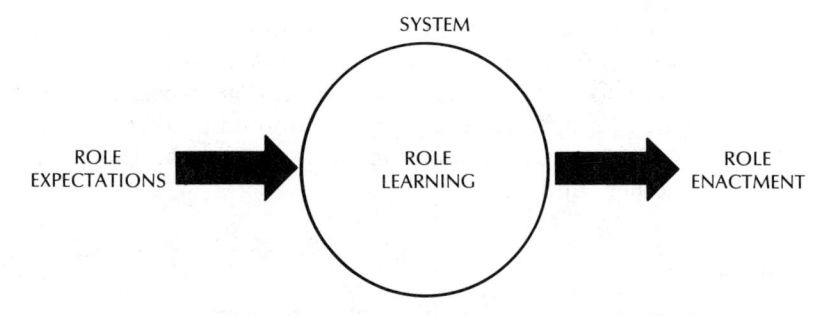

Figure 10-1 Role Socialization.

ROLE STRESS

Role stress is the felt difficulty the role enacter experiences when trying to meet role obligations. The greater the distance between role enactment and role expectations, the greater the role stress. A term frequently used interchangeably with role stress is *role dissonance*. Several types of role stress will be presented. These types are role conflict, role shock, and role ambiguity.

Role Conflict

Role conflict is a type of role stress which arises when role demands or expectations are difficult or impossible to meet. These expectations or demands are usually contradictory or mutually exclusive. For instance, as a staff nurse you are expected to conform to hospital policies and procedures; however, a specific physician demands behaviors contradictory to a policy, and at the same time you as the patient advocate are expected to protect the rights of the patient, which would be violated by following either the hospital expectation or the physician expectation. In another example, you as a nursing student are expected to use a conceptual approach to learning. This takes time and theory classes. At the same time your own expectation is that you want to learn specific procedures. You are in temporary conflict in being a nursing student in a specific program. La Rocco (1978) has identified four types of role conflict. These are intersender role conflict, intrasender role conflict, interrole conflict, and person-role conflict.

Intersender role conflict involves conflicting expectations from two or more people. For example, you as a nursing student are expected by your teacher to complete a total assessment for each assigned client as well as provide individualized care. You decide your patient would rather not be awakened for breakfast but would prefer a small snack about 10:00 AM. There seems to be no real reason for waking the patient at 8:00 AM. The expectation of the staff nurses on the unit, on the other hand, is that all patients will be awakened at 7:30 AM, have their faces and hands washed, temperature taken, and be ready for breakfast at 8:00 AM. You are now in conflict because you cannot meet the expectations of both your teacher and the staff nurse.

Intrasender role conflict involves conflicting expectations sent by the same person. The typical example illustrating this type of conflict is the supervisor inquiring why all beds, baths, and treatments aren't done by 11:00 AM and then turning around and questioning you about the incomplete care plans. Most nurses respond to this type of message with frustration and anger. How can I do both at the same time?

Interrole conflict involves role expectation from multiple roles occupied by the same role enactor which are incompatible. All of us occupy simultaneous multiple roles. Sometimes these roles have conflicting expectations. A person who is a nursing student will have specific role expectations communicated by others. At the same time you are also a volunteer paramedic for the local ambulance service. You come across an emergency situation during your clinical nursing experience. You have not yet been taught emergency procedures in your nursing program. You will probably experience some role conflict at that moment—are you a nursing student or a paramedic?

The fourth type of role conflict is the person-role type. This involves internalized values you learned and external values communicated to you by others. This is probably one of the most frequent types of role conflict experienced by new graduates. You were taught in nursing school and internalized the values of individualized care planned to meet the needs of individualized patients, yet when you are employed the institution communicates a value of bureaucratic rules and regulations over individualized care.

Role Shock

Role shock is "... the stress accompanying either major discrepancies between anticipated and encountered roles or the sudden and significant departure from familiar roles which are 'played differently' in the new setting..." (Minkler & Biller, 1979, p. 125). Role shock generally results from discrepancies in anticipated and encountered roles and from changes in the level of role ambiguity. For example, you may experience role shock as a new graduate. As a student you were dependent on your teacher and staff nurses. If you had questions and/or decisions to make you may have consulted them. You were taught how to be a competent, "good" nurse—the ideal. You were told what a nurse does. When you graduated you took a job in the local health clinic. You are the only nurse employed there. The working conditions are less than ideal. The manager of the clinic expects you to manage the appointment book and "run" the desk. In this setting you may experience role shock.

Role Ambiguity

Role ambiguity is a type of role stress which results from lack of clear role expectations. Your expectations are either ill defined or unclear. You become unsure as to what is expected of you. Role ambiguity is when the organization or environmental expectations are not clear. Subjective ambiguity is when the role enacter feels the expectations are unclear when indeed they are clear.

La Rocco (1978) has identified three sources of role ambiguity. These are the size and complexity of the organization, the rapid rate of change, and the restricted channels of communication. While these sources are institutionally oriented, they still apply to human systems. A family member may experience role ambiguity as a result of rapidly changing societal morals and values, restricted or nonexisting communication lines in the family, and the complexity of the community the family lives in.

Though the examples discussed in this section relate mainly to the nurse, role theory can also be applied to clients. For example, recall Mrs. Smith in the opening situation. Mrs. Smith presents us with symptoms of stress. From the data in this situation we suspect the stress is related to her many roles. To pursue this situation further, additional data need to be collected. Some of that data include how Mrs. Smith perceives her current roles, what were her expectations related to these roles, how have these expectations changed, and what are her beliefs regarding how others perceive these roles. To obtain this information, first have Mrs. Smith describe herself as mother, wife, nurse, and student. Next, have her relate how her enactment of these roles differs from her previous and current expectations. Finally, have her describe her beliefs about what others expect from her. Once this information is obtained, the following questions will facilitate the analysis of these data. As Mrs. Smith described these roles, how clear and specific was she? Did she exhibit role ambiguity? Did she relate any conflict between roles? For example, did she relate any problems with scheduling classes, work, and babysitters? How realistic are her expectations for each of these roles? How much adjustment has she made between what she anticipated and what she encountered in these roles? Does conflict exist between her own expectations and what she perceives as the expectations of others? As you can see, role theory can be used as a basis for assessment and can assist you in arriving at a nursing diagnosis and planning individual client care.

SUMMARY

As long as there are two people interacting, there will be roles. Roles serve the purpose of dividing the tasks which need to be done as people live together. This chapter defined role, position, and role theory. Three major approaches to studying role theory were presented. Role structure was then discussed in terms of persons, acts, or behaviors and positions. Role expectations, role learning, and role enactment were presented as components of a process called role socialization. The last section presented types of role stress.

Key points to remember about role theory are

1. For each role a counter-role exists.
2. There is no one theory of role.
3. Definition of role is determined by the perspective of the definer.
4. The obtainment of a new role requires learning.
5. Conflict develops when there is a difference between role expectation and role enactment.

REFERENCES

Baker, V. "Retrospective Explorations in Role Development." *Nursing Digest* 6 (1979): 56–63.

Banton, M. *Roles: An Introduction to the Study of Social Relations.* New York: Basic Books, Inc., 1965.

Benne, K., and Bennis, W. "The Role of the Professional Nurse." *American Journal of Nursing* 59 (1959): 196–198.

Biddle, B. J., and Thomas, E. J. *Role Theory: Concepts and Research.* New York: John Wiley and Sons, 1966.

Brief, A., Sell, M. V., Aldag, R., and Melone, N. "Anticipatory Socialization and Role Stress among Registered Nurses." *Journal of Health and Social Behavior* 20 (2) [1979]: 161–165.

Goode, W. "A Theory of Role Strain." *American Sociological Review* 25 (1960): 483–496.

Hardy, M., and Conway, M. *Role Theory Perspectives for Health Professionals.* New York: Appleton-Century-Crofts, 1978.

Heiss, J. *Family Roles and Interaction: An Anthology.* Chicago: Rand McNally College Publishing Co., 1976.

Kramer, M. *Reality Shock.* St. Louis: The C. V. Mosby Co., 1974.

La Rocco, S. "An Introduction to Role Theory for Nurses." *Supervisor Nurse* 9 (12) [1978]: 41–45.

Lindgren, H. C., ed. *Contemporary Research in Social Psychology: A Book of Readings.* New York: John Wiley and Sons, 1969.

Miller, G. A., and Wagner, L. W. "Adult Socialization, Organizational Structure and Role Orientations." *Administrative Science Quarterly* 16 (1971): 151–163.

Minkler, M., and Biller, R. "Role Shock: A Tool for Conceptualizing Stresses Accompanying Disruptive Role Transitions." *Human Relations* 32 (1979): 125–140.

Oeser, O. A., and Harary, F. "A Mathematical Model for Structural Role Theory, I." *Human Relations* 15 (1962): 89–109.

Sarbin, T. R., and Allen, V. L. "Role Theory." In *The Handbook of Social Psychology*, edited by G. Lindzey and E. Aronson. Reading, MA: Addison-Wesley Co., 1968.

Sullivan, H. S. *The Interpersonal Theory of Psychiatry.* Edited by H. Perry and M. Garvel. New York: W. W. Norton, 1953.

Smith, H. J., and Schuster, C. S. "Changing Roles in Western Society." In *The Process of Human Development: A Holistic Approach.* Edited by C. Schuster and L. Ashburn. Boston: Little, Brown and Company, 1980.

UNIT III

SELECTED CONCEPTS UTILIZED IN NURSING

This unit focuses on concepts used in nursing. What is a concept? For example, when someone uses the term *nurse* do you have an idea of what they mean? In other words, do you have an idea of what the term *nurse* stands for? A concept is a package of organized ideas about a set of things that have something in common. The concept of nurse, for example, stands for persons who function in various positions within the health care system. The medical-surgical nurse, the public health nurse, the nurse practitioner, the nurse researcher, and the nurse educator are all nurses.

Each of these individuals is a nurse because she shares a set of common characteristics or attributes. Each is a person who communicates, assesses, plans, gives nursing care, educates, evaluates the nursing care, demonstrates care and concern for clients, and assumes responsibility and accountability for actions taken.

Concepts exist on levels. We have high-level concepts and we have low-level concepts, also known as subconcepts. As a child you learned the concept of chair. A chair was something a person could sit on. At first you had to learn the attributes or identifying properties of this concept. Many children do this by asking if each object they see is a chair. They then group the attributes which identify the concept chair. In the case of the chair, it was the properties of back, seat, and legs. You learned that such things as color, arms, stationary or moving, and hard or soft had no bearing on whether it was a chair. These additional dimensions helped you learn the different types of chairs—rocking chair, high chair, lounge chair, easy chair, etc. You also learned that "chair" belonged to a high-level concept called furniture.

The important point to remember is that concepts must be defined in a clear and concise manner. They must also be defined so as to make them usable, observable, and testable.

In the profession of nursing, there are three high-level priority concepts. These concepts are man, health, and nursing. The concept of nursing is presented in the first unit of this book. This unit deals with the concepts man, health, and the health care system. Chapter 11 presents the concept of man. Man as an individual, family, or community is an open system interacting with his environment. Chapter 12 presents the concept of health. Health is the state of being of man as he exists in his environment.

Chapter 13 presents the health care system. The health care system is that societal institution that has evolved for the purpose of helping man meet his health care needs. These concepts taken together provide a basis for nursing to assist man in achieving his health care needs. Chapter 14 looks at the future of nursing by identifying influencing factors that are affecting the evolution of the profession.

REFERENCES

DeYoung, L. *Dynamics of Nursing.* St. Louis: The C. V. Mosby Co., 1981.

Jacox, A. "Theory Construction in Nursing." *Nursing Research* 23 (1974): 4–13.

Mitchell, P., and Loustau, A. *Concepts Basic to Nursing.* New York: McGraw-Hill Co., 1981.

11

Man as a system

Nursing is a service profession that assists man to obtain, maintain, and/or restore his maximal level of health. As impressive as this statement is, it means nothing unless the concepts of man, health, and nursing can be operationalized. In other words, unless the nurse can use these concepts in the actual practice of nursing, the statement has no value. The purpose of this chapter is to provide the framework for operationalizing the concept of man. At the completion of this chapter the reader will be able to

1. Define and describe man as an open system.
2. State the structure, function, and purpose of man.
3. Explain how man as an open system changes over time.

MAN DEFINED

In common usage, the term *man* usually refers to a male adult or to an individual—either male or female. In this text the term *man* is used as a concept composed of three subconcepts. Man is viewed as an individual, as a family, or as a community. Each of these three subconcepts (individual, family, and community) is an open system. Following the characteristics of open systems, these subconcepts each exist as a suprasystem, system, or subsystem, depending on the system level of study or focus. In other words, an individual is a unified whole consisting of a set of interrelated units within a boundary. In turn, the individual may be a unit or subsystem within the family. Like the individual, the family is a unified whole equal to more than the sum of its parts. This same approach can be applied to the community. The community is a unified whole consisting of subsystems, including families and individuals.

Because the concept man encompasses individual, family, and community, a definition of man is incomplete without a definition of the terms *individual, family,* and *community.* An individual is a single human being without reference to age, sex, or any other attribute. Although this may appear to be a simple, straight-forward definition, application of this definition, as is the case with all open systems, can be confusing. For example, the issue of abortion centers around the question When is a fetus a human being? At what point does an individual begin to exist? At the other end of the continuum is the issue of brain death. At what point does an individual no longer exist?

These questions can also be involved in a much more rare situation, Siamese twins. In some cases Siamese twins do not have the vital units or subsystems of two complete individuals. In such cases, are the Siamese twins two individuals or are they one, with excessive subsystems or body parts?

The point of this discussion is that what is a system depends on how the system has been defined. As a professional nurse working with colleagues and with clients, you will need to deal with the fact that everyone does not define a system, in this case an individual, in the same way. These multidefinitions can be a basic source of conflict.

The problems inherent in defining an individual are even more complex when defining a family. The term *family* usually refers to two or more individuals related by birth, marriage, or adoption. However, many people see themselves as members of families when marriage, birth, or adoptions are not the bases of their relationships. Some common examples of this are foster children and communal groups. Since we as nurses interact with the family as a unified whole, a working definition becomes imperative. In order to set the stage for such a definition, let's view three situations where a family relationship may or may not exist.

The Johnsons. When Mary Lou was growing up, her favorite aunt was her Aunt Sally. Aunt Sally wasn't a "real" aunt, but was her mother's best friend. As the years passed, Mary Lou married and had children. Aunt Sally, on the other hand, lost her only "real" family member, her husband. Mary Lou remained very close to her Aunt Sally and as the years went by, Aunt Sally became increasingly dependent on Mary Lou and her family. They helped Aunt Sally with her yard work, shopping, and doctor appointments, among other things.

When Aunt Sally was admitted to the hospital, Mary Lou tried to visit almost every day. When she was discharged, Mary Lou received no information from the hospital or the doctor. Since Aunt Sally was discharged on a special diet and several new pills, Mary Lou called the Visiting Nurse Association and asked for help. Does Mary Lou have the same rights to nursing help, including confidential and personal data which a daughter may have?

The Browns. Tom and Betty met in the seventh grade when they were both 12 years old. From the time they first met, their parents described them as inseparable. At times both sets of parents had tried to encourage Tom and Betty to date others or at least develop other interests, but neither set of parents was ever successful. By the time Tom and Betty started their junior year in high school, Betty's parents were very concerned. They were very much afraid an early marriage and/or pregnancy would prevent Betty, who was an outstanding student, from attending college. In response to their fears, they demanded that Betty not see Tom for at least six months.

After one month with this restriction, Betty and Tom decided to marry secretly. They altered their birth records and were married in a town about fifty miles from their homes. If you were the school nurse in the high school, would you consider Tom and Betty a family unit?

The Smiths. Jane and Ed dated during their junior and senior year of high school. Within a year after graduating, they were married. Within the next four years, Jane and Ed became the parents of three healthy boys. While the children were not planned, they were not unwanted. After the children were born, Jane and Ed decided it would be best for the family if Ed obtained a college education. During the next few years of their marriage, there was never enough money or time. Ed was constantly studying while Jane was always busy with housework and children.

The end of this time period marked a turning point for both Ed and Jane. The children were now in school and Ed had a very good job, but Ed and Jane had been growing in different directions. Attempts to rebuild their relationship were not successful. Although there was a certain acceptance, they were also both hurt and angered by their divorce.

In the next year, Ed began to share a home with Carol. Carol was a successful business woman whom Ed had first met in college. Ed continued to provide support for Jane and their children during this time. As the years passed, Ed and Carol purchased a home together and listed each other as first beneficiary in life insurance. However, they never married. After Ed and Carol lived together for several years, Ed was in a car accident and admitted to the Intensive Care Unit in a coma. As is common in intensive care units, only the immediate family may visit. If you were the nurse in the intensive care unit, whom would you identify as the immediate family?

In each of these situations a relationship clearly exists, but is this a family relationship? In deciding if these are family relationships, two factors are of prime importance. First, do the individuals involved in the relationship define themselves as family? If they do not, the nurse will find use of family theory of limited value. In other words if the nurse views these people as a unified whole, when they view themselves as individuals, the nurse will not have the basis for effective communication.

However, this is not enough to establish the existence of a family. The nurse relates to the family, not in a vacuum, but within a community; therefore, the second factor in deciding if a family does in fact exist is the community's definition of family. If the nurse fails to identify and work realistically within the community's definition of family, she will find some of her decisions ineffective. For example, in the last situation with Ed, Jane, and Carol, who would be the appropriate person to give legal permission for treatment? Or in the first situation, is giving medical information to Mary Lou about Aunt Sally different from giving the same information to any other family friend?

Earlier in this chapter we said we were setting the stage for a working definition of family. The stage is now set for a definition of family as it is used in this text. A family is two or more individuals who share a relationship identified as a family relationship by the individuals and by the community in which these individuals exist.

Now that family has been defined, community is the final subconcept within the concept of man that needs to be defined. The existence of a community, like the existence of family, is based on human relationships. The relationship for a community is usually based on a common goal and/or geographic location. This relationship is recognized and accepted as a community relationship by the people within the community and by the larger society in which that community exists. Without the recognition from both within the community and from the society, a community will not be sustained.

These ideas can be seen more clearly by looking at some examples of communities. The American Nurses' Association is a professional community. This community is composed of nurses who share common goals. If nurses in the society do not recognize this organization as their professional community, they will not be involved in the organization. Without this recognition and consequently support, the organization will cease to exist. However, if nurses and only nurses recognize this organization, the organization will not be able to meet its goals. If it is not recognized by the society, it cannot function and will cease to exist.

Many communities with which nurses interact are based on geographic location. People within these locations establish both formal and informal communication ties. These ties, in turn, establish the institutions which support the relationships of the community. For example, schools, governments, and businesses are formed. They support the relationship and meet the needs of the community. As these institutions develop, the community becomes based on the shared goals of the community, not just geographic location.

Though the existence of a community requires recognition from both within the community and from the larger society, recognition should not be confused with acceptance. Within the American society there are communities in which the relationship is based on the use of illegal drugs. These communities usually do not receive full acceptance from the larger society but their existence is recognized.

At this point in the chapter, the concept of man has been defined as an individual, a family, and a community. Utilization of this concept in the practice of nursing requires more than a definition. The remainder of this chapter will analyze man as an open system. The framework for this analysis is based on the characteristics of an open system as they are demonstrated in the purpose, structure, function, and change of open systems.

THE STRUCTURE OF MAN AS AN OPEN SYSTEM

In all systems, structure is the arrangement of the parts within the system. Man, be he an individual, a family, or a community, is composed of subsystems. The arrangement of these subsystems into a unique unified whole is the structure of man. Therefore, an analysis of the structure of man involves a systematic identification of the subsystems and their arrangement.

With man the subsystems exist in three overlapping interwoven dimensions. The dimensions are termed the physiological, the psychological, and the sociocultural dimensions. One way of conceptualizing this idea is demonstrated in Figure 11-1. A more concrete example of this same idea is demonstrated by your hand. Look at your hand. It is clearly a physical part or subsystem of you. Now close your eyes and picture your hand in your "mind's eye." The picture in your mind's eye is a part of your body image and, in turn, a part of your psychological dimension. Now look at your hand again. Is it smooth with manicured nails or do you see the signs of hard labor? Is this not

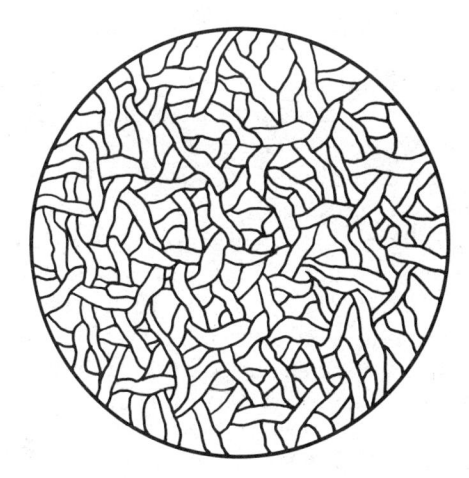

Figure 11-1 Man's Subsystems.

information about your sociocultural dimension? What this example demonstrates is that in the analysis of man, one must always remember that man is a unique whole composed of overlapping interwoven dimensions. The pattern produced by the interwoven dimensions produces the uniqueness as well as the common characteristics of each individual, family, and community. Using the structural characteristics of a system, the nurse can identify both the uniqueness and the common characteristics. These structural characteristics are the presence of attributes, a hierarchical arrangement, a boundary, and an environment.

Attributes

As a nurse, you will be collecting data as a basis for your decisions. In order to collect data about the structure of man, the attributes of the various dimensions provide a framework for a systematic format. This type of format uses the common features of man in identifying the uniqueness of each individual system. This idea will become clearer when it is applied, for example, to an individual. We have identified that all individuals have a physical, psychological, and sociocultural dimension. The physical dimension is composed of the body systems. Data collection about the individual's physical dimension reviews and examines each of these systems. This data collection about each system is commonly called a history and physical. The psychological dimension of man includes the cognitive and affective subsystems. Characteristics such as knowledge, IQ, memory, or problem-solving ability are more cognitive in nature; characteristics such as self-concept, personality, and emotional tone are more affective in nature. The sociocultural dimension of man identifies man as a social being relating to others in the environment. It includes such characteristics as income, religion, ethnic group, level of education, occupation, and roles in one's life style. What we have identified in this example are the common features of the individuals. These are the areas about which structural data is collected. The specific information collected will describe the uniqueness of each individual.

The collection of data in the practice of nursing is done as part of the first step of the nursing process. This first step is referred to as assessment. Therefore, forms utilized by nurses for data collection are usually referred to as assessment forms. As a nurse, you will see and use a variety of assessment forms. These forms will vary in both organization and in the specific content requested; however, aspects of each of man's dimensions will be reflected in the forms. When utilizing these forms for data collection, it is important to be cognizant of the fact that, of necessity, the forms separate data which exist in a unified whole. While we are at this point discussing structure, assessment forms also deal with the function and purpose of man.

As we have said, the assessment form itself identifies factors that man has in common with all others. The data that are collected by the nurse identifies the uniqueness of each individual system. These are the attributes of the system. Table 11-1 identifies examples of commonalities that are found on many assessment forms for man as individual, family, and community. As you review the examples in Table 11-1, note the overlap. This is because we are dealing with open systems which exist in a hierarchical arrangement.

Hierarchical Arrangement

The second structural characteristic of man is his hierarchical arrangement (see Figure 11-2). The complexity of each hierarchical arrangement is mainly a function of size. For example, a one-cell organism has a simpler arrangement than a human being. An individual nurse in private practice is a less complex arrangement than the nursing service in a hospital. As systems increase in size and in turn complexity, the parts of the system differentiate and specialize. Note the degree of differentiation and specialization we see in the human being as opposed to that in a one-cell organism.

Now apply this same idea to the family. In a family of two people, all functions are performed by these two. If, on the other hand, these two people have ten children, a significantly different family structure develops. Usually certain responsibilities and tasks are delegated to the children. This sets up a pattern of differentiation and specialization within the family. It is this concept you are dealing with when you as a nurse note the position of each individual in the family. You are in fact looking at the specific hierarchical arrangement within that family.

This same idea, hierarchical arrangement, may also be applied to the community system. Consider, for example, nursing service arrangements appropriate in small community hospitals as opposed to those in large medical

TABLE 11-1
Classification of attributes into the three dimensions

Dimensions	Individual	Man as a Family	Community
Physiological	Body systems	Number of family members	Organizations and agencies
		Physical characteristics including genetic characteristics	Physical setting
Psychological	Cognitive structure	Position and roles	Formal and informal power structure
	Personality	Value systems	Communication structure between various agencies
	Emotional tone	Power structure	
Sociocultural	Ethnic group	Family religion	Cultural and ethnic groups
	Religion	Ethnic group	Religious groups
	Education	Role in the community	Government groups

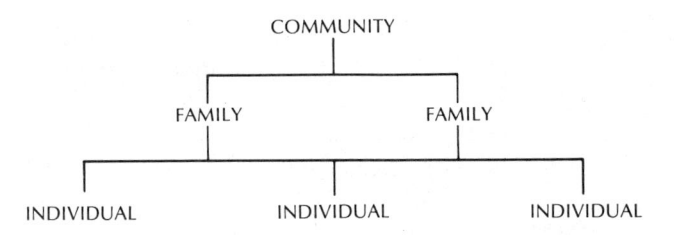

```
         COMMUNITY
        ┌────┴────┐
      FAMILY    FAMILY
     ┌──┴──┐      │
INDIVIDUAL INDIVIDUAL INDIVIDUAL
```

Figure 11-2 Man's Hierarchical Arrangement.

centers. In a small community hospital, the nurse may provide nursing care for a wide range of patients and report to one supervisor who reports directly to the director of nursing. In a large medical center, nursing care is increasingly specialized and the organization more complex, with possibly three or four levels of administration. The degree of differentiation and specialization offered in various nursing positions is a factor you should consider carefully in your initial job search.

Because open systems are arranged hierarchically with differentiation and specialization, loss or injury to any part, as well as the addition of any new part, requires a readjustment in the functioning of the whole system. If one parent in our family of twelve becomes ill and dies, a major readjustment needs to occur within the family. This adjustment is different from what it would be if the youngest child in this family dies. On the other hand, if an aging grandparent or a new baby moves in, adjustments are also necessary. How man as a system compensates for losses or adjusts for additions depends on how vital the part lost is and on the resources within the system boundaries and its environment.

Boundaries

So far in this discussion of man's structure, we have considered the parts of man and how these parts are arranged. The subsystems or units of man are arranged hierarchically within a boundary. As in all systems, this boundary is not easily identified. If you review the material related to a definition of man you will note that much of the difficulty in defining man is related to defining the boundary. Where does a community, family, or individual begin and end? It is very closely related to how we define these subconcepts. If we say that nursing is to assist man to obtain, maintain, or regain his maximal level of health, then we must clearly identify what is within the system's boundaries and what is the environment with which man interacts.

Environment

The last structural characteristic of man deals with the fact that man exists within an environment. In the study of man two types of environments are identified: the extrapersonal and the intrapersonal. Of these, the one you are most familiar with is the extrapersonal. This environment is composed of everything that exists outside the boundary of the system. For example, it is everything that exists outside your own person. The extrapersonal environment is usually identified as the suprasystem in which the target system exists. Consider, for example, a weight-control group as a community with a common purpose. Its suprasystem would be the neighborhood(s) from which its members came. This weight-control community might publish successes of its members in a local weekly newspaper, part of the suprasystem.

Although this is the environment you are more familiar with, many times in nursing we fail because we do not work with the influence of this environment. Over the years, as you use nursing assessment forms, pay attention to the amount of data asked for about the external environment. Many of these forms focus almost exclusively on the intrapersonal environment. The intrapersonal environment consists of everything which exists within the boundary. This is the environment which exists within the individual, within the family, or within the community. It is this environment on which many of your nursing courses focus.

THE FUNCTION OF MAN AS AN OPEN SYSTEM

A discussion of functioning focuses on how man operates; how he goes about the tasks of living. Three issues will be investigated in order to discuss the functioning aspect of man. First, one must differentiate between the functioning of man and the purpose of man. Second, one must identify how man utilizes energy in the process of functioning, and, third, one must identify what the functions of man are.

Purpose Versus Function

The title of this subsection could very well have been "means versus the end," as in does the means justify the end. Purpose refers to why a system exists. For what reason does it exist? Function refers to how it achieves this purpose. What tasks are involved in achieving the purpose? Let's take your school of nursing as an example.

Your school exists in order to prepare professional nurses. In fact, if you look at your school bulletin you will find this in the statement of purpose. How it achieves this purpose is the functioning of the school. In other words, all of the classes, the tests, the clinical experiences are means to the end. They are the way that the school goes about achieving its purpose.

This example with your school may leave you with the impression that it is easy to separate purpose from function; however, this is not always the case. Purpose interfaces directly with the functions much like the interface between boundary and environment. The same kind of questions about where one ends and the next begins can be asked. At this point we are going to defer these questions until you have investigated how man functions. Once you have considered how man functions, you will be better able to consider why he functions.

Man's Use of Energy

Man, as a multidimensional entity, takes in, utilizes, and puts out matter, energy, and information in order to perform the functions of life. Maintaining man's functions requires energy. Each system allocates its energy resources to meet basic survival needs first. In doing this, the system maintains itself within survival limits. Each system also strives for efficient use of this allocated energy so that the remaining energy can be allocated for nonsurvival needs. Failure to allocate sufficient energy to take care of survival needs results in death. Failure to become efficient in the use of energy results in nonsufficient energy remaining to provide for growth and development, for self-actualization.

Those inputs which man must have for life, especially for life in its fullest sense, have been defined as needs. Maslow is one researcher who focused on identification of these needs. The needs he describes as "basic" or "survival needs" are needs which reflect the physiological dimension. These are oxygen, food, fluids, elimination, rest, activity, shelter, and sex. The needs he described as "secondary or social needs" are needs which reflect the psychological and sociocultural dimensions. These are safety, love, esteem, and self-actualization (Maslow, 1970). Although the secondary needs are not usually defined as basic for life, man functions as an integrated whole. One of the most dramatic examples of this is the infant who will fail to thrive—in fact, die—from lack of love. Though Maslow's findings relate to the individual, families and communities also have needs. For example, families and communities cannot exist if they do not receive recognition from the community or the society. This idea was part of our discussion of definitions earlier in this chapter.

Earlier in this chapter we used the structure of man as a basis for data collection. Once the nurse has collected data, the data will be analyzed to determine actual or potential problems. In many cases, the nurse is identifying what needs are not being met and why. This forms the basis for the nursing diagnosis. For this reason, much of the information you will study during your nursing education reflects the needs of man; as an individual, as a family, and as a community. So far, we have established that man has a set of basic needs that requires a dynamic exchange of energy with the environment. But we have not discussed what functions man actually performs in fulfilling these needs.

Man's Functions

As man goes about the business of living, he is constantly performing a variety of activities. The activities usually involve a variety of the functions as they are classified here; boundary functions and critical processes. In order to assist your learning we will present each function and give several examples. In reading the examples, remember that they can reflect more than just the function being explained.

Boundary Functions. The four boundary functions of all open systems were discussed in Chapter 5, "Systems Theory." In that chapter these functions were explained with several examples given for the individual. However, families and communities also perform all four boundary functions. They also take in, keep out, keep in, and put out, matter, energy, and information. Table 11-2 gives several examples of these functions for man as a family and as a community. As you look at these examples, you should be able to think of several others.

As you review these examples you may not find all of them as behaviors which you accept. Keep in mind they reflect how a family or community might carry out the boundary functions. Other communities or other families might approach these functions in different ways, depending on their beliefs and values. Man, whether we are referring to an individual, a family, or a community, demonstrates these functions.

TABLE 11-2
Examples of boundary functions in a family and in a community

Boundary Function	Family	Community
Taking in	Taking in new family member by marriage, adoption, or birth	Providing special tax breaks for new business
	Acceptance of food from neighbors and friends when there is a death in the family	Accepting a federal grant for a community project
		Accepting new people via immigration
Keeping out	Refusing children permission to date members of a different religion or race	Zoning and building requirements
	Not permitting the neighbors' children to play in the house	Refusing new people with immigration laws
Keeping in	Saving old toys, money	Refusing exit visas
	Requiring a small child to play in his own yard	Tax on materials leaving the country—export tax
Putting out	Family garage sale	Waste disposal
	Turning a difficult child over to the courts	Deportation

Critical Processes. As with the boundary functions, the critical processes were introduced in Chapter 5. To refresh your memory, the three critical processes are integration, adaptation, and decision making. Although these processes are constantly ongoing we will begin here with integration. In order for man to maintain a steady state of dynamic homeostasis, all of the subsystems within each of man's dimensions must constantly be integrated to work together. When the total system fails to work together, fails to function as an integrated whole, conflict occurs. As a result, the system becomes increasingly less effective in achieving its purpose. Take as an example a traditional family where one of the "breadwinners" becomes unemployed. The family can work together to identify new sources of income as well as ways to conserve money or they can pull apart, fighting over how to make the necessary adjustments.

The problem involved with poor integration can also be clearly seen in many public school systems. As various groups with vested interests refuse to work together, the school systems become less and less effective in achieving their purpose—the education of students. The same idea can be applied to conflict within the health care system. For example, do you believe the American Nurses' Association and the American Medical Association are working together to achieve quality patient care?

In the examples given to explain integration, we talked about situations requiring adjustments or adaptation. Man is constantly confronted with the need to adjust. He must adjust to changes both within the internal and within the external environment. Think of this idea with our previous family example. The change in income originates in the external environment, but produces changes within the family. Adjustments then will require adjustment not only in how the family interacts with the external environment but also in how the family interacts among itself.

How man goes about the process of adaptation is discussed in detail in Chapter 6, "Stress Theory." It is important that you realize that when we discuss adaptation under the heading "Man as an Open System," we are not discussing something different from adaptation in "Stress Theory." It is the same process. At times the changes made in the process of adaptation are effective, but in other cases they are ineffective. An adaptive change is effective if it helps man achieve a goal and is ineffective if it does not help man achieve a goal. If our family with the decreased income continues to function in a healthy manner, these adjustments would be considered effective. What is required to achieve effective adaptation is effective decision making.

Decision making occurs when man chooses from a variety of options. This is done on both a conscious and an unconscious level. By this time in your life you have made many conscious decisions, but you have also made many more unconscious decisions. Unconscious decisions add greatly to the efficiency of man. For example, you do not consciously decide to breathe. Families and communities also make unconscious decisions as they function.

The family may eat at the same time every day without consciously planning this. Although these types of decisions add greatly to efficiency, they frequently are patterned and very difficult to change. A family may consciously decide they want to have one night a week where everyone is home for a family night. Since this is a new pattern which changes previous patterns, there will be some adjustments necessary to get this decision implemented. Many times when we work with clients we ask them to make a conscious decision to change from the patterned unconscious decision making. These kinds of changes require increased energy and effort.

In looking over the three critical processes and the four boundary functions, there are three key factors to keep in mind. First, as pointed out earlier, any one activity can reflect a variety of functions. Therefore, the examples for the boundary process could also be used to discuss critical processes. The second factor to remember is that energy is required to function. To function is to work. Many times when we work with clients we are quite aware of how tired we feel, but we must also be cognizant of how tired the client can be. The third factor is that man, as he functions, is in a constant state of change. The change is in both the intrapersonal and extrapersonal environments.

CHANGE AND THE SYSTEM OF MAN

Man as an individual, a family, and a community is—through change—always in the process of becoming. The research and other literature which has investigated this process of change in man is found under the broad heading of growth and development.

Much of this research, especially the earlier research, related to man as an individual and considered the time span from conception until the early adult years. However, since the 1950s the research on change in man as an individual has begun to consider the time from early adulthood through the total life span. Today most nursing programs require courses on the growth and development of man as an individual through his total life span. Within these courses as well as other college courses, you can anticipate learning about changes which occur in each of man's dimensions. For example, you will learn the normal temperature, pulse, respiration, and blood pressure changes throughout the life span as the physiological dimension of man changes. You will also learn about how the personality and cognitive skills grow and develop as man's psychological dimensions mature. One example of these changes is Piaget's theory of learning, which is introduced in this book in Chapter 7, "Learning Theory." As you study changes within the psychological dimension, you will discover the process by which man becomes an increasingly social being. This process develops and expands his sociocultural dimension. The "self-actualizing" individual of Maslow (1970) or the "fully functioning" person of Rogers (1961) is an individual who has moved beyond a focus on self—and is now able to fully reach out to the world around.

If you look back at the last few paragraphs you will note we have discussed the fact that man grows and develops in each of his dimensions. However, it is important to keep in mind that no one dimension develops in isolation. Man functions and changes as a whole being.

Man as a family also goes through a life cycle with several developmental stages. One widely used description of these stages was updated by Duvall in 1977 (Duvall, 1977). In this description eight stages are used. The presence of children is assumed in that the age of the oldest child is used as the guidepost. The family cycle begins with the marriage of two individuals. Growth and development occurs as children are born, grow, and are launched from the home. The final stages describe the family after the children have left through old age.

Communities, like individuals and families, also go through a life cycle. New communities are formed, grow, develop, and then die. As a nurse, you will function in communities at all stages of development. You will discover a variety of differences between new communities, established communities, and old and dying communities.

Therefore, man as an individual, a family, and as a community experiences a constant process of change. To identify the characteristics of this change process in man, we will use the characteristics of change in an open system. These characteristics are dynamic homeostasis, negentropy, entropy, equifinality, and reverberation.

Dynamic Homeostasis

The concept of dynamic homeostasis is usually used in current literature to describe physiological functioning in living organisms. However, man constantly adjusts in each of his dimensions in order to maintain himself within the limits of his steady state. For example, a family which experiences the birth of a first child will adapt in each dimension in order to maintain their steady state. The use of money within the family is an excellent demonstration of this. Money, which affects each dimension of man, will be reallocated with the birth of a child, but the family will try to stay within the limits of the funds available.

Negentropy

The process of dynamic homeostasis requires the use of energy. Man has a finite amount of energy, which is available for use. This energy is used first for maintenance and then for growth. For example, when you take in food you will gain weight only when you have exceeded the amount needed for maintenance. However, if you take in only the amount needed for basic metabolism, there will be no energy for other activities, including the activity of adaptation. In such a situation the system can easily be stressed to the point of death. This then is entropy. If a child fails to gain weight, it is a serious symptom. The child is at high risk for death. All of his energy is being used to maintain the systems with no energy to adjust, grow, and develop.

The tendency of man is to take in more than is needed for maintenance and to use this energy for increasing growth and development. This tendency is well demonstrated in the individual's growth from conception to birth and in the family as it takes in new members. It can also be seen in the growth and development of communities.

Entropy

Man not only has a finite amount of energy which he uses for maintenance and growth, but he also has energy which is bound and not available for use. This is demonstrated in the tendency of individuals, families, and communities to come to an end, to die. However, when an individual dies, not all of his cells die at the same moment. If they did, organ transplants would not be possible. This gradual process of dying can also be seen in families and communities. Subsystems will exist and function after the system has died; they represent the bound energy which is in the system but cannot maintain the system.

Reverberation

As the system uses energy, changes occur throughout the total system. The fourth characteristic of how man changes is reverberation. Because man is a functioning whole equal to more than the sum of his parts, a change in any part of his dimensions will produce change within the total system. This concept is easy to see with major changes. For example, it is not difficult to anticipate reverberation in a family with the loss of a family member as described earlier. However, minor changes also affect the total system. If you have a pimple on your nose you have a small local infection. While the physiological dimension of the system has responded to this infection, this pimple has also affected your psychological and sociocultural dimensions. You feel everyone is looking at your nose and you alter your response to people as you worry about this pimple.

As nurses who try to encourage change in order to improve health, we need to anticipate planned and unplanned results from the change. Reverberation provides a basis for considering the total effects of a planned change. How reverberation will actually occur is affected by equifinality.

Equifinality

Equifinality, the final change characteristic, refers to the fact that man reaches his final state by starting at different points and by different means.

For example, a family can be formed by a marriage which is arranged, by two people who decide to live together, or by a single person who decides to have or adopt a child. In each of these examples, a family starts at different points. The life cycle of each of these families will also differ.

This same characteristic of change is also demonstrated by communities. For example, some communities have formed overnight when gold has been found. Other communities have been carefully planned before anyone moved in. Still other communities have built up over a number of years around a major waterway. In each case the communities began at different starting points and have different life cycles. The characteristics can also be seen in your own life as you move into the role of professional nurse. Some of you started in a baccalaureate program directly out of high school. Others have completed an associate degree or diploma program first. Each of you will move through your program in different ways and in many cases at different rates. Yet each of you will reach that final end point of professional nurse.

As we talk about man reaching a final end point, what we are beginning to talk about is his purpose. What is the reason, the purpose for the structure, the functioning, and the changing of man? Why does man exist?

PURPOSE OF MAN

The fact that man exists for a reason is generally accepted, but the reason itself varies with different beliefs and value systems. In the discussion of function it was established that man will first strive to maintain the intactness of the system; in other words to survive. This goal of maintaining the system is identified by some as the main purpose of man. Following this same line of thinking, growth and development become the second purpose of man. In other words, first man will strive to survive and then to grow. Others would say these are functions; that man grows for a higher purpose. Some argue this purpose is within man; for example, to develop one's self or to become self-actualizing. Others argue the purpose is outside man; for example, to help others or to be with God.

What is important for the nurse to realize is that purpose, whatever the specific purpose, is reflected in the beliefs and values which guide individuals, families, and communities. What we as people believe about the purpose of life will influence the decisions we make as we live our lives. This idea can be more clearly understood by looking at a specific example.

Let us suppose you are assigned to care for a twenty-six-year-old woman who is currently four months pregnant. This woman has a disease which requires treatment with cortisone. The disease is not fatal in itself, but left untreated, may cause permanent lung damage. The drug required for treatment can produce abnormalities in the baby. This client must decide if she wants an abortion and treatment, treatment without an abortion, or no treatment until after the delivery.

In working with this client, both you and the client will be influenced by what you and she believe is the purpose of life. You will not only be influenced by your beliefs about an individual life, you will also be influenced by your beliefs about the family and your beliefs about the health care community in which you function.

Again, we are not talking about the functions of an individual, or a family, or a community, we are talking about purpose, the reason for the functioning. We have already discussed purpose in terms of the individual, but what is the purpose of the family? Friedman in her book, *Family Nursing*, begins her first chapter with a discussion of this very issue (Friedman, 1981). In the hierarchy of man the family unit exists between man as an individual and man as a community. In this position, Friedman identifies the family as having two purposes. First, the family exists to meet the needs of the individual within the family and, second, it exists to meet the needs of the community. In both of these purposes the family exists in order to meet needs. However, since there are a variety of needs, both within and between these purposes, Friedman identifies the basic purpose of the family as "mediation—taking the basic societal expectations and obligations and molding and modifying them to some extent to fit the needs and interests of its individual family members" (Friedman, 1981, p. 3). The family achieves this purpose of mediation through what it does—its functions. See Table 11-3 for a classification of family functions.

As you look at Table 11-3 you can analyze the content in many ways. First of all, the functions overlap because we are dealing with an open system. Functions which meet the sociocultural needs also involve the physiological and psychological needs. A second way you can analyze this information is to go back to the discussion on functions in this chapter and apply those principles to this classification of functions. For example, how do the principles related to boundary functions apply to the classification of provisions for physical necessities? And, finally, one can analyze this classification of functions in terms of purpose. As the family carries out functions in each of these areas, how does the family mediate the needs of the individual members and the needs of the community?

TABLE 11-3
Classification of functions within the family

1. Provisions for physical necessities (food, clothing, shelter, etc.)
2. Provision for psychological needs (stability, love, status, recreation)
3. Provision for sociocultural needs (socialization, education, religious activities)
4. Economic functions
5. Reproductive or procreative functions

As families function in order to meet their purposes, they interface with a variety of communities and, in turn, a variety of community purposes. Take your own situation as an example. You exist within the community of your school, the community of your profession, the community where your family lives, and with a number of other communities. Each of these communities has a different purpose. However, there are common elements which can be found within the purposes of all communities. Communities exist to meet the needs of its individual members and to meet the needs of the society in which they exist. It may be obvious to you at this point that the basic purpose of communities, like families, is to mediate. Or to paraphrase Friedman—taking the basic societal expectations and needs and molding and modifying them to fit with the needs and expectations of the members of the community.

SUMMARY

Within this chapter you have learned that man is composed of three subconcepts—the individual, the family, and the community. Three dimensions make up the structure of these subconcepts—the physiological, the psychological, and the sociocultural. These dimensions overlap and interrelate as the boundary and critical functions are carried out. As man carries out his functions he is constantly evolving and developing to reach his purpose. As a nurse this information is used to assist man to obtain, maintain, and/or restore his maximal level of health.

The key points to remember about man as a system are

1. Man, because he is an open system, demonstrates each of the characteristics of systems.
2. Man, as an individual or group, can be analyzed in terms of his dimensions.
3. Boundary and critical process functions are demonstrated in all of man's activities.
4. General agreement on the purpose of man does not exist. Disagreement on the purpose of man or disagreement between purpose and function can cause conflict.
5. Man is in a constant state of becoming; he is constantly changing.

REFERENCES

Braden, C. J., and Herban, N. L. *Community Health: A Systems Approach.* New York: Appleton-Century-Crofts, 1976.

Carter, E. A., and McGoldrick, M., eds. *The Family Life Cycle: A Framework for Family Therapy.* New York: Gardner Press Inc., 1980.

Clemen, S., Eigsti, D., and McGuire, S. L. *Comprehensive Family and Community Health Nursing.* New York: McGraw-Hill Co., 1981.

Grunebaum, H. V., and Cohler, B. J. *Mothers, Grandmothers, and Daughters.* New York: John Wiley and Sons, 1981.

Dever, G. A. *Community Health Analysis: A Holistic Approach.* Germantown, MD: Aspen Systems Corporation, 1980.

Duvall, E. M. *Marriage and Family Development.* Philadelphia: Lippincott Co., 1977.

Freeman, R. B., and Heinrich, J. *Community Health Nursing Practice.* Philadelphia: W. B. Saunders, 1981.

Friedman, M. M. *Family Nursing: Theory and Assessment.* New York: Appleton-Century-Crofts, 1981.

Fromer, M. J. *Community Health Care and the Nursing Process.* St. Louis: The C. V. Mosby Co., 1983.

Getty, C., and Humphreys, W., eds. *Understanding the Family: Stress and Change in American Family Life.* New York: Appleton-Century-Crofts, 1981.

Hall, J., and Weaver, B. *Distributive Nursing Practice: A Systems Approach to Community Health.* Philadelphia: J. B. Lippincott Co., 1977.

Hanchett, E. S. *Community Health Assessment: A Conceptual Tool Kit.* New York: John Wiley and Sons, 1979.

Howard, J. *Families.* New York: Simon and Schuster, 1978.

Jarvis, L. L. *Community Health Nursing: Keeping the Public Healthy.* Philadelphia: F. A. Davis Co., 1981.

Knofl, K. A., and Grace, H. K. *Families Across the Life Cycle: Studies for Nursing.* Boston: Little, Brown and Co., 1978.

Leahy, K., Cobb, M., and Jones, M. C. *Community Health Nursing.* New York: McGraw-Hill Co., 1982.

Maslow, A. *Motivation and Personality.* New York: Harper and Row, 1970.

Nelson, R. *Concepts Basic to Man, Health, and Nursing.* 1980. (Available from University of Pittsburgh Extended Studies Program, Pittsburgh, PA.)

Reiss, D., and Hoffman, H. A., eds. *The American Family: Dying or Developing.* New York: Plenum Press, 1979.

Rogers, C. R. *On Becoming a Person.* Boston: Houghton-Mifflin Co., 1961.

Tufte, V., and Myerhoff, B., eds. *Changing Images of the Family.* New Haven: Yale University Press, 1979.

12

Health

For the past two days, Betsy and Mary have had colds. Although neither Betsy nor Mary has a fever, both have been coughing and their noses have been congested. Betsy decides she is sick and must rest more than she has been. She calls her employer and says she is ill. She then makes an appointment with her physician. Mary, on the other hand, decides the cold is just a little inconvenience. She is not really sick, at least not sick enough to go to the doctor's or to call in sick. Why? The behaviors of these two individuals are directly influenced by their definitions and beliefs about health.

How do we define health and why is this important to nurses? Nurses in the practice of their profession perform a variety of activities. The ultimate goal of these activities is to promote and maintain health. If nurses are to achieve this goal, then nurses must have a clear understanding of the concept *health* and the impact definitions and beliefs about health have on our clients' health behaviors.

The purpose of this chapter is to sensitize you as a nurse to the dimensions of the concept *health*. Two classical definitions of health will be presented and analyzed. We will look at some ways for measuring and assessing health. Then we will examine factors that influence an individual's definition of health and ultimately his health behaviors. The examination of this concept will conclude with discussing the nurse's role as it relates to health.

At the completion of this chapter, the reader will be able to

1. Define the concept health.
2. List and describe three characteristics of the health continuum.
3. Identify specific examples of how health is measured and assessed.
4. Identify variables which influence health behavior.
5. Relate nursing role to the concept health.

DEFINITIONS

Many individuals and organizations have attempted to define the concept *health*. At first glance this seems like an easy task. After all, health is a universal phenomenon. The term is used every day. How many times have you heard or used the words health, health promotion, health care, health oriented, health care system? How many times have you heard "he looks healthy" or "isn't that a healthy looking baby?" What do we mean when we say this? We all know what health is, don't we? Not until one is asked to define and examine the concept health do the dimensions and complexities emerge.

Many attempts at describing and defining health have been made, yet no universally accepted definition of this phenomenon has emerged. Early definitions and interpretations have set the stage for the variety of current meanings. These early definitions of health reflected a soundness or wholeness of the body (Dolfman, 1973; Keller, 1981). This soundness or wholeness represented not only physiological intactness and efficiency but also included spiritual, moral, and mental soundness. These definitions were often modified by adjectives such as: good, bad, or poor. These early definitions not only influenced current definitions of health, but also influenced some of our current health practices. Health practices are directly related to the religious and cultural interpretations of disease and health. Many people view disease and health as punishment and reward for their behavior. Another common belief is that disease represents the "Lord's" testing of one's faith.

Dictionary definitions of health usually relate health and illness to an individual's ability to function normally in society. Questions arise as to what is normal. Is having a cold in the winter and going to work normal? Is being sick ten days out of the year normal? Is spending time and money on healthful activities normal? As you can see, "normal" varies from society to society. Some dictionary definitions go further and reflect a disease free state or condition.

These types of definitions leave the concepts of health and disease unclarified. Is a diabetic person who is functioning effectively in society and is happy with his life, healthy? If you can go to work but feel down and lack energy, are you ill? Another problem that quickly emerges with these types of definitions is that health is presented as an either/or situation. Either you are healthy or you are ill. There is no in-between.

In 1946, the World Health Organization (WHO) presented one of the most widely quoted and accepted definitions of health. Health is "a state of complete physical, mental, and social well being, not merely the absence of disease or infirmity" (WHO, 1947, pp. 1–2). Many people today believe this definition is really a goal—an idealistic, unreachable goal. This definition does not allow for degrees of health or illness. It gives an illusion of perfect health. Some people further believe that complete freedom from stress and disease is incompatible with life. In other words, a certain amount of stress is necessary for a person to maximize his potential and achieve self-actualization. Evidence can be found from our past that some of our great leaders did not obtain their greatness until after suffering from a disease.

The next most frequently quoted definition of health was presented by Dunn, who stated that health is a disease-free state or condition (Dunn, 1961). He introduced a new concept, high-level wellness. According to Dunn, good health is a passive state of being related to adaptation to the environment. Since good health is a passive state then an individual's health is directly related to his environment. If he lives in a poor environment, his health will be poor. Health status does not require active participation by the person. High-level wellness, on the other hand, is a dynamic growth to one's full potential (self-actualization). It represents a direction toward optimal being and requires active participation.

As can be seen from this discussion, no generally accepted meaning of the term health exists. The reasons for this lack of agreement on one definition can be summarized as follows:

1. Health is a value judgment which can vary from individual to individual.
2. Health is subjective and abstract. We currently have no definitive measurement of health.
3. Health is culturally determined and defined.
4. Health is dynamic. Some definitions represent health as static.
5. At times the difference between health and illness is difficult to see. (Siegel, 1973)

Although no definition of health that deals with all these problems exists, one definition which the authors believe considers these issues is as follows: "Health is a dynamic state which exists on a continuum from optimal well being to death." This definition implies that health has three basic characteristics: (1) health involves constant change; (2) health exists on a continuum; and (3) health involves total man.

Health involves constant change. We are constantly experiencing varying degrees of illness and wellness. Man, as an open system, is in constant interaction with stressors from his environment. As man strives to adapt to these stressors, his health status fluctuates. This interaction with stressors causes a constant movement on the health continuum.

Health exists on a continuum. The health continuum has two dimensions. One dimension reflects time, from the beginning of life to death. As we move along the time continuum our health status fluctuates from optimal well-being to degrees of deviation, and finally to death. What this means is that as we strive for optimal wellness as defined by each individual, we will not always experience wellness, but will experience degrees of deviation and finally death. The other dimension represents health from optimal well-being or wellness to death. How one defines the optimal well-being end of the health continuum differs depending on the model of health being utilized. Table 12-1 summarizes four main health models as identified by Smith (1981). These models can be viewed as a hierarchy. Both the clinical and role performance models focus on the maintenance of stability of the system through, first, considering physiological functioning and, then, including social homeostasis. The adaptive model focuses on change, and the final model is oriented toward growth. This eudaimonistic model is the most comprehensive recognizing the total being of man.

Health involves man as a total being. This holistic view of man means that well-being involves wellness in all of man's component parts or dimensions. Whether you define dimensions as physiological, psychological, and sociocultural or whether you view man as a biopsychosocial being, the point is that man reacts as a whole. Achieving optimal wellness means wellness in all dimensions of man.

Let's look at an example to help clarify these points. When you were born someone rated you as healthy, not so healthy, ill, or seriously ill. As you moved along the time dimension, you experienced varying degrees of wellness. At two years of age, you were teething, had a temperature, and were irritable. You did not sleep well or eat normally. After the tooth emerged, you felt better and continued learning, developing, and reacting to your environment. Your physical needs were met as well as your needs for love, attention, stimulation, and interaction; you were healthy or well. Now suppose at age six you fall and break your leg. The fact that your psychological and

TABLE 12-1
Health models as identified by Smith

Model Name	Definition of Health	Definition of Illness
Eudaimonistic	The realization of man's best potential	A condition that impedes self-actualization
Adaptive	Man engaged in effective interaction with the physical and social environment	Failure of man to cope with changes in his environment
Role performance	Occurs when man is able to perform his social roles	An incapacity that prevents people from "doing their jobs"
Clinical	The absence of morbid physical or mental conditions	The presence of disease or disability

From: Smith, J. "The Idea of Health: A Philosophical Inquiry." *Advances in Nursing Science* (3) [1981]: 43-50.

sociocultural dimensions are well provides a better environment for recovery and achievement of wellness. Suppose, however, that in addition to your broken leg, your love and attention needs are not being met. Your reaction to the broken leg would be quite different and your movement toward the death side of the continuum greater. In other words, wellness in one or two dimensions provides a more positive environment for achieving wellness as a whole.

Why do some people move along the continuum at different rates and different degrees? Why when exposed to the flu virus, do some people develop flu and others do not? Why do some people experience illness after the death of a family member and others do not? Man's health status is dependent on the ability of his system to interact with stressors. The parts of man which interact with stressors have been called lines of defense (normal and flexible), line of resistance, and basic energy core (Neuman, 1982). These lines of defense and resistance help explain the variation in rates and degrees of movement along the continuum. The stronger these defense and resistance lines, the more resilience man has in coping with stressors.

Lines of defense prevent stressors from penetrating the system. When stressors are interacting with the system, we are dealing with decreasing levels of wellness on the health continuum. One of your normal lines of defense is your intact skin. It prevents microorganisms from entering the body. However, while the skin remains intact, it undergoes constant change—it may be drier in the winter. This dryness is represented by the flexible lines of defense. In other words, the normal lines of defense are the more constant factors in your defense against stressors, and the flexible lines represent the constant change in the normal lines of defense. The example just given is a physical one related to the individual. These defenses also operate in other dimensions. For example, you have all heard the statement "The family which prays together stays together." This statement implies that a family can provide support to its members so that stressor penetration is minimal.

Sometimes stressors do penetrate the lines of defense. It is at this point that the system experiences illness or further movement toward the death side of the continuum. Illness is a failure of the normal lines of defense of man to adequately counteract the stressors, which results in a disturbance in structure and function. Once a stressor has penetrated and illness occurs, the interaction is now with the lines of resistance. The idea of man's resistance to stressors is discussed in Chapter 6, "Stress-Adaptation Theory." Many times the signs and symptoms of illnesses are also signs and symptoms of resistance. For example, you cut your finger, and a few days later the cut is reddened, warm to touch. Your white blood cell count is elevated. Your temperature is 101°F. These signs and symptoms of an illness, infection, are also your body's way of resisting the foreign-body invasion.

If man is effective in his resistance, reconstitution occurs and a new level of wellness is established. A new level of wellness emerges because the system changes as a result of this experience. This new level may be above or below the previous level on the continuum. Man, however, is not always successful in his resistance. A stressor may penetrate the basic energy core. This energy core is the very basis of life. When stressors penetrate this basic energy core, man slides further toward the death end of the continuum and at some point dies.

As you can see from this discussion, the concept of health as defined by professionals is abstract and somewhat complex. The defense and resistance lines help the nurse understand the variations among man as he interacts with stressors and strives for health. Individuals view health, especially their own health, in much more personal terms. This subjective perception influences how individuals live their lives and, in turn, their health behaviors. The nurse, in order to help individuals develop positive health behaviors, must first assess their health status.

ASSESSING HEALTH

Since there is as yet no one guide for measuring health, we currently measure health in bits and pieces. To facilitate changing man's health practices, the nurse must assess man's health status. Emphasis on assessing health has been on measuring the absence of disease, i.e., no cancer, no mental illness, no hypertension. An assumption is made that if there is no disease, the person is "healthy." The fact that health has been defined by many as the absence of disease has encouraged this focus when assessing health. This is considered a clinical focus or medical model of health.

Now that people are reexamining and expanding their definitions of health, concern is being expressed about how to measure or assess a person's health status. Dunn (1961) believed much can be done to quantify positive health. Some of his suggestions included refinements in determining incidence and prevalence rates and developing susceptibility indices for different groups which are most likely to develop specific diseases. He believed that this would help us with assessing and implementing preventative strategies with clients. However, before you can look at specific techniques for assessing health, the following limitations of our current measures must be considered: (1) an ideal assessment of health will determine the amount of stress the whole of man could tolerate—this assessment tool does not currently exist; (2) most current assessment techniques measure the absence of disease; (3) the current assessment techniques tend to measure parts of the whole, not the whole. Keep these limitations in mind when analyzing some of the techniques which are available for assessing man, the individual, family, and community.

Individual

Many personal health profiles or health-risk appraisals exist today to help in assessing health practices, beliefs, and risks. (See Table 12–2 for sample ques-

TABLE 12-2
Sample questions found in health risk profiles or appraisals

Assessment Area	Sample Questions
Personal information	How old are you? What is your sex? With whom do you live? What is your level of education? What is your marital status? What is your religion? What is your ethnic background? What is your height? What is your weight?

Attitudes toward health	How concerned are you about your health?
	How often do you visit the doctor?
	How concerned are you about getting heart disease, hypertension, diabetes, and cancer?
	How often do you see the dentist?
	How much time and energy are you willing to devote to maintaining your health?
	What has been your experience with the health care system?
	Do you believe the following can help prevent serious illnesses?
	    Eating properly
	    Not being overweight
	    Not smoking
	    Taking vitamins
	    Getting enough rest
	    Avoiding tension, etc.
	Do you perform self-breast or self-testicular exam?

Health habits
A. Nutrition
	Do you eat foods such as fruits and vegetables, whole grain breads and cereals, lean meat, and dairy products such as milk and cheese?
	How much do you eat of the following:
	    Eggs Cream
	    Fatty meats Organ meats
	    Butter
	How much salt do you eat?
	Do you snack between meals? On what?
	Do you drink? What? How much?

B. Exercise	Do you exercise? How often? How long?
	Do you do any of the following:
	    Run Swim
	    Brisk walk Bicycle
	Do you participate in exercises to enhance muscle tone, yoga, calisthenics, etc.? How often? How long?

C. Smoking	Do you smoke? If yes, cigars, cigarettes, or pipe? How much? How long ago did you start? stop?
D. Alcohol	Do you drink? If yes, what type of alcohol? How much? How long ago did you start? stop?

(Continued)

TABLE 12-2 (Cont.)

Assessment Area	Sample Questions
E. Safety	Do you wear seat belts? If yes, what type (lap or lap-shoulder)? How many accidents have you been in? Describe. Have you received driving tickets? Describe. Are poisons in your home labeled and out of reach of children? Are there gates to steps? Are there smoke alarms? where?
F. Stress control	Do you have a stressful job? Do you have friends you can talk to about personal matters? How many stressors have you experienced in the past year? Do you have hobbies or leisure activities you enjoy? Do you use stress management techniques?
Family and health history	Does anyone in your family have diabetes, cancer, tuberculosis, heart trouble, mental illness, or high blood pressure? Do you have any of the above? How do you generally feel? How happy and satisfied are you with your life?

tions found on these profiles or appraisals.) Generally these profiles are completed by the individual. Some of them are scored by the individual, but others require you to send the completed profile to them for scoring and interpretation. A fee is usually involved when profiles are sent for scoring and interpretation. The contents of these health profiles vary in length but generally include personal information, such as age, sex, education, residence; attitudes about health, such as, "I don't like to bother the doctor," "I go to the doctor's for yearly exams"; health habits dealing with nutrition, exercise, smoking, alcohol, safety, and stress control; and family history. Some profiles that are sent for scoring provide information for improving your health status, such as, suggested changes in health habits, whether you are high risk for developing a disease, what you need to do about it, and places you may go to help reduce stress. For further information about these health profiles you can inquire at health education centers, wellness centers, and the federal government. Table 12–3 contains some of these centers along with their addresses. Whether you choose to use a prepared health profile or not, you should include questions about these areas in the assessment of the individual's health status.

Another technique for assessing an individual's health status is the traditional history and physical examination. This exam provides data useful in determining existing diseases and potential problems. Many books are on the

TABLE 12-3
Selected education and wellness centers

Center*	Address
The Center for Consumer Health Education	380 West Maple Avenue Vienna, VA 22180 (703) 281-5893
Center for Health Promotion and Education c/o Charles A. Althafer	Centers for Disease Control Atlanta, GA 30333 (404) 329-3415
Health Education Center	200 Ross Street Pittsburgh, PA 15219 (412) 392-3160
The Institute for Personal Health	2100 M Street, N.W. Suite 316 Washington, DC 20063 (202) 872-5379
Public Relations Department Blue Cross/Blue Shield of Michigan	600 East Lafayette Detroit, MI 48226 (313) 225-8430
Wellness Associates	42 Miller Avenue Mill Valley, CA 94941 (415) 383-3806
Wisconsin Center for Health Risk Research	University of Wisconsin Center for Health Sciences 600 Highland Avenue Room 84/414 Madison, WI 53792 (608) 263-3010

* This list is not meant to be exhaustive nor does inclusion mean endorsement.

market to aid the nurse in learning the necessary skills for performing this exam. No matter what reference is used it is important for efficiency and thoroughness that the nurse develop a systematic way of proceeding with the exam.

Since man also has a psychological and sociocultural dimension, no health status evaluation would be complete without information about these dimensions. Many nurses assess these dimensions during the history and physical by noting appropriateness of the client's response to questions, vocabulary used, affect, and mood. In addition, the nurse asks questions about normal coping strategies and self-concept, including sexuality. In some cases you may also have such information as personality tests and IQ tests collected by others which add to your assessment of the individual's health status. In the sociocultural dimension, assessment data include information about the environment (home, community, and work), family as a support system, economic status, occupation and educational history, ethnic and cultural background, religion, and leisure activities. When collecting these data, the nurse should also observe communication and interaction patterns. Although some nurses believe this information is not necessary for giving care in acute care settings, this information influences how the client reacts during his illness and recovery.

The last area that needs to be assessed to help determine an individual's health status is the developmental continuum. For children, the Denver Developmental Screening Test (DDST) is an example of a test for determining if the client is moving along appropriately for his age group. For adults, the nurse refers to adult developmental theories. Most of you have been or are currently being exposed to normal developmental tasks through human development courses. There is general agreement that each age group has developmental tasks that need to be accomplished before moving along the life span. Recently, attention has been focused on identifying more specifically the developmental stages for adults and elderly. The nurse needs to remember that the norms used for comparison are tied to our culture. Although there are many similarities, what is normal for one culture may not be in other cultures. Knowing the developmental tasks can aid the nurse in anticipating and preparing clients for positive experiences as they move along the life continuum.

During the total assessment process the nurse must remember that concern is with assessing the client's health status, not just illness status. This requires that the client be assessed in all dimensions. The information from this assessment provides the data for identification of strengths, potential stressors, and current problems.

Family and Community

While most health care providers focus their attention on individual clients, more health care providers are beginning to also include families and communities as clients. As we expand the number of people who are our clients, assessments become more complex. Much of the information collected on individuals is helpful when assessing the health status of families or communities. Although assessment of these complex systems may seem like an overwhelming task, approaching it systematically helps.

As with the individual assessment, the dimensions of man are useful in family assessment. In the physiological dimension data are collected about family history of disease, physical status of each member, how health status of each member affects total family, and family profile of health habits. In the psychological dimensions information is collected about interaction patterns, affect of family, self-concept, family values, and family beliefs. Socioculturally, data include family involvement in the community, economic status, educational and work values, environment, leisure activities, religious involvement, and ethnic background. Also included in an assessment are data about the developmental continuum. Data to be collected relate to the age of the family and the developmental tasks facing families of this age. For example, young families face decisions around having or not having children. Older families face planning for retirement, adjusting to death of spouse, etc.

In assessing communities, data are once again collected in all dimensions. In the physiological dimensions information about pollution, life expectancy, infant mortality, and occupational hazards are included. Psychologically, the nurse would be concerned about the self-concept of the community, i.e., "good" community vs. "bad" community, "wealthy" community vs. "poor" community, communication among people and businesses, etc. Additional data needed in the sociocultural dimension would include type of government, services available, community norms, social problems, crime rate, employment, and finances. Lastly, you assess the developmental continuum. Is this a new or old community? What additional problems face new communities, old communities?

What was presented here was a brief look at some of the data the nurse collects in order to assess the health status of man. Table 12-4 summarizes this information. With this information, the nurse is in a better position to examine factors that influence man's health behaviors.

FACTORS INFLUENCING HEALTH BEHAVIORS

Many health professionals are increasingly concerned with the lack of positive health behaviors in today's society. Many nurses believe that they should have a great impact in changing an individual's health behaviors, but they find themselves frustrated when they attempt to. Much of this frustration results because nurses do not always understand what motivates health behaviors and, in turn, what will stimulate change.

Striving for optimal well-being generally requires a willingness to change your normal way of life. For example, a healthy life style includes balancing work and play, reducing stress, exercising, and proper nutrition. In other words, obtaining health requires time, energy, motivation, and, in many cases, money. Positive health behaviors require the individual to become actively involved with himself.

Why are many people unwilling to make these changes? To make these commitments? An individual's definition of health and ultimately his health behaviors are closely related to perceptions. Perception is an awareness of something through our senses. Examination of what influences perception as related to health behaviors will help in understanding and possibly motivating an individual's health behaviors. When a person perceives a need

TABLE 12-4
Summary of assessment areas to help determine health status

Man	Dimension	Content
Individual	Physiological dimension	Body systems review
	Psychological dimension	Support systems
		Coping patterns
		Self-awareness
		Intellectual development
		Mental skills
		Perceptions and attitudes toward health
	Sociocultural dimension	Demographic data (residence, occupation, relation, marital status, etc.)
		Educational and economic status
		Cultural background
		Leisure and recreation activities
		Environment
		Family history
	Developmental continuum	Age
		Past health history
		Developmental tasks
Family	Physiological	Systems status of members
	Psychological	Interaction and communication patterns
		Educational level
		Support systems
		Values, beliefs, perceptions
	Sociocultural	Interaction with community
		Economic status
		Educational status
		Environment
		Leisure activities
		Cultural and religious background
	Developmental	Age of family
		Family developmental tasks
Community	Physiological	Pollution indices
		Life expectancy
		Infant mortality
	Psychological	Suicide rates
		Feeling tone, i.e., safety
		Support systems
		Coping patterns
		Educational level
	Sociocultural	Type government services available
		Community norms
		Social problems—employment, crime
		Financial condition
	Developmental	Age of community
		Developmental tasks of the community

for health this serves as a motivational factor to health behaviors. Motivational factors can be classified as intrapersonal, interpersonal, and extrapersonal (see Table 12-5).

Intrapersonal Factors

Intrapersonal factors are those beliefs and values, which exist within a system, that influence health behaviors. The first of these factors is the importance of health to the individual. How much does the person value health? While most people will tell you health is important to them, health behaviors more closely reflect this importance. Some people believe that health is important as long as it doesn't inconvenience them, take a lot of time, or cost money. Other people believe that health is so important that they commit long hours to strive for optimal well-being and spend whatever money is needed. Some people commit their total lives to striving for health.

The second intrapersonal factor is the person's perception of his own vulnerability or susceptibility to disease and illness (Mikbail, 1981). If you see yourself at high risk of developing a disease or becoming ill, you are more likely to take preventive actions. A person who experienced severe chest pain is more likely to stop smoking than a person who feels fine and whose father smoked and lived to be ninety. When a family member has cancer this generally makes other members of the family more aware of warning signs and possible preventive behaviors.

This leads us to the next factor—the value placed on early detection of disease. Some people are procrastinators when it comes to their health. They take the attitude of, "If I ignore it, it will go away." The attitude is reinforced

TABLE 12-5
Summary of factors influencing health behaviors

Classification	Specific Factor
Intrapersonal	Importance of health
	Perception of vulnerability
	Value placed on early detection
	Perception of action benefits
	Perception of degree of control over self
	Perception of seriousness of various illnesses
Interpersonal	Significant others
	Family health patterns
	Friends (peers)
	Professionals
Extrapersonal	Cultural acceptance behaviors
	Societal norms
	Information from nonpersonal sources

by the fact that many illnesses are self-limiting. In other words, they go away with no extra effort on the individual's part.

The value placed on early detection relates to the fourth intrapersonal factor. This factor reflects the perceived benefits derived from action, especially early action. Have you ever heard the statement "If I have cancer I would rather not know"? These people delay receiving treatment because they believe it is hopeless. "Everyone who has cancer dies." I must see that changing my health behavior in a positive direction will result in decreasing the threat of this illness. If I run and eat properly, what are my chances of not having a heart attack? The hard part in dealing with this influencing factor is that there are no guarantees. Even if you change your health habits positively, you may still develop heart problems. Your chances of staying healthy increase by proper health habits but not to 100 percent.

The benefits of action relate to the fifth intrapersonal factor influencing your health behavior—the degree of control you believe you have over your own destiny. Some people believe that they have limited control over their lives. Some people are referred to as having an external locus of control. Other people, who see themselves as having a great deal of control, are referred to as internal locus of control people. Although locus of control exists on a continuum, most people tend toward one or the other end of the continuum. A health locus-of-control scale has been developed to measure this personal characteristic (Wallston, Wallston, Kaplan, & Maides, 1976). The degree of control perceived by individuals influences how amenable they are to changing their health behaviors.

The final influencing intrapersonal factor is how the system perceives the seriousness of various illnesses. The perceived seriousness of a disease is usually influenced by the visible changes resulting from the illness, whether it is life threatening, and how it affects your life style. For example, some people do not perceive an elevated blood pressure as serious. Many times there are no symptoms or visible changes in the body and there are no alterations in life style. However, individuals whose family member has suffered a stroke related to high blood pressure see high blood pressure as a potentially serious problem. They have seen the life-threatening changes in their family member, the alterations in life style, and possibly other residuals from the stroke.

Interpersonal Factors

Interpersonal factors are those things existing between you and other people that influence your health behaviors. There are four of these interpersonal factors. In the usual order of influence these are significant others, family health patterns, friends, and professionals.

The concern that significant others have for your health can motivate you to more positive or negative behaviors. Recent television commercials attempted to use this factor to motivate parents to stop smoking. They made rather dramatic appeals to the children to encourage their parents to stop smoking. Many commercials showed scenes with and without a parent. Many times people seek assistance of health professionals because they promised their husband, wife, sister, etc.

Generally your pattern of using health facilities, i.e., seeking help with your health, closely resembles those of your parents. Think about your own behaviors. What do you do when you have an upset stomach? Call the doctor? Eat chicken soup? Drink ginger ale? Do you get yearly physicals? How often do you see a dentist? Do you go to school or work when you have a cold? Do you exercise routinely? Do you eat a balanced diet? Now reflect back and answer these questions as your mother or father would. Do you see similarities? This is not to say that we don't or can't change from the way our parents do things, but changing does indicate some other factor was more influential. The new factor required you to examine how important achieving optimal well-being is. Most of the time we don't stop and think about it. We take our health for granted.

The third interpersonal factors are your friends. Peer pressure plays an important part in the development of your health habits. Many teenagers smoke and take drugs as a way of gaining acceptance by peers. Others go on fad diets. Still others are active in sports or join various clubs. Today exercising and joining health spas seem to be gaining in popularity.

The last influential factor in this category is professionals. Professionals generally have the least impact on influencing health behaviors. Part of this lack of influence is related to their failing as role models of health. Many health professionals take an attitude of "Do as I say, not as I do." This approach has a negative influence on clients changing their health behaviors. Another reason for this lack of influence is the limited contact professionals have with their clients. How much time do you spend with family versus professionals? Another contributing factor to this lack of influence relates to the hesitation of some health professionals in telling someone else how to live his life, especially when there are no guarantees the change will produce good health. In addition to the above, the focus in the health care system has been on illness, not health promotion. We have concentrated our efforts on getting sick people better. This focus is changing, and more people are concerned with promotion of health behaviors. Professionals can have a positive influence on health behaviors by serving as a credible source of information and serving as role models.

Extrapersonal Factors

Extrapersonal factors are those things that occur in our environment and influence our health behaviors. Three of these are especially important. The first extrapersonal factor is cultural acceptance of health behaviors. The

United States is a mixture of cultures and ethnic backgrounds all with their own health beliefs and practices. Your cultural and ethnic background influences your health beliefs and practices. The more important the culture and ethnic background is to the individual, the stronger the commitment to these beliefs and practices. This commitment may result in clients resisting opposing views from health professionals. For example, birth control has been described as "Black genocide" by some members of the Black community. There has been a proliferation of textbooks, articles, and courses addressing health beliefs and practices of a variety of cultures to aid health professionals in increasing their understanding of cultures and their potential influence on health practices.

While every individual exists with a cultural and ethnic background, they also exist in a society. The society may be composed of people from more than one culture and ethnic background. Societal group norms may be different from the cultural and ethnic norms. An individual is then caught in a position of conflict. For example, in some cultures the norm is no drinking; the societal norm is social drinking. What do you do? The person is forced to make a decision.

Another influential extrapersonal factor is information from nonpersonal sources, i.e., TV commercials and health insurance. Many television commercials promote nonhealthful behaviors. One example is sugar-coated cereals. Traditional health insurance also conveys the message that it is not acceptable to seek preventive health care, i.e., prenatal classes, well-baby check-ups, immunizations. These activities are not covered by many traditional health insurance carriers, only by carriers such as health maintenance organizations.

You may be wondering what is the point of all this information? What can I do with it? As you can see, health beliefs and practices are formed over a period of time and through a variety of factors. Health beliefs and practices are intertwined in our life styles. In order to work effectively with clients, nurses need to assess their clients' beliefs and practices and use these factors to help in the change process. Changing health practices means changing life styles and that takes time, energy, and commitment.

NURSING ROLE

Bruhn (1977) believes wellness behavior is a learned behavior. Certainly what is known about health perceptions supports this belief. If health behavior is learned then health professionals can help people learn positive health behaviors. Health behaviors include both illness and wellness behaviors.

There are three activities that the nurse engages in in order to change health behaviors. The first is acquiring a knowledge base about health and illness. The nurse must define health and identify her beliefs and values about health. Self-analysis will aid the nurse in identifying the impact her value system may have on her client and his reaction to her. The nurse must also become knowledgeable about the latest information on high risk and actions necessary to promote health. In addition to the knowledge base, the nurse also needs to develop skills related to facilitating change and learning. (For details, see Chapters 9 and 7.) For example, if you know that change is a slow process, then you know that to have your client change his health behaviors will take time. You would also know that identifying existence of some stress in the system could help motivate the system to want to change. In addition, you would need to understand factors that prompt or inhibit health behaviors. Understanding these factors could be helpful in identifying forces that could inhibit the client's movement toward health.

The second activity the nurse engages in is related to identifying factors which will motivate the client to change behavior. Motivation is the key to assisting clients to change health behaviors. Without motivation, the client will not be willing to spend the time and energy needed to make the change. How can the nurse motivate clients to change? First, the nurse needs to identify principles and techniques useful for this client. A careful assessment of the client will help accomplish this. Knowing that this client's mother is a major influence on this client could alert you to trying to aim your change at the mother, who would then influence the client to change. Secondly, in stimulating motivation, the nurse needs to provide the client with proper information. Providing clients with information about consequences of illness for which the person is at high risk gives the client an opportunity to make intelligent decisions. This information may increase anxiety which could serve to motivate the client to action. Next, the nurse provides the client with time to reflect, clarify his thoughts, and make decisions, i.e., make a commitment to change. Providing clients with specific information about amount of change needed and the time, effort, and money which may be involved can help them make their decision. Sometimes seeing things in writing also helps. The nurse supports and encourages the client throughout the decision-making process.

The third and last activity the nurse engages in related to helping clients change their health behaviors is the development of protection or wellness plans. After you have assessed your client's health state, identified areas that need assistance, and motivated your client to want to change, you develop a wellness plan with the client. Wellness plans generally include what the client will do in relation to nutrition, exercise, rest, stress, detection and screening programs, seeking medical assistance, and hygiene. A properly done wellness plan includes measurable goals and specific approaches for achieving them. (A sample wellness plan is included in Table 12-6.) When

TABLE 12-6
Sample wellness plan

LONG-TERM GOAL: OBTAIN A HEALTH LEVEL HIGHER THAN THE CURRENT ONE WITHIN ONE YEAR

AREA OF CONCENTRATION	GOAL	APPROACH
Nutrition	I will improve my dietary habits by increasing my fruit and vegetable consumption and decreasing my meat consumption	Eat three fruits per day. Eat vegetables two times per day. Limit beef consumption to four times per week. Try one new vegetable each week
Exercise	I will improve my cardiovascular function and muscle tone as evidenced by no sore muscles and no shortness of breath when exercising	Participate in aerobic dancing one-half hour three times per week. Isometric exercises for thirty minutes three times per week

FUTURE AREAS OF CONCENTRATION	GOAL	APPROACH
Rest	To be completed after attainment of above goals	
Stress		

developing these plans the nurse needs to be sensitive to the client and the amount of change requested. Persistence, patience, and acceptance go a long way in working with the client.

SUMMARY

Many definitions of health exist. This chapter examined several definitions and presented one of its own. In order for nurses to assist their clients to achieve a goal of optimal well-being, the difficulties in measuring or assessing health status were discussed. To date, assessing health status is both difficult and complex. We tend to measure the absence of disease, not health. Since health behaviors are learned, factors which influence these behaviors were presented. These factors can assist the nurse in planning and facilitating a change in health behaviors. The chapter concluded with a discussion of the three major activities of the nurse related to facilitating positive health behaviors. These three activities involve knowledge and skill, motivational strategies, and development of wellness plans.

Key points to remember are

1. Health is difficult to define because it involves value judgments; it is subjective, dynamic, and abstract; and it is culturally bound.

2. Health is seen as a dynamic continuum involving constant change and total man.
3. Most assessment guides measure absence of illness, not health, but efforts are being made to assess health.
4. Intrapersonal, interpersonal, and extrapersonal factors influence one's health beliefs and practices.
5. The nurse is responsible for assessing the client's health status and for developing wellness plans to maintain health.

REFERENCES

Bruhn, J. G., and Cordova, F. D. "A Developmental Approach to Learning Wellness Behavior, Part 1: Infancy to Early Adolescence." *Health Values* 1 (1977): 246-254.

Doerr, B. T., and Hutchins, E. B. "Health Risk Appraisal: Process, Problems, and Prospects for Nursing-Practice and Research." *Nursing Research* 30 (1981): 299-306.

Dolfman, M. L. "The Concept of Health: An Historic and Analytic Examination." *The Journal of School Health* 43 (1973): 491-497.

Dunn, H. L. *High Level Wellness*. Arlington, VA: Beatty, 1961.

Dunn, H. L. "High Level Wellness for Man and Society." *American Journal of Public Health* 49 (1959): 1901-1905.

Grasser, C., and Craft, B. J. G. "The Patient's Approach to Wellness." *The Nursing Clinics of North America* 19 (1984): 207-218.

Keller, M. J. "Toward a Definition of Health." *Advances in Nursing Science* 4 (1) [1981]: 43-64.

Mikbail, B. "The Health Belief Model: A Review and Critical Evaluation of the Model, Research, and Practice." *Advances in Nursing Science* 4 (1) [1981]: 65-80.

Moore, P. V., and Williamson, G. "Health Promotion: Evaluation of a Concept." *Nursing Clinics of North America* 19 (1984): 195-206.

Neuman, B. *The Neuman Systems Model: Application to Nursing Education and Practice*. Norwalk, CT: Appleton-Century-Crofts, 1982.

Shillinger, F. L. "Locus of Control: Implications for Clinical Nursing Practice." *Image: The Journal of Nursing Scholarship* 15 (1983): 58-63.

Siegel, H. "To Your Health—Whatever That May Mean." *Nursing Forum* 12 (1973): 280-299.

Smith, J. "The Idea of Health: A Philosophical Inquiry." *Advances in Nursing Science* 3 (3) [1981]: 43-50.

Wallston, B. S., Wallston, K. A., Kaplan, G. D., and Maides, S. A. "Development and Validation of the Health Locus of Control Scale." *Journal of Consulting and Clinical Psychology* 44 (1976): 580-585.

World Health Organization. *Chronicle of the World Health Organization* 1 (1947): 1-2.

13

The American health care system

Although Mrs. Smith was 73 years of age, she was a self-sufficient, independent woman who maintained her own home. In fact, she was sweeping the rug in that home when she tripped over the sweeper cord and injured her hip. As soon as she fell she realized she was in real trouble. She crawled across the room, pulled her phone to the floor, and called her daughter. Mrs. Smith's daughter, who lived on the other side of town, called an ambulance and went directly to the emergency room. Later they were to learn that Mrs. Smith's insurance would not cover the cost of the ambulance since it was not ordered by a physician. Within less than one-half hour, Mrs. Smith was being admitted to her local community hospital via the emergency room. Mrs. Smith was examined by the emergency room physician, medicated for pain, had blood drawn, and was sent to the X-ray department.

Shortly after she returned from X-ray, an orthopedic surgeon arrived. By this point, Mrs. Smith was overwhelmed by the pain, the pain medication, the fracture, and the strangeness of the hospital. She was so glad to have her daughter there and was really relieved when the surgeon seemed more than willing to talk with her daughter. The physician was certainly reassuring to Mrs. Smith's daughter. While Mrs. Smith would need surgery, the doctor believed the results would be excellent since there was a good blood supply to the fracture area. Neither Mrs. Smith nor her daughter realized that the physician now considered the daughter the responsible adult with whom he should deal. Throughout the rest of her hospitalization, Mrs. Smith always found the physician very polite but it became obvious he communicated only with her daughter. On the days that Mrs. Smith's daughter was not there when the surgeon made rounds, there was little communication. As a result Mrs. Smith and her family often felt they did not know what to expect or what was happening.

Three weeks after her fracture, the surgeon announced that Mrs.

Smith's hip was healing well and she was ready to go home. Mrs. Smith and her family were shocked. Although she could feed herself, she needed help with her bath. She could not get out of bed without help and could walk only a short distance with a walker. She had a small bed sore on her heel and, furthermore, she had gotten used to a bed with side rails. The surgeon was sympathetic but felt there was nothing he could do. Since her bone was healing well, he could not justify Mrs. Smith's staying in the hospital. He felt sure a nice family like this would manage somehow; after all they had just received fast and effective care from the American health care system.

The American health care system is a large and complex system undergoing constant and dynamic change. As can be seen from this example, clients who interact with the system can get caught in the system and, in turn, fail to achieve quality health care. Nurses, if they are going to assist clients in dealing with these types of problems, need to understand this health care system. The purpose of this chapter is to provide the student of nursing with a framework for analysis of the American health care system. The objectives of this chapter are based on the three key points of this framework. At the completion of this chapter, the reader will be able to

1. Explain the evolving purposes of the health care system.
2. Describe the organizational structure of the health care system.
3. Discuss the functions of the health care system in American society.

PURPOSE

All open systems have a purpose, a reason for their existence. In the case of the American health care system, the purposes have evolved over time and continue to change. Historically this system had its roots in Europe. Beginning after the fall of Rome and through the Middle Ages, hospitals developed which provided custodial services for individuals who could not care for themselves or be cared for by their families.

As the sciences began to develop, changes occurred in the health care system. With knowledge from developments in the sciences (i.e., anatomy, physiology, and microbiology), the purpose of the health care system began to move from providing custodial care to a second purpose, providing treatment for illnesses and injuries. The pattern of the move from custodial care to treatment follows in many ways the pattern of scientific discovery. For example, scientific discoveries related to understanding physical diseases occurred earlier than the understanding of psychological disorders. In turn, those parts of the health care system which focused on physical disorders became effective treatment centers before those areas dealing with psychological disorders. This pattern of moving from custodial care to effective treatment continues today. One example of this pattern can be seen in nursing homes. In many cases nursing homes provide custodial care; however, as more is being learned about the problems of patients in these settings the move toward effective treatment is beginning.

Although custodial care is no longer the primary purpose of the health care system it will remain a significant purpose as long as there are health care problems that cannot be prevented or effectively treated. Treatment, on the other hand, has become in many ways the dominant purpose of the health care system. Scientific knowledge as well as treatment itself has also produced other significant purposes. These purposes include prevention and rehabilitation.

Knowledge about what produces or causes health care problems has provided a basis for preventing these problems. For example, several infectious diseases are now prevented by childhood immunizations. Currently, major discoveries are being made concerning the initiating events in chronic diseases. From these types of discoveries concerning initiating events a third major purpose for the health care system is evolving—the prevention of disease or the maintenance of health.

The fourth purpose of the health care system results from the fact that effective treatment does not always mean the client's problems are cured. For example, a client who experiences paralysis due to a spinal cord injury may be treated but never cured. He will still be paralyzed. Such situations require that individuals learn to make adjustments to the limitations that result from their health problems. The need of these individuals and their families to learn how to make the necessary adjustments has resulted in the fourth major purpose of the health care system—rehabilitation.

Like prevention and treatment, effective rehabilitation is dependent upon a knowledge base. This knowledge, which forms the basis of these purposes, is not limited to pathophysiology or to knowledge of disease process but includes knowledge of how people learn, adjust, develop, and live their lives. In other words, all knowledge about man as a living system can be used to assist in providing effective care.

STRUCTURE

Once purposes are identified, open systems do not automatically achieve them. Systems function within a structure. In studying the structure of the American health care system, one must deal with the fact that ideally purposes are stated first and then the system is structured to meet the purposes. With the American health care system, structure, like purpose, is evolving and is constantly influenced by changes in society itself.

In a system as large and as complex as the American health care system, several interacting subsystems exist. These subsystems can be organized and discussed in a variety of ways. In this discussion, these subsystems will be divided into four types. The first two types will be classified according to their administrative control. These are the governmental and nongovernmental subsystems. The second two types of subsystems are classified according to roles. These are the health care recipients (consumers) and health care providers (workers).

The Governmental Subsystem

Health care systems which are under the administrative control of the government are usually referred to as official, tax supported, and/or public. Such systems are authorized and governed by law. Their services and activities are supported by tax funds. Since government is structured in this country on three levels, federal, state, and local, the governmental health care organizations are structured around these levels. No matter which level is involved, the functions of government organizations tend to focus on the general population and groups as opposed to individuals.

Federal Health Care Organizations. The organization of the health care structure on the federal level demonstrates some variation with each political administration; however, the basic structure does follow the branches of the federal government. The function and organization of the federal health care system is authorized by federal law and financed by Congressional appropriation. Currently, the majority of Congressional involvement originates in seven committees, three in the House of Representatives and four in the Senate. Table 13–1 identifies each of these committees as well as the appropriate related subcommittees.

TABLE 13–1
Congressional committees dealing with health

Branch of Congress	Committee	Subcommittee
Senate	Labor and Human Resources	Health and Scientific Research
	Finance	Health
	Appropriation	Labor, Health, and Human Services
	Budget	No subcommittees
House of Representatives	Interstate and Foreign Commerce	Health and Environment
	Ways and Means	Health
		Labor, Health and Human Services
	Budget	Human and Community Resources

From: Banta, D. "The Federal Legislative Process & Health Care." In Jonas, S., *Health Care Delivery in the United States,* 2nd ed. New York: Springer Publishing Co., 1981, p. 356.

Once federal laws have been passed and appropriations authorized, implementation occurs in the executive branch of the federal government. While many departments within the executive branch are involved with health, the most visible is the Department of Health and Human Services. This department "touches the lives of more Americans than any other federal agency" (U.S. Government Manual, 1980, p. 299). As can be seen in Table 13-2, there are four main divisions within the Department. For three of these divisions the administrative responsibilities are straightforward. These are outlined in Table 13-3. The administrative activities of the fourth division, the Public Health Service, are much more complex. It is "charged by law to promote and assure the highest level of health attainable for every individual and family in America and to develop cooperation in health projects with other nations" (U.S. Government Manual, 1980, p. 299). To achieve this charge the Public Health Service performs seven major functions

1. Assists with development of local health resources.
2. Assists with education for the health professions.
3. Assists with improvement of the delivery of health services.
4. Conducts and supports research.
5. Disseminates scientific information.
6. Protects the health of the nation against impure and unsafe foods, drugs, and cosmetics.
7. Provides leadership for prevention and control of communicable disease.

While the U.S. Department of Health and Human Services is one of the most important federal agencies, several other agencies are involved in health care activities. For example, the Department of Defense and the Veterans' Administration are active in research, education, and construction, as well as providing care in their various facilities. Many of these federal programs and organizations are referred to in professional and lay literature without any indication that they are federal agencies. The National Institutes of Health are frequently in the news; yet, many people, including health personnel, do not realize these are federally financed and controlled. For this reason professional students of nursing need to be aware of the names and activities of the major federal agencies.

State and Local Health Care Structure. Within each of the fifty states exists a state health department which has the legal responsibility for the health of the people within its jurisdiction. The actual structures of these departments are as varied as the fifty states; however, most include the following six basic functions: (1) vital statistics, (2) communicable disease control, (3) health education, (4) maternal and child health, (5) environmental sanitation, and (6) laboratories (Leahy, Cobb, & Jones, 1977). The specific tasks

TABLE 13-2
Organizational chart: Department of Health and Human Services

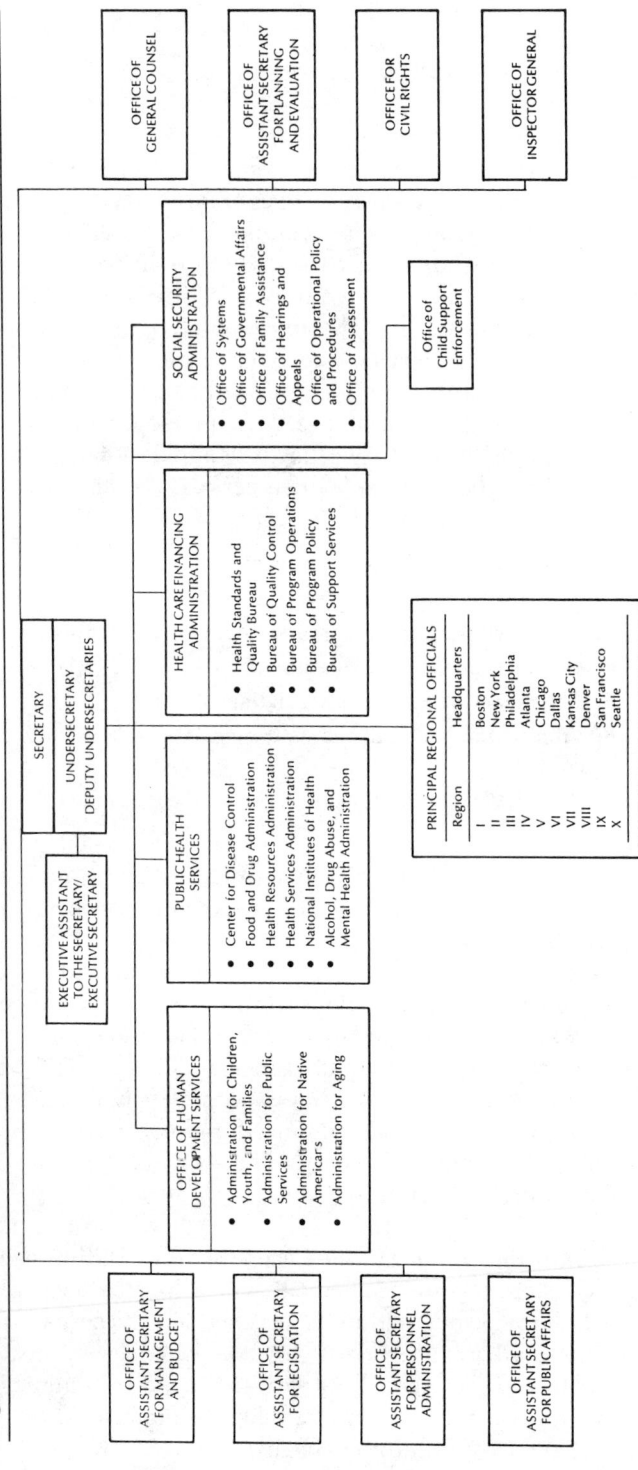

SECRETARY
UNDERSECRETARY
DEPUTY UNDERSECRETARIES

EXECUTIVE ASSISTANT TO THE SECRETARY / EXECUTIVE SECRETARY

Reporting to the Secretary:

- OFFICE OF GENERAL COUNSEL
- OFFICE OF ASSISTANT SECRETARY FOR PLANNING AND EVALUATION
- OFFICE FOR CIVIL RIGHTS
- OFFICE OF INSPECTOR GENERAL
- OFFICE OF ASSISTANT SECRETARY FOR MANAGEMENT AND BUDGET
- OFFICE OF ASSISTANT SECRETARY FOR LEGISLATION
- OFFICE OF ASSISTANT SECRETARY FOR PERSONNEL ADMINISTRATION
- OFFICE OF ASSISTANT SECRETARY FOR PUBLIC AFFAIRS

OFFICE OF HUMAN DEVELOPMENT SERVICES
- Administration for Children, Youth, and Families
- Administration for Public Services
- Administration for Native Americans
- Administration for Aging

PUBLIC HEALTH SERVICES
- Center for Disease Control
- Food and Drug Administration
- Health Resources Administration
- Health Services Administration
- National Institutes of Health
- Alcohol, Drug Abuse, and Mental Health Administration

HEALTH CARE FINANCING ADMINISTRATION
- Health Standards and Quality Bureau
- Bureau of Quality Control
- Bureau of Program Operations
- Bureau of Program Policy
- Bureau of Support Services

SOCIAL SECURITY ADMINISTRATION
- Office of Systems
- Office of Governmental Affairs
- Office of Family Assistance
- Office of Hearings and Appeals
- Office of Operational Policy and Procedures
- Office of Assessment

Office of Child Support Enforcement

PRINCIPAL REGIONAL OFFICIALS

Region	Headquarters
I	Boston
II	New York
III	Philadelphia
IV	Atlanta
V	Chicago
VI	Dallas
VII	Kansas City
VIII	Denver
IX	San Francisco
X	Seattle

250

TABLE 13-3
Administrative responsibilities of the four main divisions within the Department of Health and Human Services

Division	Responsibilities
Office of Human Development Services	Administers a wide range of programs designed to deal with the problems of specific populations
Health Care Financing Administration	Administers medicare, medicaid, and related federal medical care quality control staffs
Social Security Administration	Administers the national program of contributory social insurance
Public Health Service	See text

From: *U.S. Government Manual 1980.* Washington, D.C.: Office of the Federal Registrar, National Archives and Records Service, General Services Administration, 1980, p. 296-309.

performed within the various state health departments also vary, but four general divisions can usually be identified in each of the states: (1) statewide planning and evaluation, (2) state and federal relations, (3) interstate agency relations, and (4) statewide regulatory functions.

The size, structure, and specific functions of *local* health departments vary even more than state health departments. There is a tendency for local health departments to be patterned after their state health departments. Most develop their programs around the six basic functions of the state health department. Historically, these specific programs are based on the health care needs of the community. Along with the development of the programs, the local health departments provide facilities and qualified staff to carry out the programs (Leahy, Cobb, & Jones, 1977).

Although government, especially at the federal level, is increasingly involved in the financing of health care, it provides only a small proportion of the actual supplies and services utilized for health care. Most of the supplies and services, whether financed by the government or not, originate in the private segment of the health care system.

The Private Subsystem

Health care organizations which are not under the administrative control of the government are referred to as private. The term *administrative control* is essential to understanding this concept. The term means that the individual(s) with the final administrative responsibilities for the organization are not government employee(s). It does not mean that government funds are not used by the organization or that the government does not impose rules and regulations on them.

Many community hospitals offer an excellent example of this concept.

A board of trustees or directors is responsible for the operation of the hospital. The individuals on the board are private citizens. Patient care, on the other hand, may be financed by federal funds (Medicare), state funds (Medicaid), private insurance (Blue Cross), or the patient's own private funds. The hospital itself is classified as private because of who has administrative control, not because of who pays for the patient care delivered.

Private health care organizations are usually classified in two different and overlapping ways. First, they may be classified as profit or nonprofit. Profit health care organizations are developed and exist to return a profit to the owners or investors in that business. They vary from one-man operations, for example, a physician in private practice; to major multinational corporations, for example, a drug company.

In contrast nonprofit organizations are developed and exist to provide a community service. There are no investors in the business; in fact, nonprofit organizations are required by law to invest all returns back into the organization. Like profit organizations, nonprofit organizations vary greatly in size from small local groups to multinational organizations (i.e., the Red Cross).

A second way of classifying private health care organizations is in terms of what they produce: services or supplies. Although it is possible for an organization to offer both, at the present time most organizations focus on either supplies or services. Table 13-4 demonstrates these overlapping classification systems and some of the specific types of businesses involved.

All of these various health care organizations have an influence on the practice of nursing. Therefore nurses need to understand how these organizations function and what some of the health care issues involved in their operation are. A review of all these organizations is beyond the scope of this book. Two of the more pertinent health care organizations, for nurses, are reviewed in more detail here. These are hospitals and voluntary organizations. While

TABLE 13-4
Classification of organizations by product and profit motive

Types of Organizations	Product or Output	Profit Motive
Drug companies	supplies	profit
Medical equipment companies	supplies	profit
"Rent a Nurse"	service	profit
Proprietary hospitals	service	profit
Private practices (i.e., physicians)	service	profit
Voluntary organizations	service	nonprofit
University medical center	service	nonprofit
Visiting nurse associations	service	nonprofit

the great majority of hospitals are private, not every hospital is private. This point will be further explained in the discussion on hospitals.

Hospitals. Hospitals are formal organizations where health care and illness treatment have been institutionalized. Their growing role in health care has paralleled the growing complexity of health care technology. In today's society, hospitals are considered the "cornerstone" or "hub" of the health care system (Somers & Somers, 1977; Freeman, Levine & Reeder, 1979). Over half of employed nurses work in hospital settings.

Though hospitals have a basic core of common features, they differ in size, type of service offered, administrative control, and numerous other features. Usually they are classified by two of these features: type of service offered and administrative control.

Type of service offered deals with the type of health care problems treated by the employees of the hospital. Many hospitals provide care for a wide variety of acute illnesses or flare up of chronic illness. These are commonly referred to as general or acute care hospitals. Such hospitals are almost always short term, which means that over 50 percent of the patients stay less than thirty days (VerSteeg & Croad, 1979). Other hospitals are prepared to deal only with specific diseases or clients. These are referred to as specialty hospitals. Pediatric, maternity, orthopedic, and psychiatric are some examples of this type of hospital.

Although general hospitals are short term, specialty hospitals can be either short or long term. For example, a children's or maternity hospital is usually short term while psychiatric or orthopedic hospitals tend to be long term. Long-term institutions can vary in one other important factor: the amount of emphasis the institution places on rehabilitation vs. custodial care.

The second way hospitals are classified is in terms of administrative control. Hospitals are first of all governmental or nongovernmental. Government hospitals may be either federal (i.e., Veterans hospitals and Public Health Service hospitals), state (i.e., psychiatric or tuberculosis hospitals), or local hospitals (i.e., geriatric hospitals). Nongovernmental institutions are either profit or nonprofit. Profit hospitals are referred to as proprietary. While there are some excellent proprietary hospitals, one should keep in mind these hospitals focus on the production of a profit and will tend to limit their services to those areas which show good potential for producing a profit.

In looking at the classification of hospitals by service and by control it is important to remember these are overlapping classification systems. Therefore, all hospitals fit in both groups. For example, the great majority of hospitals are acute care, nonprofit institutions. Any nurse working or planning to work in a hospital should know how the hospital is classified.

Voluntary Organization. The second group of health care organizations with special significance to nurses are the voluntary agencies. Nurses continuously utilize these agencies as resources for themselves and for their clients. Voluntary organizations are nonprofit agencies. They are usually formed by a group of individuals who are interested in a specific problem or set of related diseases. A few examples of well-known voluntary agencies are the American Heart Association, American Cancer Society, and Planned Parenthood. In the United States there are about 70 national agencies, and it is estimated that there are about 100,000 local agencies. The older, larger, and more established of these agencies tend to have federal, state, and local divisions while smaller groups may only be local. In most communities a listing of these agencies can be found in the yellow and/or blue pages of the phone book under the heading "social services."

Although there is a great deal of variation in the actual services provided by voluntary agencies, the types of services provided can usually be classified under one of three headings

1. Providing educational materials and programs for both the public and health care providers.
2. Conducting research or providing grants for research.
3. Providing direct services to clients and their families.

As private, nonprofit, voluntary organizations these agencies have experienced a great deal more flexibility and freedom than many other parts of the health care system. This freedom has provided them with a great advantage as well as a source of criticism. Flexibility permits them to establish demonstration projects and experiment with new ideas. At the same time they can collect and spend a great deal of money with limited accountability. Nevertheless, these agencies have proven to be a vital part of the American health care system.

Though there are numerous organizations within the health care system, each of these organizations can be classified with the basic structure presented here. First, organizations are either private or governmental. If they are governmental, their classification is discussed in federal, state, or local terms. If they are private, they are classified as either profit or nonprofit. Overlapping this basic structure is a second structure. This second structure focuses on people and the roles they fill in the system. These roles can be divided into two basic types, those roles related to providing health care services and those related to receiving the services.

Health Care Providers

As one of the fastest growing industries in the United States, the health care system has become a major employer of an increasingly diverse group of workers. Three factors related to the growth of the health care system have encouraged both the increasing number and types of workers. First, increasing the size of a system requires not only more workers but also induces a need for administrators and planners. Second, the health care system is growing because of the increase in the types of effective services which it can provide. These services are the result of the knowledge explosion which in turn results in increased specialization. There are now, for example, not only more physicians than ever before, but also more types of physicians than ever before. A final factor, which is part of the knowledge explosion, is modern technology. Modern technology brings with it its own manpower requirements along with a need for workers who are able to apply the technology to patient care.

The confusing variety of providers or workers that results from the above factors encourages severe problems with communication and coordination within the health care system. To begin to deal with these problems nurses need—not a list of all possible workers—but a framework of analysis that can be applied to a variety of settings. The framework proposed here focuses on three questions

1. What type of service does the provider emphasize?
2. What degree and type of education is required for the provider?
3. Does the provider represent specialization in an identified area?

Specific activities a particular health care provider does can be referred to as a job description. However, in considering a large variety of providers, initial analysis begins on a more general level. Based on the services provided, health care workers can be divided into three groups

1. Those that emphasize provision of direct services to individuals and their families.
2. Those that emphasize support services to groups either in the community or the health care system.
3. Those that emphasize utilization of technology (See Table 13-5 for some examples).

These three groups provide a basis for discussing the emphasis of various health care jobs. Specific job descriptions can and do show interesting combinations across these groupings. For example, a physician may function as the administrator in a medical laboratory, thereby belonging in all three groupings.

You might be wondering why this information is important. Individuals within the three groups will have a different focus. They see different problems or even see the same problems in different ways. Nurses, as well as other health care providers, often function without any awareness of these differences and therefore cannot understand the source of some of their conflicts within the health care system.

A second factor, which adds to these conflicts of understanding these

TABLE 13-5
Examples of types of health care providers by emphasis of service provided

Emphasizes Direct Service	Emphasizes Support and/or Group Service	Emphasizes Technological Service
Ambulance Attendant	Environmentalist	Dialysis Technician
Dentist	Health System Analyst	Medical Computer Specialists
Dental Assistant	Hospital Administrator	Medical Laboratory Technician
Dietitian	Medical Librarian	Radiologic Technologist
Mental Health Aide	Medical Record Administrator	Respiratory Therapist
Nurse	School Health Educator	
Occupational Therapist	Unit Clerk	
Physical Therapist		
Physician		
Speech Pathologist		
Social Worker		

many roles, is the wide variations which exist in education and, in turn, status, self concept, and power among people who need to work and function closely. Note the differences which exist in years of education as well as the other factors between a physician who has finished his residency and a nurse's aide with an eighth-grade education. The same pattern of difference exists when a nurse with a PhD communicates with the same aide. Many times individuals are uncomfortable with this difference and the result is noncommunication. This discomfort and resulting self-imposed silence can do more to inhibit communication than actual differences in vocabulary level or comprehension.

A clear example of this problem occurred with Mrs. M., who was admitted to the local community hospital for surgery. Mrs. M was terrified if anything was placed over her mouth or nose. She was embarrassed to tell her doctor or her nurse but did gain enough courage to tell the nurse's aide. Neither the nurse, physician, or aide communicated about this problem. The reasons for not sharing information can be seen in the following mental dialogue:

Nurse or Doctor: I have already talked to Mrs. M. and have all the pertinent data; therefore, there is nothing significant an aide can tell me.

Nurse's Aide: They have already talked with the patient, so this must not be that important.

OR	OR
I know that I am supposed to collect all pertinent data, so I feel "dumb" when the aide points out something I don't know about a patient.	There is no use saying anything. Everyone will just act like I am wasting their time.

A final factor which adds to the complexity of understanding the roles of workers within the health care field is specialization. There are about 180 types of health care occupations if listed by primary title (e.g., physician). However, if secondary titles (alternative or specialties) are considered this increases to about 500 (French, 1979). For the physician alone there are 22 specialties recognized by the American Board of Medical Specialties (Somers & Somers, 1977). However, it doesn't stop there; there are also recognized subspecialties. For example, endocrinology, gastroenterology, and nephrology are a few examples of the recognized subspecialties of the specialty, internal medicine.

One effect of this growing, confusing variety of health care providers is the expansion in the numbers of professional organizations. The development of professional organizations has paralleled in many ways the development of labor unions. A professional organization is a formal organization that represents the views of a group of professional workers. Each organization has a written purpose and a set of goals. In a professional organization this statement reflects a concern with the needs of society; however, the concern will be stated in terms of the group represented. When a professional organization takes a position on an issue one must assume some degree of "vested interest." A good example of this is seen in the conflicting views of the American Nurses' Association and the American Medical Association on what method(s) of health insurance with which the government should be involved.

Taking a position on issues of concern to the profession is only one of the ways that a professional organization supports the beliefs and values of that profession. They may exert strong influence over the educational programs as well as the scope of professional practice. They do this by involvement in school accrediting programs and in the procedures utilized to obtain and maintain a state license to practice. The amount of influence professional organizations are able to exert varies greatly from one group to another. Some groups are well established and very influential in the health field, for example, the AMA. On the other hand, some groups are fairly new and represent a small specialty group of professionals. As the number of groups grow there has been an increase in the variety of formal opinions concerning health care within the health care field itself. The result is that the older, more established professional organizations are finding the need to adjust to a new variety of influences from a growing number of related professional organizations. These adjustments must be made when these organizations and the variety of health care workers they represent interact with their counterrole, the health care recipient.

Health Care Recipient

The final subsystem in the health care system's structure is the health care recipient. The recipient is the counterrole of the provider. He is the individual, family, or group who is receiving the services of the health care provider and is paying either directly or indirectly for those services.

Like all roles, the role of health care recipient has both rights and responsibilities. In the past the recipient role was a more passive role, but today's society is learning that for its own benefit and protection, the recipient must be more active in exercising both his rights and his responsibilities. The responsibilities of the recipient for his own health became clearer as society gained a better understanding of factors involved in the production of disease. One analysis by a group of American experts identified four contributing elements to the causes of death and disease (Table 13-6).

This analysis indicates that half of these elements are under the influence of individuals within their families. Or in other words

> Of the ten leading causes of death in the United States at least seven could be substantially reduced if persons at risk improved just five habits: diet, smoking, lack of exercise, alcohol abuse, and use of antihypertensive medications. (*Healthy People*, 1979, p. 14)

This does not mean that health care providers have no responsibility with these 50 percent of the problems. In fact, it means providers have a great deal of responsibility to find specific and realistic methods of prevention and health education. This search for methods should be focused on those behaviors that have already been related to improved health (see Table 13-7).

TABLE 13-6
Contributing elements to death and disease in America by percent

Contributing Element	Percentage
Inadequacies of existing health care system	10
Behavioral factors or unhealthy life style	50
Environmental factors	20
Human biological factors	20

From: U.S. Department of Health, Education, and Welfare. *Healthy People: The Surgeon General's Report on Health Promotion and Disease Prevention.* Washington, D.C.: U.S. Public Health Service, 1979, pp. 8-9.

TABLE 13-7
Behaviors related to improved health

Elimination of cigarette smoking
Reduction of alcohol misuse
Moderate dietary change to reduce intake of excess calories, fat, salt, and sugar
Periodic screening for major disorders such as hypertension and certain cancers
Adherence to speed laws and use of seat belts
Adequate exercise

From: U.S. Department of Health, Education, and Welfare. *Healthy People: The Surgeon General's Report on Health Promotion and Disease Prevention.* Washington, DC: U.S. Public Health Service, 1979.

Though the health care provider is responsible for providing this information to recipients, the recipient maintains the responsibility for his own behavior. Health care providers must recognize that they cannot be effective if they attempt to usurp the responsibility of the recipient for his own behavior.

As society has become more aware of recipient responsibilities, it has also become more aware of recipient rights. This awareness has been demonstrated both in the general press as well as in the professional literature. In reviewing recipient rights the nurses must realize that some key words have been used interchangeably, yet do not have the same meaning. Three of these key words are health, health care, and medical care. Medical care is one part of health care, that part provided by the physician. Health care is any service provided to a recipient by a health care provider. Health is the state of being of that recipient. Providing for the right to medical care does not ensure recipients of health care. On the other hand, providing for the right to health care does not ensure health. In discussing the issues related to recipient rights, it is important that these points not be confused.

With the discussion related to recipient rights, three sets of rights are evolving. The first set of rights relates to the rights of recipients who are clients within the health care system. The "Patient's Bill of Rights" (see Table 13-8) is a good example of this type of rights (Quinn & Somers, 1974). Controversy around this set of rights deals with the issue of control. For example, does a client have the right to read the medical records concerning himself?

The second set of rights deals with the rights of society for services related to health. For example, do clients have the right to have a physician available to them? Controversy around this set of rights deals with the issue of money. Who is responsible for paying for these services? National health insurance is an example of this issue.

The final set of rights evolving relates to the rights of individuals with health handicaps within the society. For example, what are the rights of an individual with a handicap to an education or to a job? Again, the issue in this controversy is money. How much should society pay and in what form to insure these rights? This whole area of recipient rights is an evolving, controver-

TABLE 13-8
Patient's Bill of Rights

The American Hospital Association presents a Patient's Bill of Rights with the expectation that observance of these rights will contribute to more effective patient care and greater satisfaction for the patient, his physician, and the hospital organization. Further, the Association presents these rights in the expectation that they will be supported by the hospital on behalf of its patients, as an integral part of the healing process. It is recognized that a personal relationship between the physician and the patient is essential for the provision of proper medical care. The traditional physician-patient relationship takes on a new dimension when care is rendered within an organizational structure. Legal precedent has established that the institution itself also has a responsibility to the patient. It is in recognition of these factors that these rights are affirmed.

1. The patient has the right to considerate and respectful care.

2. The patient has the right to obtain from his physician complete current information concerning his diagnosis, treatment, and prognosis in terms the patient can be reasonably expected to understand. When it is not medically advisable to give such information to the patient, the information should be made available to an appropriate person in his behalf. He has the right to know, by name, the physician responsible for coordinating his care.

3. The patient has the right to receive from his physician information necessary to give informed consent prior to the start of any procedure and/or treatment. Except in emergencies, such information for informed consent should include but not necessarily be limited to the specific procedure and/or treatment, the medically significant risks involved, and the probable duration of incapacitation. Where medically significant alternatives for care or treatment exist, or when the patient requests information concerning medical alternatives, the patient has the right to such information. The patient also has the right to know the name of the person responsible for the procedures and/or treatment.

4. The patient has the right to refuse treatment to the extent permitted by law and to be informed of the medical consequences of his action.

5. The patient has the right to every consideration of his privacy concerning his own medical care program. Case discussion, consultation, examination, and treatment are confidential and should be conducted discreetly. Those not directly involved in his care must have the permission of the patient to be present.

6. The patient has the right to expect that all communications and records pertaining to his care should be treated as confidential.

7. The patient has the right to expect that within its capacity a hospital must make reasonable response to the request of a patient for services. The hospital must provide evaluation, service, or referral as indicated by the urgency of the case. When medically permissible, a patient may be transferred to another facility only after he has received complete information and explanation concerning the needs for and alternatives to such a transfer. The institution to which the patient is to be transferred must first have accepted the patient for transfer.

8. The patient has the right to obtain information as to any relationship of his hospital to other health care and education institutions insofar as his care is concerned. The patient has the right to obtain information as to the existence of any professional relationships among individuals, by name, who are treating him.

9. The patient has the right to be advised if the hospital proposes to engage in or perform human experimentation affecting his care or treatment. The patient has the right to refuse to participate in such research projects.

10. The patient has the right to expect reasonable continuity of care. He has the right to know in advance what appointment times and physicians are available and where. The patient has the right to expect that the hospital will provide a mechanism whereby he is informed by his physician or a delegate of the physician of the patient's continuing health care requirements following discharge.

11. The patient has the right to examine and receive an explanation of his bill regardless of source of payment.

TABLE 13-8 (Cont.)

12. The patient has the right to know what hospital rules and regulations apply to his conduct as a patient. No catalog of rights can guarantee for the patient the kind of treatment he has a right to expect. A hospital has many functions to perform, including the prevention and treatment of disease, the education of both health professionals and patients, and the conduct of clinical research. All these activities must be conducted with an overriding concern for the patient, and, above all, the recognition of his dignity as a human being. Success in achieving this recognition assures success in the defense of the rights of the patient.

Reprinted with the permission of the American Hospital Association, copyright 1972.

sial area in which nurses will play an active and important role in the coming years.

For the purposes of discussion the structure of the American health care system was divided into four substructures. As with all open systems, these substructures must be viewed as the functioning whole for analysis to be accurate. The open system is always more than the sum of the subsystems. This interaction of the subsystems is most clearly seen when one analyzes the functioning of the whole system.

FUNCTION OF THE HEALTH CARE SYSTEM

As an open system the functioning of the American health care system can be analyzed in terms of input, throughput, and output. The inputs into the system consist of money, knowledge, and skill. The throughputs are the activities or processes which utilize the inputs. Outputs are the results that the health care system has on society.

System Inputs

Both the health care provider and the health care recipient bring to the health care system knowledge and skill about health and illness. As indicated, health care workers are reasonably well prepared to perform their own particular functions. What can interfere with their effectiveness is their lack of knowledge about the whole system and, in turn, their lack of knowledge about other practitioners in the system. A major factor in perpetuating this weakness is that most, if not all, of the educational preparation of health care workers occurs in a segregated environment. There are very few, if any, courses in the country where health care students are integrated, i. e., taking the same courses and covering content and concepts needed by all health care providers.

Besides knowledge and skill, money is also an input into the health care system. In the case of the American health care system it is an increasingly large amount of money (see Table 13-9). The money which is spent on the

TABLE 13-9
Health care costs in the United States

Year	Total Spent in Billions of Dollars	Average Spent per Person in Dollars	Percent of Gross National Product
1935	$ 3.6	$ 22.65	4.0
1965	43.0	217.42	6.2
1975	131.0	604.57	8.5
1977	170.0	768.77	9.0
1980	223.0	855.00	9.2
1981	256.0	975.00	9.4

From: Gibson, R. M., 1979; Waldo, D., 1981.

health care system comes from four basic sources: (1) private insurance, (2) direct payment for individual services, (3) federal government, (4) state and local government.

The percentage of the total cost covered by these sources has been changing since the 1930s (see Table 13-10). Two factors have had the greatest effect in producing these changes. The first factor was the introduction of private insurance plans, especially since these have become in many cases a fringe benefit of employment. The second was the introduction of Medicare and Medicaid in 1965. The overall result was an increase in the percent of health care cost covered by the federal government and private insurance. Since much of the health care costs are covered through insurance programs, nurses are increasingly interested in direct payment for services via third party payment. (See Table 13-11 for a summary of types of insurance.)

A third factor is currently evolving which will also influence the percentage of payment from these various sources. In April 1983, President Ronald Reagan signed into law H.R. 1900 (P.L. 98-21). This law, which became effective October 1, 1983, changes the way the government pays for hospitalized Medicare patients. The provisions of the law apply mainly to

TABLE 13-10
Changes in source of payments for personal health care expenditures

Source of Payment	Change in Percentage of Total Cost Covered
Federal government	Steady and significant increase starting in 1965
State and local governments	No significant change
Private insurance	Slow steady increase starting in 1930s
Direct payment	Decrease since 1930 Decrease since 1965

From: Jensen, L. E., 1978, p. 1-26.

TABLE 13-11
Summary of insurance types

GOVERNMENT INSURANCE

Medicare—is a program of federal governmental insurance administered through the Social Security Administration for individuals over 65 years of age and covered by Social Security. This insurance has two parts: Part A is required and pays mainly for the setting in which care is delivered. It is similar to Blue Cross. Plan B is voluntary and pays for the physician and other related costs. It is similar to Blue Shield.

Medicaid—is a joint federal and state governmental insurance program set up to cover health care costs of the poor. The federal government matches state funds and provides general regulation. Each participating state writes the specific regulations of that state. The result is a different program in each state.

PRIVATE NONPROFIT INSURANCE

Blue Cross—is a nonprofit private health care insurance offering a variety of programs set up mainly to cover health care costs related to hospitalization costs. Blue Cross trademark is owned by the American Hospital Association. Hospital administrators make up the majority of the directors in almost all the seventy-four Blue Cross Plans.

Blue Shield—is a nonprofit private health care insurance offering a variety of programs set up mainly to cover certain physician costs. The majority of the covered costs are associated with hospitalization (e.g., surgery). The relationship of Blue Shield and the American Medical Association is similar to the Blue Cross Plans and the American Hospital Association.

PRIVATE FOR PROFIT INSURANCE

Commercial—is made up of a large number of private, profit-making insurance companies. Their rates and coverage vary greatly as well as their quality. Some are outright frauds, though others offer an important alternative for services.

PRIVATE SERVICE AND INSURANCE COMBINED

Health Maintenance Organization—is an organization which combines the services of the insurance carrier and health care provider. The recipient prepays a set fee and is guaranteed he will be provided as needed with health care services by the organization.

---

acute care hospitals and are to be phased in over a four-year period. This new method of payment establishes a prospective payment system based on a diagnosis related group. In other words, the payment that a hospital will receive for providing care is predetermined and is based on the DRG of each patient. If the hospital provides care for less than the predetermined amount, the hospital may keep the difference. If on the other hand, it costs the hospital more, the hospital is expected to pick up the extra costs. It is believed a prospective system such as this will provide an incentive for cost containment. But just what techniques hospitals utilize in holding down costs is of concern to many. The full effects of this new system are not yet known. How prospective payment based on DRG's will reverberate throughout the health care system is yet to be determined.

Throughput Activities

Since a lot of money is taken into the health care system from a variety of sources the next question becomes, for what? Over 80 percent of the money is

264 SELECTED CONCEPTS UTILIZED IN NURSING

spent for personal health care costs. Hospitalization comprises the largest proportion of this money (see Figure 13-1). This is of special significance to nurses since the majority of nurses work in hospitals. Current accounting methods frequently leave hospital administrations with no accurate information concerning what nurses add to the efficiency of the organization nor what they cost the organization. This can be unfair to both sides when salaries are negotiated.

Health care activities can be analyzed not only in terms of cost but also in terms of services provided. Services in the health care system are divided into three levels. It should be noted that these levels of care refer to care within the health care system. They do not refer to levels of nursing care or levels of prevention. The first level is referred to as primary care. Primary care provides for prevention and for care related to most routine illnesses.

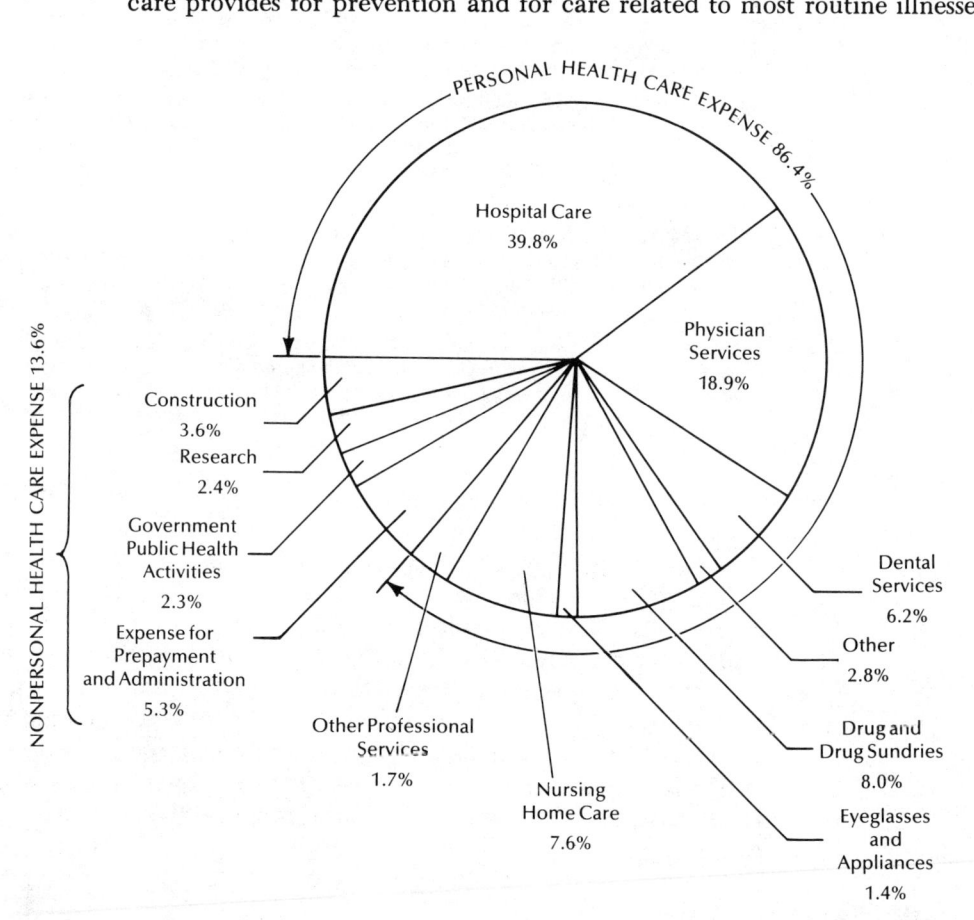

Figure 13-1 How Health Care Money Is Spent (1976). (From: Somers, A. R., and Somers, H. M., *Health and Health Care: Policies in Perspective.* Germantown, MD: Aspen Systems Corporation, 1977, p. 509.)

These providers are usually referred to as generalists. They are in reality a unique type of specialist who focuses on the whole client. Some common examples of primary providers are pediatricians, family nurse practitioners, and family physicians.

Primary level of care is given in a variety of settings such as well-baby clinics, doctors' offices, neighborhood health centers, and hospital outpatient departments. Rarely is hospitalization required. Ideally, most ill clients would be seen first in one of these settings by a primary care provider then referred to the appropriate specialist if necessary. At this point the client enters the secondary level of the health care system.

Secondary level of care provides for the treatment of specific disease problems. These providers who see the patient only for a specific illness tend to have a narrow perspective of the client. Usually secondary care is provided in the specialist's office, and in general or community hospitals.

Though all people should have available the services of a primary care provider and many patients will at some point benefit from the services of a specialist, only a limited number of patients will require tertiary care. Tertiary care is provided by "superspecialists" who have an understanding of complex medical technology, are highly skilled in their specialty, and are concerned with rare and complex medical conditions (Rosser & Massberg, 1977, p. 85). The provisions of tertiary care by these superspecialists occur only in large medical centers.

System Outputs

Although there is no question the health care system has an effect on the American society, what specific effect it has is open to great debate. The problem is a lack of measurement techniques and instruments. In Chapter 12 on health it is pointed out that there are no current techniques for measuring health. Furthermore there is no general agreement that health is what one would want to measure. The need for criteria and for measuring techniques of health care output has only lately been identified.

Even though the concept of measuring the health care outputs of the total system is new, there are some indications of what effect the system has on society. Measures of mortality, morbidity, and life expectancy indicate that the American health care system is producing an improved level of health. Life expectancy has been increasing as death rates for most of the major causes of disease have been decreasing.

Although there is some question whether these results are due to the health care system or other factors in society, a closer look at these statistics also indicate there are problems. Several countries experience a longer life expectancy than the United States. Certain populations within the United States have a life expectancy much lower than the national norms.

Society's expression of satisfaction and/or dissatisfaction is another indication of what effects the health care system has. Demand for health care has been increasing. This would indicate some degree of satisfaction since people logically would not increase demand for services they see as of little or no value. On the other hand, the increase in malpractice suits would indicate people are not always satisfied with the services they receive. Dissatisfactions have been expressed about the availability of health care, the quality of the care, and the cost of the care. These kinds of outputs are producing feedback to the system and pressuring the health care system as it responds to the pressure from society.

SUMMARY

This chapter has presented the American health care system as an open system through an analysis of the purposes, structure, and functions of that system. The initial purpose of the health care system was custodial care. Today, there are four evolving purposes: prevention, treatment, rehabilitation, and custodial care. The health care system attempts to meet these purposes in a continuously changing structure. This structure consists of four types of subsystems: governmental and nongovernmental agencies, health care recipients, and providers.

Finally the American health care system functions within this structure. Money, knowledge, and skills are taken into the system; these are utilized in the provision of health care services. The result is a change in the health status of the American society. Some key points to remember are

1. The system is in a constant state of change from pressures within the system and from environmental pressures.
2. The health care system functions as a whole. Changes in any part produce changes throughout the system.
3. The purposes of the health care system are evolving as a result of new knowledge and skills.
4. The government has become increasingly involved in all aspects of health care.
5. Along with a recognition of recipient rights has come a recognition of recipient responsibility.

REFERENCES

Bobula, J. D., and Freshnock, L. J. "The Supply of Medical Services and the Cost of Medical Care." In *National Commission on the Cost of Medical Care 1976–1977 Vol III, Literature Review and Data Base.* Monroe, WI: American Medical Association, 1978.

Bower, F. L., and Bevis, E. O. *Fundamentals of Nursing Practice: Concepts, Roles and Functions.* St. Louis: The C. V. Mosby Co., 1979.

Brown, J., and Upton, H. *The Politics of Health Care*. Cambridge, MA: Ballinger Publishing Co., 1978.

Chesari, F., Nakamura, R., and Thorup, L. *The Consumers Guide to Health Care*. Boston: Little, Brown and Co., 1976.

Curtin, L. "Determining Costs of Nursing Services per DRG." *Nursing Management* 14 (4) [1983]: 16-20.

Editors of Consumer Reports. *The Medicine Show*. Revised edition. Mount Vernon, NY: Consumers Union, 1974.

Freeman, H., Levine, S., and Reeder, L. G. *Handbook of Medical Sociology*. 3rd ed. Englewood Cliffs, NJ: Prentice-Hall, Inc., 1979.

French, R. M. *Dynamics of Health Care*. 3rd ed. New York: McGraw-Hill Co., 1979.

Gibson, R. M. "National Health Expenditures, 1978." *Health Care Financing Review* 1 (1) [1979]: 1-37.

Jenson, L. "Trends in Health Care Costs and Prices." In *National Commission on the Cost of Medical Care, 1976-1977. Vol. II. Report of Presentations Before the Commission*. Monroe, WI: American Medical Association, 1978.

Jonas, S. *Health Care Delivery in the United States*. 2nd ed. New York: Springer Publishing Co., 1981.

Judd, L. *A Supplement to a Handbook for Consumer Participation in Health Care Planning*. Chicago: Blue Cross Association, 1979.

Judd, L., and McEwan, J. *A Handbook for Consumer Participation in Health Care Planning*. Chicago: Blue Cross Association, 1977.

Iglehart, J. K. "Health Policy Report." *The New England Journal of Medicine* 307 (20) [1982]: 1288-1292.

Leahy, K. M., Cobb, M., and Jones, M. C. *Community Health Nursing*. 3rd ed. New York: McGraw-Hill Co., 1977.

Leopold, J., and Langwell, K. M. "The Demand for Health Care with Special Emphasis on Cost Containment: A Review of the Literature and Data Base." In *Literature Reviews and Data Base* by National Commission on the Cost of Medical Care. Monroe, WI: American Medical Association, 1978.

National Commission on the Cost of Medical Care, 1976-1977. *Volume I: Final Reports of the Full Commission. 1977. Volume II: Report of Presentations Before the Commission, 1978. Volume III: Literature Reviews and Data Base, 1978.* Monroe, WI: American Medical Association, 1978.

Navarro, V., ed. *Health and Medical Care in the U.S.: A Critical Analysis*. Farmingdale, NY: Baywood Publishing Co., 1975.

Newhouse, J. P. *The Economics of Medical Care: A Policy Perspective*. Reading, MS: Addison-Wesley Publishing Co., 1978.

Parson, T. "Definitions of Health and Illness in the Light of American Values and Social Structure." In *Patients, Physicians and Illness*, edited by E. G. Jaco. New York: The Free Press of Glencoe, 1959.

Quinn, N., and Somers, A. "The Patient's Bill of Rights: A Significant Aspect of the Consumer Revolution." *Nursing Outlook* 22 (4) [1974]: 240-244.

Rosser, J., and Massberg, H. *An Analysis of Health Care Delivery*. New York: John Wiley & Sons, 1977.

Shaffer, F. A. "DRG's: History and Overview." *Nursing & Health Care* 4 (1983): 388–396.

Shaheen, P. "National Health Care: A Humanitarian Approach." *Nursing Outlook* 29 (1981): 358–363.

Somers, A. R., and Somers, H. M. *Health and Health Care: Policies in Perspective.* Germantown, MD: Aspen Systems Corporation, 1977.

U.S. Department of Health, Education and Welfare. *Healthy People: The Surgeon General's Report on Health Promotion and Disease Prevention.* Washington, DC: U.S. Public Health Service, 1979 (Pub. No. 79-55071).

U.S. Department of Health, Education and Welfare. *Health of the Disadvantaged Chart Book.* Washington, DC: U.S. Public Health Service, 1977 (Pub. No. HRA 77-628).

United States Government Manual, 1980-1981. Washington, D.C.: Office of the Federal Registrar, National Archives and Records Service, General Services Administration, 1980.

Waldo, D. "National Health Expenditures and Related Measures." *Health Care Financing Trends* 2 (3) [1981]: 1–7.

VerSteeg, D. F., and Croog, S. H. "Hospitals and Related Health Care Delivery Settings." In *Handbook of Medical Sociology*, edited by Freeman, H., Levine, S., and Reeder, L. 3rd ed. Englewood Cliffs, NJ: Prentice-Hall, Inc., 1979.

14

Nursing's future

During his high school years, Mark became interested in nursing. He knew several nurses and had spoken with them about the nursing profession at different times. One of his neighbors, Mrs. Johnson, was a night nurse and usually pulled into her driveway at the time Mark started for school. They often exchanged a few words about nursing; Mark talking about speakers' topics he had heard at the future nurses' club and Mrs. Johnson reflecting on where she thought nursing was heading. Both agreed that nursing was changing but what it would be like by the year 2000 was a mystery.

How can nurses learn to look ahead and gain a direction for the future? What can be expected in the upcoming years? One way to answer this question is to examine relationships among prior events and attempt to make projections based on identified patterns of activity and outcomes. Activities internal to nursing relate to those outside the profession and external events relate back to nursing. Each activity or event affects the other. What does this actually mean? Basically, this means you identify great influencing factors and then identify how these factors are influencing nursing and are being influenced by nursing. For example, one of the great influencing factors in today's world is an expanded knowledge base. This factor is in turn influenced by a second factor, limited resources. Nursing is experiencing an increase in knowledge base and is contributing to the growth of knowledge. How nurses go about the job of organizing this information and utilizing the knowledge is influenced by limited resources. Limited resources in turn set the direction for expanded knowledge, i.e., research.

Another important factor that also affects nursing is the accelerated rate of change in today's world. Many impacts and discontinuities are felt, and there is a pervasive feeling of needing to catch up. One of the more visible examples of this feeling occurs with computer skills, especially within the adult population. Among the diversity of nurses there has been a surge of work toward computer literacy, of being able to use computers effectively in their daily work.

To deal with factors such as vast knowledge, limited resources, and rapid change, nurses are helped by theories that relate to the state of man. The six theories presented earlier in this book provide a rational, systematic way for you to view man, his health, and his environments. The use of theories helps you gain a sense of how to proceed with health problems and matters of living. Theories also assist in promoting selected predictions of outcomes and, in this way, help to guide your thinking for future events. This is exemplified through information concerning societal trends, economic pressures, education, and technological advances.

At the completion of this chapter the reader will be able to

1. State social and economic influences relating to health needs and health care that will impact on nursing's future.
2. Identify trends in education that are exerting effects on the profession of nursing.
3. Examine technological advances that are influencing man, health, and nursing.
4. Identify professional practice issues impacting on nursing's future.
5. Describe ways to make projections based on past and present events.

SOCIETAL TRENDS

Societal changes can be classified into two types. There are those changes that are more objective in nature. These changes are the ones we can measure with current instruments. For example, we can count the number of children born in a year or we can calculate the average age of the population. Two major objective societal trends are aging and rate of chronic illness. There are also a group of societal changes that are not so easily measured but are more experiential in nature. These changes are reflected by changing values, beliefs, and expectations. Although these changes are not easily measured, their influence can be clearly seen in individual life styles.

Aging

Population and community shifts are being seen across the United States. Not only are there more individuals over sixty-five but also more over seventy-five and eighty. In addition, there are 147 women for every 100 men over age sixty-five. Population trends demonstrate steady increases in the percentage of the population over sixty-five (see Table 14-1). The estimated acceleration in the number of elderly people expected to occur after the year 2010 reflects the baby boom, which extended from approximately 1945 to 1960. Health manpower will have to accommodate for the changing numbers and special health needs within this population.

TABLE 14-1
Percent of the population over 65 (1900-2040)

Year	Percentage of Population
1900	4
1920	5
1940	6
1960	9
1980	11.5*
2000	12*
2020	14*
2040	16*

*Projected data.
From: Weller, R. H., and Bouvier, L. F. *Population: Demography and Policy.* New York: St. Martin's Press, 1981, p. 266.

As an individual ages, each of his dimensions demonstrates the cumulative effects of stressors encountered over the years. These changes can be viewed on an individual level. For example, an older person is more likely to have experienced losses through the death of loved ones. The changes of aging can also be viewed on the community level. Note the increasing rate of chronic illness as the average age of the population increases. This relationship is just one demonstration that influencing factors or trends do not exist in isolation, but interact as they operate.

Chronic Illness

The elderly who are more prone to develop chronic illnesses, such as heart disease, stroke, emphysema, and cancer, need prolonged health care for their illnesses. This care is often provided in the home or in ambulatory centers close to home. When no family member remains to assist in the care, more institutional resources are required. At present in the United States, about 80 percent of all health resources are used for chronic disease services and research (Cluff, 1981).

An additional concern for the elderly comes from environmental toxins and thermal extremes. Toxins have been increasingly discovered in the air, water, soil, and common materials used around the home. The older person is more vulnerable to air pollution, exposure to cold temperatures, and the diversity of toxic materials. This vulnerability can be compounded by the variety of medications that might be needed in the treatment of chronic illness. Although the older person is more apt to acquire chronic diseases, younger persons now able to survive such health problems as serious congenital defects or infectious diseases are displaying conditions requiring long-term care. Nursing must prepare practitioners to work competently in this complex area of long-term care.

Societal Expectations

Economics, the political arena, and the increasing educational level, among other factors, have produced changes in societal expectations and the behaviors of its members. One clear example of this change in society is demonstrated by diverse role changes for men and women. Some so-called traditional roles have become fluid, with counterpart roles for both sexes such as housewife-househusband. More men have taken on roles formerly assumed by women and vice versa. These factors are interacting to produce changes in who applies for admission to schools of nursing. In the past the great majority of applicants were white females, ages eighteen to twenty-two. Today we are seeing increasing numbers of men, older students, students of various ethnic backgrounds, and second degree students. These students come with different educational preparation, value systems, and expectations of the nursing schools and the profession. The increasing variety of backgrounds provides nursing with a challenge and a reward. The challenge is to adjust the educational program to meet the needs of these students and to adjust the practice world for more knowledgeable, assertive practitioners.

The reward is in the knowledge, values, and skills the students bring with them. These students will be of major value as nursing deals with another societal trend originating from changing values: consumerism.

Consumerism

A fourth major social trend is seen in consumer activity. Recipients of all types of health services are making their ideas, requests, and complaints known. A number of factors have led to the consumer movement. The general increase in the educational level of the public is considered a major factor. Part of this comes from the overall educational system and part is a result of communication through mass media—mostly TV, radio, and news publications. As a result, consumers are not only more knowledgeable about health, but are placing a higher value on good health.

What indicators exist that the consumerism trend will continue? An important indicator comes from the many consumer-oriented messages. Not only are goods and services reported in general, but health information provided by editors, experts, clients, and their families has increased substantially. Television newscasts often include a health spot. Popular magazines and newspapers frequently emphasize health topics. Some libraries now employ a nurse to handle calls for health information. Health education centers have begun operating dial-access systems for audiotaped health messages designed to handle questions frequently raised.

In addition to the increase in public information access through mass media, telephone systems, and library networks, the presence of consumer support groups in increasing numbers is an indication of the strength of consumerism. Supportive consumer organizations permit an exchange of views and discussions about complaints. They serve as an escape valve and can prevent an explosive build-up from troubled consumers. Nursing needs to keep alert to consumerism and the dynamics involved in order to provide leadership in informing and instructing the public about health topics.

ECONOMIC PRESSURES

General economic factors and health care costs share a continuing relationship. With every pressure experienced in the overall economy, there is pressure felt in health care costs. Energy bills are higher, food prices have increased, and the cost of materials has risen sharply. Along with these rising costs are pockets of high unemployment; bankruptcy, especially of smaller companies; and high interest rates for home mortgages and other loans. When people are unemployed and without insurance coverage they may elect to postpone nonessential health care normally covered by insurance. This postponement results in a decreased demand for care, with some empty hospital beds and reduced waiting time to see physicians and dentists.

Although individuals have fewer resources to spend on health care, the cost of health care continues to increase at an alarming rate. In an attempt to control those costs, Medicare payments have recently become based on diagnostic related groups instead of the previous retrospective cost-based system. With DRG's just beginning, the situation is less familiar and less fixed.

There has also been a reduction in other federally funded health care programs. Fewer funds have been available through the National Institutes of Health for research purposes. Grant writing for federal funds has become increasingly competitive. Distributing available funds to the most useful services and research projects has been a challenging task.

Each of these economic problems and trends exerts an influence on the others. The complexity and intricacy of attempts to balance and adjust these problems foretells a continued struggle with them in the decades ahead.

While changes bring a certain amount of instability, they also bring opportunities to try new approaches to health care. For example, with fewer medical resources coming into the hospital system, increased outputs are needed, such as the early discharge of patients. Patients and their families will need more instruction to provide care after discharge. As more patients go home on IV's, liquid diets, nasogastric tubes, in-dwelling catheters, or other equipment requiring special knowledge, family members will need to be taught acute care procedures prior to the patient's discharge. Nursing needs to stay abreast of the situation to facilitate the highest quality care.

Nurse educators and researchers will have much to examine and to make recommendations about. With funding sources not as readily available for research, innovative problem solving will need to be done. Interdisciplinary teams and intradiscipline networking may offer help.

EDUCATIONAL TRENDS

Our educational system is one component of society that has and will continue to influence nursing. Societal trends that influence the educational system, as well as educational trends themselves, will impact on faculty, students, and the educational process. This in turn will impact on nursing education and practice.

Environment

Environmental influences are demonstrated in terms such as retrenchment, cost containment, unionism, and quality. In one way education has been bursting at the seams and in another way it is retrenching. There has been a vast growth in knowledge and in faster ways to store and access that knowledge. The general population has acquired greater knowledge from formal and informal means, primarily television. Now with abundant computers, another large educational wave is being seen. At the same time, due to lowered birth rates, enrollment in schools at all levels has been declining. This has caused a number of schools to close, teacher ranks to decrease, and subject matter to be prioritized.

While the educational system is contracting, the cost of education continues to increase. Questions regarding what is essential content and what should public schools be responsible for teaching, are being asked. Issues of cost versus quality are current headlines in the media. These headlines are reflecting a movement that has been termed "Back to Basics." This trend began in elementary and secondary schools and is now seen in all levels of education. Although quality nursing education has always been expensive, the question of how many schools are needed and what they should teach is becoming a major issue as we move into a period of potential nursing surplus. As environmental trends influence educational systems, the characteristics of students moving from one educational system to another also change.

Students

Since the 1960s, the educational preparation of high school students for the experience of higher education has been interpreted as decreasing. One commonly cited evidence of decreasing quality in early education has been noted in reading problems. At the same time, the *percentage* of high school graduates entering higher education has been increasing. Today higher education stands at a crossroads with conflicting pressures on which way to turn. As the potential student population decreases, pressure is exerted on institutions of higher learning to decrease admission criteria. However, a conflicting pressure is being exerted to maintain the quality of the educational programs. One response to the decreasing population pool has been to recruit from a diverse body of potential students. For example, in nursing there has been increased activity in recruiting minorities, encouraging RN's to return for more education, and recruiting second degree students. One clear implication of these trends for nursing is the potential for a decreasing number of nursing students.

Faculty

Retrenchment in education has also had an impact on the faculty. As educational systems contract there is decreased need for the numbers of educators. As a result, the average age of faculty is increasing. Individuals within the system have limited opportunities for promotion or transfer to other institutions. New faculty are recruited less frequently and new ideas are not developed or crossfertilized as thoroughly. Educational institutions that do not deal effectively with these trends will experience a stagnant faculty. This has special significance in nursing, which is dependent on new educational ideas but also on faculty with current practice skills.

If nursing fails to deal effectively with these trends (environment, student, and faculty), the quality of the graduates in nursing will also change. We will then probably see increasing consumer complaints about the quality of nursing care received and more comments such as, "Where are the caring, concerned nurses?"

Nursing

While educational trends influence how we educate nurses and, in turn, nursing practice, changes in the nursing role also have an impact on how nurses are educated. Two major changes in the nursing role that are influencing nursing education are specialization and consumer education.

Specialization is the direct result of the knowledge explosion. While specialization is blamed for much of the fragmentation of health services, it has also been recognized as necessary for in-depth work in a particular field. As a discipline's knowledge base grows, it becomes more difficult to remain a generalist, to continue to be in touch with all aspects of the profession. At the turn of the century, there were just a few nursing journals to help disseminate nursing knowledge. Today there are many dozens of journals, a number of which are in specialty areas. There is great interest among specialty nurses to focus on narrower subdivisions of information involving patients and their health. The question usually raised is, How much can one person learn about everything there is to know in nursing? With continued biomedical technological advances and increased nursing research, knowledge will continue to grow.

In recent years along with interest in specialty education, there has also been a movement toward family health practices by nurses. These two phenomena seem to be at opposite poles, yet family practice requiring more general knowledge is accepted as a specialty area, too. Adult health practitioners have moved into family practices in some cases. Psychiatric mental health practitioners have also developed family practices. These signs point the way for further work in family health. Research relating to family practices by various practitioners and community health nurses will be studied by nurses carefully, especially in light of the prevailing interest in primary prevention. Although specialization produces a narrow area of practice, all nursing practice areas will still have some common elements to their roles. One of these common elements is the teaching role.

Given complaints about fragmented information, the possibilities of patients being discharged earlier, and the receptivity of the public to know about their health, the role of teacher in nursing continues to evolve as important. In some institutions all the nurses on staff are expected to teach patients and are oriented through in-service education means. Other institutions have emphasized the teaching role of a specialist nurse whose role involves patient education. No matter which way institutions structure patient teaching in the future, the need for teaching will exist and nurses will need to have a foundation of teaching learning theory in order to practice. In addition, nurses of the future will need to be prepared to work with educational technology in carrying out their teaching responsibilities.

Technological changes will continue, some with amazing speed. The equipment that nurses are often now called upon to interact with is highly sophisticated. If nurses are to instruct patients about the equipment, they need to have a thorough grounding beforehand. Computer-assisted video instruction programs or in-house cable television may become routine ways of offering patient education in hospitals and other health settings. Standing microcomputers or minicomputers may be interfaced with home television sets thereby providing health education programs in the home. A video phone system may permit dialing up prerecorded topics on videotape, much as audiotapes are used today.

TECHNOLOGICAL ADVANCES

Predicting future technological advances and their influences begins by looking back to the beginning of technological change, which resides in the development of scientific thought. Many efforts in science have served as building blocks for technological applications over the centuries. In the area of health care, noticeable advances relate to World War II and subsequent periods. Today evidence of technological influence can be seen frequently in health settings. Hospitals are primary examples of this phenomenon. Anyone who has been in a hospital lately is well aware of the impact of technology on health care. A commonly encountered scene is a viewing screen with a keyboard. In addition, various instrumentation systems have been developed to provide precise data indicating the slightest changes in the patient's condition. It is a challenge to consider how nurses can be prepared to meet growing technological demands for tomorrow's work environment. Let us look at significant influences of technology on nursing education.

Influences on Nursing Education

The first and most important influence of technological advances on nursing education is that technology raises some serious questions. How can the nursing student be prepared to provide competent nursing care in a technical environment? What does the nurse need to know and how can it best be learned? These and similar questions just scratch the surface when attempting to determine the task of present-day nursing schools that are preparing students for future responsibilities. There are no simple answers. Though nursing education must introduce the student to computers and provide a frame of reference for their use, it is unrealistic and unnecessary to think that a student can be prepared for all particulars of electronic hardware. Innovations in technology are happening so fast that by the time the student has graduated, the equipment may have a whole new look or a number of different functions. A certain amount of instruction will come from in-service programs by the institution giving care. In instances of new equipment, the vendor may be expected to provide instructions. There will have to be various approaches to assist nurses in upgrading technological competence.

The second major influence is felt in the process of education. Nursing education is beginning to change quite a bit due to automation. Computer-driven programs have been designed to offer instruction, for example, through patient data-base simulations. Computers also enable rapid literature searches, statistical analyses, text processing, and management tasks. How much programming knowledge is needed by nurses will vary according to their interests and work responsibilities. Figure 14-1 shows different ways which nurses may choose to go in acquiring levels of computer knowledge.

A beginning level of computer knowledge results from operating existing computer software programs. No matter the brand of equipment or program, the concepts of logging in, issuing a password, and running a program remain similar. Once the nurse has executed a program on one system, applying the knowledge to another system can often be tackled with success. The second level of computer knowledge involves beginning programming skills. You learn how to write an introductory program and input it on a

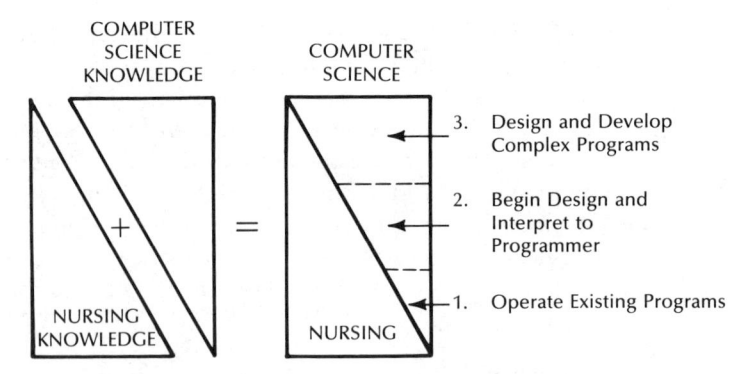

Figure 14-1 Three Levels of Computer Knowledge.

keyboard. To prepare the program, some knowledge of flowcharting is needed. You may be exposed to the word *algorithm*, which means a series of predetermined steps through decision points. In flowcharting the logic of the computer program, algorithms begin to evolve. Although some have opposed the idea of algorithms, stating they go against intuitive approaches which are part of a discipline, algorithms are credited with organizing information clearly. This is an important factor in these years of expanding information. The third level of computer knowledge is in-depth and includes an ability to design and program a complex computer job. At this point you may have learned a number of computer languages and would be well acquainted with which language would fit a given purpose best.

Once you have acquired computer literacy, you can read and interpret information and use the functions just as you would with any other carrier of information such as a book or newspaper. The knowledge becomes combined with nursing knowledge and this synthesis helps you in applying computer capability to nursing situations. Figure 14-2 shows the process and lists applications commonly used in nursing today.

All kinds of data can be collected and stored on the computer. The data can be moved about, manipulated if you will, and maintained in a documentation format for others to review. Data can be shifted from one computer location to another, and it can be printed out if a paper copy is needed. Information can also be exchanged between two or more computer systems, a process commonly referred to as "networking."

The ability of the computer to manipulate data with ease makes it an ideal instrument for instruction. The computer is capable of handling many decision points and has unlimited patience for reviewing details. Traditionally, the use of computers for instructional purposes has been classified in three ways: drill and practice, tutorial, and simulation or problem solving. Drill and practice is generally used for learning that involves repetition and rote memorization. The student is able to receive continuous feedback while

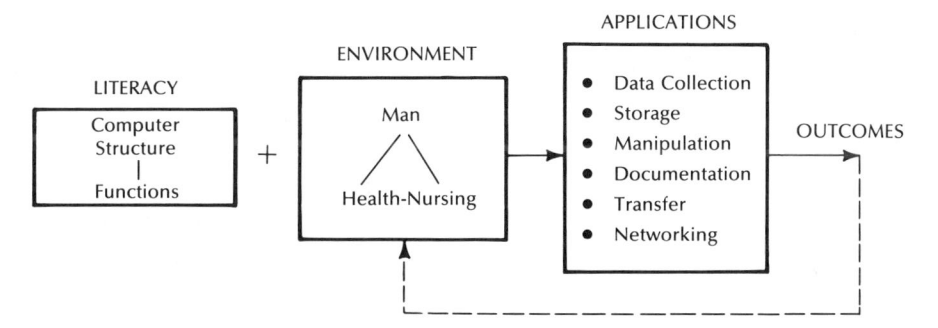

Figure 14-2 Computer Applications in Nursing.

involved in unlimited practice. In tutorial instruction, material is presented and the student is queried. Based on his response, he is branched to an area where readiness and need have been demonstrated. Branching permits a certain amount of self-pacing even in a group-paced course. In simulation or problem solving the student interacts with a real-world problem or situation and attempts to determine solutions. Simulations can be used for both the individual student or groups of students.

An example of a sophisticated instructional computer program has been developed by David Hon, of the American Heart Association, and other specialists. Emphasizing cardiopulmonary resuscitation (CPR), the system includes an adapted microcomputer, a videodisc player, two monitors, a random-access audio machine, and adult and infant mannequins wired with sensors to detect key CPR skills. This system combines elements that would be included in a live teaching situation such as: (1) an orientation to the instructional setting, (2) ways to attract and restimulate attention, (3) a dictionary of new terms, (4) organized information reflecting objectives, (5) redundancy, (6) practices, and (7) testing segments (Hon, 1982).

The challenge today is to catch up with the need for instructional software programs. Publishers and other companies are beginning to produce floppy discs or tapes on nursing subjects. Books, journal articles, and newsletters are disseminating much information about computer equipment and programs. Professional conferences in nursing have also begun emphasizing computer applications in nursing.

Progress has been demonstrated in the development of on-line data bases. This has been useful in research and service, as well as in education. For any nurse interested in writing a professional journal article, an adequate literature search is essential. Two such data bases are MEDLINE, of the National Library of Medicine, and ERIC, Educational Resources Information Center. While MEDLINE focuses on medical literature, it does have a subdivision for nursing topics. The ERIC emphasizes educational topics, and many of these will be of interest to nurses. Accessing the data bases is usually done with the assistance of a librarian. There is a charge for on-line searching. You will want to learn how to search efficiently leading to identification of relevant documents and savings of time that will offset the cost.

Besides actually providing instruction, computers can maintain management activities for instruction, such as student schedules, records, and test analyses. Statistical analyses can also be handled well by the computer, giving a promise of great help to future nursing research. Nursing education is in a position to create fresh approaches with the aid of computer technology to realistically prepare the nurse for practice in the 1990s.

Impact on Service

Future projections show that technological changes will probably continue at a rapid rate in the 1980s, especially with the computer. In nursing, where human caring is central, applications of technology have to include the effects on the patient. For example, if the computer has contact with the patient for purposes of physiological monitoring and multiparameter displays, there is a need to prepare the patient for invasiveness and an ongoing need to keep the patient informed about each intervention. Currently, almost all patients in acute care settings will have some contact with microprocessor units. These units are utilized for everything from temperature monitoring to sophisticated intensive-care-type monitoring. In all of these situations, the nurse needs to be cognizant of the patient and his reaction to the equipment.

The range of computer information systems installed in hospitals and other health agencies varies. Nurses need to explore types and assist with decisions made. Separate systems may be used by the laboratory, pharmacy, nursing, and other departments of the hospital. On the other hand, a coordinated system may be possible. The pros and cons of each type of system need to be understood. The more complex hospital systems store the patient record and permit entries into this record by professionals working with the patient. They also are used for a number of management areas such as admitting or billing, and they can send transactions to different departments. The size of the computer depends on whether the system will be an overall one or if separate systems for departments will be used. Budget and future needs are primary considerations. Planning committees are needed to get ready for information systems; they must include a knowledgeable nurse to assist in identifying computer needs regarding nursing care. Care plans and other documentation on the computer require consistency of format, and this needs to be discussed in advance. If some nurses have not used terminals before, an orientation plan needs to be devised.

The storage and ready access of vast information permits nurses to document complex nursing activities and to analyze interventions with precision and comprehensiveness not possible before the computer. Nurses may be able to see more quickly the effects of interventions on patient care. Think what this could mean for clinical research. Data could be selectively called up and calculated.

An example of computer work in nursing service can be seen at the Clinical Center in the National Institutes of Health. A computer system using codes of nursing content has been used for a number of years. In this system, services for patients are entered in the computer, including nurse's notes and nursing care plans. Nursing information has been organized according to a framework of patient needs and corresponding nursing responses (Romano, McKormick, & McNeely, 1982). A second example involves an administrative system that maintains an operating room inventory of resources (Hayes & Smith, 1981). Other nursing settings could also use computer inventories. Programs could focus on manpower needs, material and space resources, and time schedules for planning purposes.

As the student of tomorrow graduates, there must be at least beginning computer skills developed. There must be a base of knowledge about bioinstrumentation systems. Knowledge of flowcharting would be useful as well as ways of evaluating electronic equipment used in patient care. The process involved in deciding criteria to evaluate new equipment can give the student greater security when exposed to it in clinical settings. There is no indication that biomedical hardware will become less complex. There is every indication that technological applications will continue as extensions to health care. New issues will accompany biomedical and technological progress. For example, improved techniques of resuscitation and other methods of life support have created a need to look at the point at which death occurs.

THE PROFESSION MOVES FORWARD

As the nursing profession moves forward into the next century, technology is only one of the issues that must be addressed. Other issues include how nursing controls its practice, defines its role, cares for its practitioners, and interacts with others in the health care system and in total society.

Attention to Policy Making

Recently the American Nurses' Association supported a national agenda for a health policy intended to benefit the health and welfare of the population. The policy emphasized access to care, financing health care, funding basic needs, funding nursing education and nursing research, protecting human rights, providing for the economic and general welfare of nurses, and decreasing health hazards. The agenda calls for actions to assist the poor and elderly and for federal support of nursing education programs. Access to quality health care included services, such as long-term care services and maternal child health care services; mechanisms for the unemployed, urban, and rural Americans; and expansion of community based nursing services (ANA, 1983). The agenda is broad in scope and describes priorities for actions related to health care in the future. It will be advanced by an ANA project called "Nurses: Visible in Politics." Workshops will be held for nurses across the country. The project represents a major thrust of activity in role development, that of policy maker, which is a growing trend in nursing today. The idea is to be more proactive politically. We are beginning to see much more literature about nurses and politics. However, effective functioning in the American political system requires further work in the development of nursing autonomy.

Autonomy

Autonomy means to be self-governing; in other words, control arises from internal forces. Total autonomy would not likely be possible for open systems since external inputs are always entering the system. Although much control may be possible by a given system, a certain amount of interdependency is needed by viable systems. Because nursing in the past often reported powerlessness in situations, many efforts have been directed to gaining power and autonomy. What accounts for the struggle in this area? One factor blamed has been sex-role stereotyping. Historically, nursing has consisted mostly of women who learned passive behaviors: being kind, showing emotions, feeling inferior, and needing to be accepted by others. Today, many more nurses are taking on independent behaviors, but centuries of traditional role taking continue to linger.

The second factor that has limited nursing autonomy in the past has been inadequate economic self-governance. Today, attempts to define and price actual nursing care is helping nursing move toward autonomy. In many settings, nursing care is included in room and board or other general charges. In the future, nursing care may be a separate item charged to consumers, like X-rays, drugs, and physician services. In addition, some nurses have begun moving into entrepreneur activities. Nurses have established consulting firms, private practices, and interdisciplinary team arrangements. Attempts to establish economic independence will be greatly influenced by nurses' ability to negotiate for third party payments. Control of nursing practice and, in turn, the development of autonomy will also be influenced by the nurse's ability to deal with issues of credentialing.

Credentialing

Different types of credentials are earned by nurses, for different purposes. The usual credential thought about by a beginning nurse is the credential given upon completion of an educational program, a degree, or a diploma. The legal credential is the one which permits the nurse to practice in the profession by law. The RN awarded after successful completion of state board examination and described in nurse practice acts is an example of a legal credential. A third type of credential is the type given by a professional organization and is exemplified by certification programs provided through the American Nurses' Association since 1975 (Sammons, 1983). Future control of credentialing is seen as an important issue. Problems arise when two nursing organizations attempt credentialing for the same specialty or when other disciplines exert control over credentialing for nursing practice. The overall purpose of a professional credential is the protection of the public. Only individuals prepared to practice according to standards of safety are accorded appropriate credentials. Professional standards are best known by the expert professionals in practice. As practitioners increase and continue to advance practice, nursing will need an effective mechanism for credentialing. Without an effective credentialing mechanism, other professions or institutions with fewer qualifications or knowledge about nursing will step in. This leads us to the next issue, how does the nursing profession handle conflict?

Conflict

Credentialing and economic independence are only two of many possible areas of conflict. The health care system consists of numerous interrelationships and communication networks. There are many opportunities for successful transactions as well as for conflicts. Conflicts have been identified in interactions between nurses and physicians, nurses and nurses, and nurses and administrative officials (NLN, 1982). The conflicts tend to stand out since they are problematic, present an element of risk, and require energy and time for problem solving. Conflicts can be resolved successfully for nursing. However, it will require that nurses have an educational background in conflict management. If nurses are left with unsuccessful conflict management skills, one consequence the profession will continue to deal with is burnout.

Burnout

If the working environment is having a negative effect on the nursing profession, what can be done? First, the nurse has to be able to read the environment and to be able to analyze constraining forces and resources that might be tapped to turn things around. Knowledge of organization and management approaches give a base line with which to compare the nurses' own settings. As an illustration, if the structure of a work setting is such that the staff nurses have little opportunity for case conference discussions and it is needed, then a specific recommendation for this type of change can be made. The key is identifying what the problem is and knowing how organizations in general use methods to solve the problem.

The nurse who continues to work in problematic settings without being able to effect constructive change is in danger of burnout from just "spinning wheels." To prevent burnout, knowledge must be gained about how to exert influence on the external environment and how to develop or use support systems. Burnout is not unique to nursing, but it is seen enough in nursing to warrant detection and preventive efforts. Your knowledge of change theory and stress adaptation theory should help to equip you as you deal with issues around burnout.

MAKING PREDICTIONS

Return now to Mark who was introduced at the beginning of the chapter. Mark tried to see into the future of nursing by reading and talking to a variety of experienced people. Although he collected a great deal of information about the profession of nursing, he was still unsure about the future. How does one go about organizing and utilizing information in order to anticipate future events?

Several suggestions that might help Mark use the collected information in a systematic manner are as follows:

1. Develop a knowledge base about nursing and related issues by reviewing the literature and by listening to what experts are saying. Oral presentations may represent newer information than written sources that may have been two or three years in preparation. Remember, however, that written sources may be better researched.
2. Study technological progress. Advancing technology forces shifts and changes.
3. Look for lags and missing elements in the data you have collected.
4. Analyze the data in order to identify long-term patterns in advancing trends. Your knowledge of theories (systems, stress, learning, role, change, and communication) will be helpful in identifying these trends.
5. Sound out your ideas with others and begin developing specific projections.
6. From your projections, identify and prioritize a list of problems and possible resources for dealing with these problems.
7. Finally, conduct research related to your predictions as well as familiarize yourself with related research conducted by others.

SUMMARY

This chapter identified a number of factors that are currently influencing nursing and will have a major effect on how nursing evolves. First, social, economic, and educational trends were analyzed in order to identify how these trends are impacting on health needs and care. Then, the specific impact on nursing was related to each of these trends. Against this background technological advances were examined. Emphasis was placed on the computers' impact in nursing education and practice. After the various trends were discussed, professional-practice issues were identified. The chapter concluded by providing a list of methods that can be utilized for making projections into nursing's future.

Key points to remember are

1. Nursing does not currently exist in a vacuum nor will it in the future. Many of the trends that influence the development of nursing originate in the external environments.
2. Social, economic, educational, and technological trends interrelate and overlap. It is impossible to analyze trends from any one of these sources without considering the others.
3. Just as the society in which it exists has changed rapidly, nursing has undergone a period of rapid change.
4. Analyzing trends systematically within nursing and within society will assist one in projecting the future of nursing.
5. How effectively nursing is able to meet health care needs of the future will be determined by how effectively nursing controls its own practice while interacting with other health care professionals and society.

REFERENCES

Ackerman, W. B. "Technology and Nursing Education: A Scenario for 1990." *Journal of Advanced Nursing* 7 (1) [1982]: 59–68.

"ANA Starts Project to Advance National Health Policy Agenda." *The American Nurse* 15 (10) [1983]: 1, 5, 20.

Banta, D. "Technology: Review of Medical Technology Policies Shows Need, Opportunities for Changes." *Hospitals* 56 (7) [1982]: 87–90.

Bird, S., and Mailhot, C. "DRGs: A New Way to Reimburse Hospital Costs." *AORN Journal* 38 (5) [1983]: 773–777.

Bird, S., and Mailhot, C. "The Impact of DRGs on OR Nursing." *AORN Journal* 38 (5) [1983]: 778–782.

Brewer, A. M. "Technology, Education and the Nurse." *The Lamp* 38 (6) [1981]: 43–47.

Cluff, L. F. "Chronic Disease, Function and Quality of Care." *Journal of Chronic Disease* 34 (1981): 299–304.

Davis, C. K. "The Federal Role in Changing Health Care Financing." *Nursing Economics* 1 (1) [1983]: 10–17.

Davis, C. K. "Nursing and the Health Care Debates." *Image: The Journal of Nursing Scholarship* XV (3) [1983]: 67.

Diers, D., and Molde, S. "Nurses in Primary Care, the New Gatekeepers?" *American Journal of Nursing* 83 (5) [1983]: 742–745.

Dunkley, P. H. "The ANA Certification Program." *Nursing Clinics of North America* 9 (1974): 403-409.

Edmunds, L. "Computer-Assisted Nursing Care." *American Journal of Nursing* 82 (7) [1952]: 1076-1079.

Evans, R. W. "Health Care Technology and the Inevitability of Resource Allocation and Rationing Decisions, Part 1." *JAMA* 249 (15) [1983]: 2047-2053.

Gartenfeld, E. "The Community Health Information Network." *Library Journal* 103 (17) [1958]: 1911-1914.

Griffith, H. "Competition in Health Care." *Nursing Outlook* 31 (5) [1983]: 262-265.

Hayes, C., and Smith, K. "A Computer Information System for the OR Suite." *AORN Journal* 33 (4) [1981]: 672-676.

Hon, D. "Interactive Training in Cardiopulmonary Resuscitation." *Byte* 7 (6) [1982]: 1-14 (reprint).

Hynes, V. B. "Nursing Education and Practice: Idealism and Reality, an Educator's Viewpoint." *Journal of the New York State Nurses Association* 14 (1) [1983]: 26-32.

Kalisch, B. J., and Kalisch, P. A. *Politics of Nursing.* Philadelphia: J. B. Lippincott, Co., 1957.

Kiley, M., et al. "Computerized Nursing Information Systems (NIS)." *Nursing Management* 14 (7) [1983]: 26-29.

Marion, R., Niebuhr, B. R., Petrusa, E. R., and Weinholtz, D. "Computer-based Instruction in Basic Medical Science Education." *Journal of Medical Education* 57 (7) [1982]: 521-526.

Marr, P. B. "Critical Issues in H. I. S. Selection." *Journal, NYSNA* 14 (1) [1983]: 19-21.

McConnell, E. A. *Burnout in the Nursing Profession.* St. Louis: The C. V. Mosby Co., 1982.

McCormick, K. A. "Preparing Nurses for the Technologic Future." *Nursing and Health Care* 4 (7) [1953]: 379-382.

Mirin, S. "The Computer's Place in Nursing Education." *Nursing & Health Care* 11 (9) [1981]: 500-506.

Muirhead, R. C. "Computers in Critical Care Nursing: The New Revolution." *Dimensions of Critical Care Nursing* 2 (3) [1983]: 133-134.

Murphy, S. A., and Hoeffer, B. "Role of the Specialities in Nursing Science." *Advances in Nursing Science* 5 (4) [1983]: 31-39.

National League for Nursing. *Survival of the Fittest: A Management Challenge for Nursing.* New York: National League for Nursing, 1982.

Romano, C., McCormick, K., McNeely, L. "Nursing Documentation: A Model for a Computerized Data Base." *Advances in Nursing Science* 4 (2) [1982]: 43-56.

Ronald, J. A. "Guidelines for Computer Literacy Curriculums in a School of Nursing." *Journal of the New York State Nurses Association* 14 (1) [1983]: 12-18.

Sammons, L. N. "Control of Credentialing for Advanced Practice Analysis Using a Lewinian Model." *Advances in Nursing Science* 5 (4) [1983]: 13-20.

Shields, E. A. "H.I.S. Implementation Approach." *Journal of the New York State Nurses Association* 14 (1) [1983]: 22-24.

Skiba, D. J. "Computer Literacy: The Challenge of the 80's." *Journal of the New York State Nurses Association* 14 (1) [1983]: 6–11.

Stoia, J. P. "Nursing Instruction: Can Data Base Searching Enhance the Practice? A Guide to the Novice User." *Journal of Nursing Education* 22 (2) [1983]: 74–79.

Sweeney, M. A., O'Malley, M., and Freeman, E. "Development of a Computer Simulation." *Journal of Nursing Education* 21 (9) [1982]: 28–38.

Tosteson, D. C. "The Right to Know: Public Education for Health." *Journal of Medical Education* 30 (2) [1975]: 117–123.

Viers, V. M. "Introducing Nurses to Computer User World." *Nursing Management* 14 (7) [1983]: 24–25.

Weller, R., and Bouvier, L. *Population Demography and Policy.* New York: St. Martin's Press, 1981.

Wilson, E. "Nursing Care in a Technological World." *Supervisor Nurse* 12 (6) [1981]: 59–62.

Wingrove, C. R. "Graying America: Demographic Trends, Health Needs, and Provider Education." *Virginia Nurse* 51 (2) [1983]: 83–85.

Index

A

Abstract symbols, 134
Achieved positions, 191–192
Accommodation, 132
Ackoff, R., 82
Adaptation
 cognition and, 131
 open systems, 87–88
Adaptive responses, 101–108
 dimension interaction, 106–108
 physiological adaptation, 101–102
 psychological adaptation, 102–105
 sociocultural adaptation, 105–106
Administrative control (of institutions), 251–252
Affect
 communication and, 159–160, 167
 learning and, 138–139
Affective behaviors, 131
Aging, 270–271
Alarm stage and reaction, 102, 104
Alcott, Louisa, 31
Algorithm, 278
Allen, D. E., 71
Allen, V. L., 190, 195, 197
Almy, M., 132, 133, 134
American Association of Critical Care Nurses, 41
American Association of Industrial Nurses, 41
American Association of Junior Colleges, 59
American Association of University Professors, 52
American Cancer Society, 254
American College of Surgeons, 55
American Heart Association, 254, 279
American Hospital Association, 55
American Indians, 23
American Journal of Nursing, 36, 40, 58
American Medical Association, 55, 66, 216, 257
American Nurses' Association (ANA), 6, 8–9, 13, 37, 39–40, 41, 42, 43, 59–60, 208, 216, 257, 281–282, 283
American Public Health Association, 55
American Red Cross, 32, 50
American Society of Superintendents of Training Schools of Nursing, 39, 51, 52
American Urological Association, 41
Anderson, N. E., 31, 66, 69
Antiquity, 22–25
Anxiety, 163
Apprenticeship, 28
Army Nurse Corps (U.S.), 32
Asprec, E., 181
Assessment
 change theory and, 178–180
 family/community, 234–235
 health, 230–235

Assessment (contd.)
  man and, 210–211
  stress states, 109–115
  See also Diagnosis
Assimilation, 132
Associate degree (AD) nurses, 58–59, 70–71
Association of Collegiate Schools of Nursing, 41
Attitudes
  change theory and, 183
  health assessment and, 231
Attributes
  man and, 210–211
  open systems, 86
Audiovisuals, 138
Autonomy, 282
Aztec Indians, 23

B

Banta, D., 248
Barton, Clara, 31, 50
Beatty, W., 22, 23, 25, 26, 27, 30
Behavior
  affective learning and, 138–139
  classification of, 131
  health and, 235–240
  role expectation and, 195
Behavioral approach, 121–124
Behavior modification therapy, 124
Beliefs
  change theory and, 183
  See also Sociocultural dimension
Bellevue Hospital (NYC), 31, 51, 53, 66
Benedictines, 27
Benne, K., 185
Bickerdyke, Mother Mary-Ann, 31
Biddiss, M., 22, 23, 24, 25, 27
Biddle, B. J., 190, 192, 193
Biggs, J. B., 122
Biller, R., 199
Bingham, S., 36
Birth control, 240
Bit (information processing), 128

Blacks
  health and, 240
  nursing and, 14, 37, 51
  nursing education and, 31–32
Blue Cross, 252, 263
Blue Shield, 263
Bolton Act, 33, 37
Botsford, E. R., 71
Boundaries
  man and, 212
  open systems and, 83–85, 87
Boundary function, 215
Bower, G., 127
Breckinridge, Mary, 31
Brewster, Mary, 36
Bridgman, Margaret, 58
Brill, E., 181
Brody, S., 27
Bronze Age, 22
Brooten, D., 172
Brown, Esther, 57
Brown Report (1948), 41, 57
Bruhn, J. G., 240
Bullough, B., 6, 15, 33, 39, 40, 69, 70
Bullough, V., 6, 15, 33, 39, 40, 69, 70
Burnout, 283–284
Byrne, M., 100, 111

C

Cannon, Walter, 102
Cantile, G., 26
Capacity, 128–129
Capelle, R., 178
Cardiopulmonary resuscitation, 279
Career decision, 3, 4, 284
Carnegie Corporation, 57
Cartwright, F., 22, 23, 24, 25, 27
Catholic University, 70
Certification programs, 42
  See also Licensure
Change
  affective learning and, 138–139
  health and, 227
  man and, 217–220

Change (contd.)
  nursing future and, 269, 270
  open systems, 89–90
Change reactions, 181–184
Change theory, 173–188
  change defined, 174–177
  change models in, 177–178
  change principles in, 184–185
  definitions in, 173
  identification of change reactions in, 181–184
  need assessment in, 178–180
  situational example of, 173–174
  strategies for implementing change in, 185–186
Changing model, 177–178
Channel, 153, 168
Chayer, M., 51
Chickering, A., 134
Child developmental learning theories, 132–134
Chin, R., 177, 185
China (ancient), 23
Christianity. See Religion
Christy, T., 52
Chronic illness, 271–272
Civil Rights legislation, 38–39
Civil War (U.S.), 31–32, 48, 50, 66
Classical conditioning, 122
Classification, 133
Client(s)
  communication and, 153, 167–168
  component of nursing, 12–13
  defined, 5
  education and, 136–144
  health care system and, 258–261
  nurses and, 16
  See also Patient(s); Recipient(s)
Closed system
  defined, 82, 83
  See also Open system; Systems theory
Cluff, L. F., 271
Cobb, M., 249, 251
Coddington, R. D., 111, 112
Code for Nurses (ANA), 9
Cognition
  change strategies and, 185

Cognition (contd.)
  communication and, 158–159
  developmental approach, 131, 132
Cognitive behaviors, 131
Collegiate education. See University education
Collegiate Education for Nurses (1953), 58
Columbia University Teachers College, 52, 53, 54, 69
Committee on the Grading of Nursing Schools, 55–57, 69
Communication
  clients and, 153, 167–168
  health care system and, 255, 256
Communication theory, 147–171
  communication definition, 149–150
  component of model of, 151–153
  definitions in, 147
  facilitators and inhibitors in, 160–169
  influences on communication, 158–160
  levels of communication, 154–158
  reasons for communicating, 150–151
  situational example of, 148–149
Community
  assessment, 234–235
  change and, 218, 220
  defined, 206, 208–209
  man and, 205–206
  purpose and, 221–222
Community College Education for Nursing (1959), 58–59
Community health. See Public health
Community hospitals, 251–252
Complex, 82
Computers, 269–270, 276, 277–281
Concept learning, 138
Concepts, 203–204
Conceptual frameworks
  defined, 72
  elements of, 72–74
Concrete operations stage, 133–134
Conditioned response, 122
Conditioned stimulus, 122
Conditioning, 122

Conflict
   health care providers, 255–256
   nursing's future and, 283
Congress (U.S.)
   health care system and, 248–249
   Red Cross and, 50
   See also Federal government; Government; Law
Connecticut Training School (New Haven), 31, 66
Connectionism, 123
Consequences, 73–74
Consumerism, 272–273
Continuum
   change and, 174–175
   health and, 227–228, 229–230
Conway, M., 192, 196, 197
Coping
   psychological adaptation, 102–104
   stress state assessment, 110–111
Costs (medical), 273–274
Cramming (learning technique), 128
Credentialing
   nursing's future and, 282–283
   See also Licensure
Crimean War, 30–31, 49
Crisis, 174–175
Critical processes, 87–89, 216–217
Croad, S. H., 253
Crusades, 29–30
Culture
   change theory and, 183
   health and, 226, 239–240
   See also Sociocultural dimension
Curriculum. See Nursing education
Custodial care, 246–247

D

Death rates, 265
Decision making, 87–88
Defense mechanisms, 104
Delano, Jane, 32
Deloughery, Grace S., 55
Demography, 270–271
Denver Developmental Screening Test (DDST), 234

Dependence, 132–133
Depression, 103
Developmental approach, 131–135
   adult learning theory, 134–135
   change theory, 177
   child development, 132–134
Developmental continuum, 99–100
Diagnosis
   change theory and, 178–180
   See also Assessment
Dickens, Charles, 28–29
Dietz, L. D., 23, 24, 25, 28
Dimensional interaction, 106–108
Disasters, 50
Disease, 226, 227
Distance zones, 156
Dix, Dorothea, 31, 48
Dock, Lavinia, 52–53
Dolan, J., 22, 23, 28, 36, 50, 55, 56, 69
Dolfman, M. L., 226
Dubos, R., 102
DuGas, B., 137
Dunn, H. L., 227, 230
Duvall, E. M., 218
Dynamic homeostasis
   man and, 218
   open systems, 89

E

Early detection, 237–238
Economy, 273–274
Education
   change strategies and, 185–186
   consumerism and, 272
   early discharge and, 273
   health care providers, 256
   nursing education and, 59
   nursing's future and, 274–276
   women and, 36, 52
   See also Health education; Nursing education; Public education
Egypt (ancient), 22–23
Ehrenreich, B., 27
Elderly, 270–271
Electronic communication, 157–158
Emitted behaviors, 124

Emotion. *See* Affect
Empirical-rational change strategy, 185
Energy
  man and, 214, 218, 219
  open systems, 86
  stress-adaptation theory, 98, 106
England, 65–66
English, D., 27
Entropy
  man and, 219
  open systems and, 89
Environment
  burnout and, 283–284
  chronic illness and, 271
  communication and, 159–160
  health and, 227
  information processing approach, 125
  man and, 212–213
  nursing's future and, 274
  open systems, 84–85
Epidemics, 25–26, 27
Equal Pay Act of 1963, 38
Equifinality
  man and, 219–220
  open systems, 90
Ethnicity
  health and, 240
  nursing profession and, 14
Europe, 49
Event-response stress models, 105
Example, 138
Exhaustion, 102, 104
Extrapersonal communication, 157–158

F

Fabiola, Saint, 26
Facilitators
  change theory, 178
  communication, 160–169
Fagen, R. E., 81, 82, 84, 90
Family
  assessment and, 234–235
  change and, 218, 220
  defined, 206, 207–208
  health and, 238–239

Family (*contd.*)
  man and, 205–206
  purpose of, 221–222
Family health practice, 276
Federal government
  budget cuts and, 273
  health care system, 248–249
  payments, 262, 263
  private health care and, 252
  See also Congress (U.S.); Government; Law; State and local government
Feedback
  communication and, 149
  health care system, 266
  open systems, 88
Fitzpatrick, M., 22, 24, 40, 59, 69
Flannagan, L., 39
Fleming, M., 137
Flexner Report, 55
Fliedner, Friederike, 29
Fliedner, Theodor, 29
Flight or fight syndrome, 102
Freeman, H., 253
French, R. M., 257
Friedman, M. M., 221
Function
  defined, 86
  man and, 215–217
  open systems, 86–89
  purpose versus, 213–214

G

General adaptation syndrome (GAS), 101, 102, 104, 105
Goals, 11–12
  conceptual framework and, 72–73
Goldmark, Josephine, 54–55
Goldmark Report (1923), 54–55
Goodwin, S., 102
Goostray, S., 40
Government
  health care system and, 248–251
  hospitals and, 253
  industrialization and, 35
  payments and, 262, 263

Government (contd.)
  See also Federal government; Law; State and local government
Graham, Davis, 57
Grant writing, 273
Great Depression, 69
Greece (ancient), 23–24
Grippando, G., 70
Gut communication level, 156

H

Hale, J. R., 26
Hall, A. D., 81, 82, 84, 90
Hall, E., 156
Hall, J. E., 82, 87
Hampton Institute (Virginia), 31
Harary, F., 190
Hardy, M., 192, 196, 197
Havelock, R. G., 178, 181
Hayes, C., 281
Hayes, J., 164
Hayman, L., 175
Hazzard, M. E., 83
Health, 225–243
  assessment of, 230–235
  definitions of, 226–230
  factors influencing, 235–240
  nursing role in, 240–242
Health Amendments Act, 38
Health care providers, 254–258
Health care system, 245–268
  conflict in, 283
  employment in, 254–258
  function of, 261–266
  purpose of, 246–247
  structure of, 247–261
Health education
  mass communication and, 157
  types of, 136
  See also Education; Nursing education; Public education
Health maintenance organizations, 263
Heap, 82
Hebrews (ancient), 23
Hein, E., 151
Helena, Saint, 26

Henderson, V., 9, 10, 12
Henry Street Settlement, 36, 53, 54
Henry Street Visiting Nurse Service, 54
Herrmann, E., 22, 69
Hierarchy
  health care providers, 255–256
  history and, 28
  man and, 211–212
  open systems, 85–86
Hippocrates, 24
History, 21–45
Holmes, T., 111, 113
Home care
  early discharge and, 273
  nursing and, 16–17
Homeostasis
  man and, 218
  open systems, 89
Hon, David, 279
Hospitals
  communication and, 160
  community hospitals, 251–252
  early discharge, 273
  health care system and, 253
  nursing education and, 39, 54–55, 57, 59, 66, 67
  nursing profession and, 17–18
  payment to, 263, 264
  technology and, 279–280
Hull, C., 122, 123–124
Hunt, E., 129
Hunter, E., 71
Hyland, P., 99, 106

I

Inanimate systems, 82–83
India, 23
Individual
  defined, 206
  health and, 230–234
  man and, 205–206
Individual differences
  developmental approach, 135
  information processing approach, 129
Industrialization, 35–36, 48
Information, 86

Information processing approach
　input, 125–127
　output, 130–131
　throughput, 127–130
Inhibitors (communication), 160–169
Input(s)
　health care system, 261–263
　information processing approach, 125–127
　open systems, 86–87
Insecurity, 182
Insurance payments, 262, 263
Integration, 87–88, 216
Intentional learning, 130, 139
Interaction
　communication theory, 151–152
　systems theory, 81–82
Interference, 128
International Council of Nurses, 37, 53
Interpersonal communication, 154–156
Involvement, 197

J

Janis, J., 106
Jennings, F. G., 132
Jensen, L. E., 262
Job descriptions, 255
Johns Hopkins Training School (Baltimore, Md.), 52, 53
Jones, M. C., 249, 251
Jones, V. A., 71

K

Kaiserwerth Institute (Germany), 29
Kalisch, B., 33, 42, 43, 49, 67
Kalisch, P., 33, 42, 43, 49, 67
Kaplan, G. D., 238
Keller, M. J., 226
Kelly, L., 41, 42
Kilts, D., 181
King, I., 10, 12, 24
Kluckholn, C., 13
Knefelkamp, L., 132
Kolb, D., 134, 135

Korean War, 34–35
Kramer, M., 190

L

Language development, 133
La Rocco, S., 198, 200
Larson, K. H., 164
Law
　Civil Rights legislation, 38–39
　licensure and, 40
　military nursing corps, 32
　nursing and, 37–38
　nursing definition and, 6–8
　nursing education and, 32, 33
　nursing profession and, 24–25, 26
　See also Federal government; Government; State and local government
Lawrence, R., 102
Lawrence, S., 102
Leadership, 15, 48–54
Leading part, 89–90
Leahy, K. M., 249, 251
Learning
　definition of, 124
　role learning, 196–197
　teaching and, 142–144
　See also Education; Nursing education; Public education
Learning theory, 119–146
　adult, 134–135
　application to practice of, 135–144
　behavioral approach, 121–124
　child development, 132–134
　definitions in, 119–120
　developmental approach, 131–135
　information processing approach, 124–131
Leprosy, 27
Levie, W. H., 137
Levine, S., 253
Lewin, K., 178
Licensure, 37, 38, 40, 42, 70, 282–283
Life Change Unit, 111
Life expectancy, 265
Listening, 165–166

Livermore, Mary, 31
Living systems, 82–83
Local adaptation syndrome (LAS), 101, 102
Local pathology approach, 67
Long-term memory, 127–130
  See also Memory
Lysaught, J. P., 60
Lysaught Reports (1970, 1973, 1981), 60

M

Mahoney, Mary, 51
Maides, S. A., 238
Malpractice suits, 266
Man
  defined, 205–209
  change and, 217–220
  health and, 228–230
  open system and, 209–217
  purpose of, 220–222
M. A. Nutting Award, 52
Marcella, Saint, 26
Marital status, 37
Marks, G., 22, 23, 25, 26, 27, 30
MASH units, 34
Maslow, A., 214, 217
Massachusetts General Hospital, 31, 66
Massberg, H., 265
Mass communication and media, 157–158
  consumerism and, 272
  health and, 238–239, 240
Matter, 86
Mayan Indians, 23
McGee, Anita, 32
McKormick, K., 281
McNeely, L., 281
Meaningfulness, 137–138
Meat Inspection Act, 35
Medical education, 55
Medical records, 259
Medicare and Medicaid, 252, 262, 263, 273

Medieval period, 26–28
Memory
  communication and, 155
  information processing, 127–130
  learning and, 139
Mental illness, 48
Message, 149, 153, 159, 167–169
Mikbail, B., 237
Military, 29–35
Miller, J. G., 86
Minkler, M., 199
Mobile Army Surgical Hospital (MASH) units, 34
Monasteries, 27
Money. See Payment
Montag, Mildred, 58, 70
Morris, W., 174
Morrison, S., 35
Mortality rates, 265
Muff, J., 4
My ideas communication level, 156

N

National Association of Colored Graduate Nurses, 41, 51
National Institutes of Health, 249, 281
National Intravenous Therapy Association, 41
National League for Nursing, 37, 41, 42, 43, 61, 68, 71, 74, 77, 283
National League for Nursing Accrediting Service, 58
National League for Nursing 1982 Position Statement, 61
National League of Nursing Education, 39, 55, 69
National Nursing Accreditation Service Organization, 58
National Organization for Public Health Nursing, 36, 40
National Organization for Women (NOW), 37
National Organization of Public Health Nursing, 36, 40
Native Americans, 23

Navy Nurse Corps (U.S.), 32
Naylor, M., 175
Need
   change theory and, 178, 180
   learning theory, 123–124
Negentropy
   man and, 218–219
   open systems, 89
Neuman, B., 10, 12, 229
Neuman model, 73, 74
New England Hospital for Women and Children (Roxbury, Mass.), 50, 51, 66
New England Hospital School of Nursing, 50
Newman, M., 66
New York Training School, 54
Nightingale, Florence, 9, 10, 11, 12, 29, 30, 31, 48–50, 65–66
Nightingale Fund, 49
Nightingale model, 67
Nightingale Training School for Nurses, 65–66
1965 Position Paper, 59–60
Nonprofit health care organizations, 252
Nonverbal communication, 149, 150, 168–169
Normative-reeducative change strategy, 185–186
Norms
   change strategies and, 185–186
   See also Sociocultural dimension
Notter, L. E., 27, 29, 66
Nurses
   clients and, 16
   conceptual framework, 73
   demography of, 13–14
   personality characteristics of, 14–15
   stereotypes of, 3–4, 48, 282
   voluntary organizations and, 253–254
Nurses Associated Alumnae of the United States and Canada, 39–40
Nursing
   career decision, 3, 4, 284
   components of, 12–19
   definitions of, 4, 5–11

Nursing (*contd.*)
   development of, 21–45
   future of, 269–287
   health and, 240–242
   introduction to, 3–20
   legal definition of, 6–8
   military forces and, 29–35
   purpose and goal of, 11–12
   religious forces in, 22–29
   secular forces and, 35–43
   status of, 50
Nursing and Nursing Education in the United States (Goldmark Report 1923), 54–55
Nursing education
   American schools (early), 66–69
   Brown Report, 1948, 57
   Civil War (U.S.) and, 31
   Collegiate Education for Nurses (1953), 58
   Community College Education for Nursing (1959), 58–59
   conceptual frameworks and, 72–74
   Dock, Lavinia and, 53
   English influence on, 65–66
   financial assistance for, 38
   Goldmark Report, 1923, 54–55
   hierarchy and, 28
   history of, 48
   hospitals and, 39
   law and, 37, 38
   Lysaught Reports, 60
   mid century, 70–71
   Nightingale and, 48–49, 50
   1965 Position Paper, 59–60
   NLN 1982 Position Statement, 61
   nursing profession and, 14
   Nursing Schools at Mid Century (1950), 57–58
   nursing's future and, 274–276
   Nutting, M. D. and, 52
   professional organizations and, 40, 41, 42, 43
   public health nursing and, 36
   quality standards in, 54, 55, 56, 58, 59–60, 61, 69
   race and, 31–32

Nursing education (contd.)
  Richards, Melinda and, 50–51
  Robb, I. H. and, 53
  student applicants to, 272
  technology and, 277–280
  training contrasted, 51
  university education and, 57, 69–70
  World War I and, 32–33
  World War II and, 33–34
Nursing for the Future (Brown Report, 1948), 57
Nursing homes, 18, 246–247
Nursing leaders. *See* Leadership
Nursing Schools at Mid Century (1950), 57–58
Nursing Schools, Today and Tomorrow (1934), 55–57, 69
Nutting, Mary Adelaide, 51–52

O

Observation, 165
Oeser, O. A., 190
Open systems
  change in, 89–90
  defined, 82, 83
  function in, 86–89
  health care system, 261–266
  man and, 209–217
  purpose of, 91
  structure in, 83–86
  subconcepts of man and, 205
  See also Closed systems; Systems theory
Orem, D., 10, 11, 12
Orem model, 73
Organizations. *See* Professional organizations
Output
  health care system, 265–266
  information processing approach, 130–131
  open systems, 87
Overlearning, 130
Overload, 126–127

P

Palmer, I., 49
Patient(s)
  communication and, 256–257
  conceptual framework and, 73
  defined, 4, 5
  education and, 136–144
  health care system and, 258–261
  nursing education and, 67, 68, 71
  stress and, 112–115
  See also Client(s); Recipient(s)
Patient history
  adaptive behavior and, 112
  health assessment and, 232
Patient's Bill of Rights, 259, 260–261
Pavlov, I., 122, 123, 124
Payment
  allocation of, 264–265
  sources of, 261–263
Peak communication level, 156
Peer pressure, 239
Peplau, H., 12
Percept, 127
Perception
  communication and, 153, 165
  developmental approach, 132
  information processing approach, 125–126
  learning and, 137
Person-centered approach, 71
Peterson, C. J., 72
Philanthropy Movement, 35–36
Phoebe of Rome, 25
Physical sciences, 121
Physicians
  nursing education and, 57, 60, 66
  patient rights and, 259
  specialization and, 257
Physicians' assistants (PAs), 35
Physiological dimension
  adaptation, 101–102
  communication, 158
  man and, 209
  response interactions, 107
  stressors, 99
  stress state assessment, 110
Piaget, J., 132, 133, 134, 135

Planned Parenthood, 254
Pluckhan, M., 150
Policy making, 281–282
Population. *See* Demography
Position, 190–191, 194, 197
Poverty, 48
Power-coercive change strategy, 186
Practical nurse movement, 70
Practice, 74
Preemptiveness, 197
Preoperational stage, 133
Prescription, 194
Prevention, 247
Primary care, 264–265
Primary nursing, 17
Print communications, 158, 272
Prisons, 48
Private health care system, 251–254
Professional definition, 8–9
Professional organizations, 39–43
  health care system and, 257–258
  Robb, I. H. and, 53
  See also entries under names of organizations
Professionals, 239
Profit health care organizations, 252
Proximity, 156
Psychiatry, 193
Psychological dimension
  communication and, 158–159
  man and, 209
  response interactions of, 107
  stressors, 99
  stress state assessment, 110–111
Psychomotor behaviors, 131
Public education, 50
  See also Education; Health education; Nursing education
Public health
  nursing profession and, 18–19
  Nutting, M. A. and, 52
  Philanthropy Movement and, 36
Public Health Service hospitals, 253
Pure Food and Drug Act, 35
Purposes, 11–12
  function versus, 213–214
  man, 220–222
Pythagoras, 23–24

Q

Quinn, N., 259

R

Race
  health and, 240
  nursing and, 14, 37, 51
  nursing education and, 31–32
Rahe, R., 101, 106, 107, 111, 113
Ransom, A., 101, 106, 107
Reagan, Ronald, 262
Reality distortion, 111
Receiver, 149, 153, 161–166
Recipient(s)
  conceptual framework and, 73
  See also Client(s); Patient(s)
Redman, B., 137
Reductionist approach, 121
Reeder, L. G., 253
Referent, 151–152, 160–161
Reformation, 28
Registered nurse, 7
Rehabilitation, 247
Reich, C., 99
Reinforcement, 124
Reinkemeyer, A., 178
Religion
  health and, 226
  nursing development and, 22–29
Religious orders, 26–28
Remembering, 127
Renaissance, 28–29
Reports others communications, 154, 156
Resistance, 102, 104, 181
Respondent behavior, 124
Reverberation
  man and, 219
  open systems, 90
Richards, Melinda Ann, 50–51
Riehl, J. P., 72
Robb, Isabel, 52–53
Roberts, M. M., 66
Rodgers, J. A., 177
Rogers, C. R., 218

Index

Rogers, M., 10
Role
  health care providers, 255–256
  nursing's future and, 272
  recipients and, 258
  specialization and, 257
Role ambiguity, 199–200
Role conflict, 198–199
Role dissonance, 198
Role enactment, 197–198
Role expectations, 195–196
Role learning, 196–197
Role shock, 199
Role stress, 198, 199
Role theory, 189–201
  defined, 192–193
  definitions in, 189
  role defined, 190–192
  role socialization and, 194–200
  role structure and, 193–194
  situational example of, 189–190
Romano, C., 281
Rome (ancient), 24, 25–26
Roosevelt, Theodore, 35
Rosser, J., 265
Roy, C., 10, 12, 72
Roy model, 73, 74
Russell Sage Foundation, 57, 58

S

Sammons, L. N., 283
Sarbin, T. R., 190, 195, 197
Saxton, D., 99, 106
Schutt, B., 43
Scientific method, 121
Secondary care, 265
Secular forces, 35–43
Selye, H., 96, 101, 104, 109, 110
Sender, 149, 152, 161–166
Sense organs, 125–126
Sensory motor stage, 132–133
Sex discrimination, 38
Sex role
  antiquity and, 24
  military and, 30
  nursing and, 13–14

Shock-depression-adaptation process, 103
Short-term memory, 127–130
  See also Memory
Skidmore College (New York), 58
Skinner, B. F., 122, 124
Smith, J., 228
Smith, K., 281
Smith, M., 104
Snelbecker, G., 122, 123, 124
Social pressure, 105–106
Social psychology, 192–193
Social Readjustment Rating Scale, 111, 112, 113
Sociocultural dimension
  adaptation, 105–106
  communication and, 159
  man and, 209–210
  response interactions of, 107
  stressors, 99
  stress state assessment, 111–115
  See also Beliefs; Norms; Values
Somers, A., 259
Somers, A. R., 253, 257, 264
Somers, H. M., 253, 257, 264
Source, 152
Spalding, E. E., 27, 29, 66
Spanish-American War, 32
Specialization, 255
  nursing education and, 276
  professional organizations and, 41
  role and, 257
Spellman Seminary (Atlanta, Ga.), 31
Spradley, B. W., 178
State and local government
  health care system, 249–251
  licensure laws, 70
  payments and, 262, 263
  See also Federal government; Government; Law
Status, 256
  See also Hierarchy
Steady state, 89
Stereotypes, 3–4
  Nightingale and, 49
  nurses and, 14–15
  Reformation and, 28
Stevens, B. J., 72

Stimulus-response (S-R) unit, 122, 124
Stone Age, 22
Stress
　change theory and, 177
　defined, 96–97
　factors influencing, 97–98
　health and, 227, 229, 232
　role stress, 198, 199
　response to, 100–108
Stress-adaptation theory, 95–118
　classification of stressors, 98–100
　definitions in, 95
　factors influencing stress, 97–98
　stress response, 100–108
　systems theory and, 108–116
Stressors
　classification of, 98–100
　defined, 97
　energy consumption and, 106
　identifying model for, 113–115
　nature of, 97–98
　stress response and, 100
　systems theory and, 109
Stress reduction strategies, 115–116
Stress response, 100–108
　adaptive responses, 101–108
　factors influencing, 100–101
Stress state assessment, 109–115
Structuralism, 192
Structure
　defined, 83
　open systems, 83–86
Structuring, 127
Suffrage, 36–37
Sullivan, H. S., 193
Surface communication, 154
Symbols, 168
System inputs. *See* Inputs
System outputs. *See* Outputs
Systems theory, 79–93
　change theory and, 177, 178
　definitions in, 79–80
　man and, 209–217
　open system change, 89–90
　open system function, 86–89
　open system purpose, 91
　open system structure, 83–86

Systems theory (*contd.*)
　stress-adaptation theory and, 108–116
　stress and, 96
　subconcepts of man and, 205
　system defined, 81–83

T

Taft-Hartley Act, 38–39
Task-oriented coping, 104
Teachers College. *See* Columbia University Teachers College
Teaching
　learning and, 142–144
　requirement of, 120
Technology, 255
　nursing education and, 275–276
　nursing's future and, 276–281
Tertiary care, 265
Theory
　criteria for, 77–78
　interactions of, 108–109
　See also entries under names of theories
Thinking. *See* Cognition
Thomas, E. J., 190, 192, 193
Thompson, J., 26
Thompson, L., 100, 111
Thorndike, E., 122–123, 124
Throughput
　developmental approach and, 132
　health care system, 263–265
　information processing approach, 127–130
　open systems, 87
Toxins, 271
Training, 51
　See also Nursing education
Travers, R., 121, 124, 129, 132
Treatment, 247
Treaty of Geneva (1882), 50
Trust, 182
Truth, Sojourner, 31
Tulving, E., 129
Tuskegee Institute (Alabama), 31

U

Unconditioned response, 122
Uniforms, 48
Unintentional learning, 139
Unionization, 39
United Nations, 34
United States Department of Health and Human Services, 249
United States Public Health Service, 33, 60
United States Red Cross, 50
United States Sanitary Commission, 48
University education, 54–55, 57, 58, 69–70
University of Minnesota, 69

V

Values
  communication and, 166
  health and, 237–238
  nursing future and, 272
  purpose of man and, 220
  See also Sociocultural dimension
Vanderbilt University School of Nursing, 55
Verbal communication, 149–150
VerSteeg, D. F., 253
Veterans Hospitals, 253
Vietnam War, 34–35
Visiting Nurse Quarterly, 36
Voluntary organizations, 253–254
Von Bertalanffy, L., 81, 91
Von Senden, M., 126

W

Wald, Lillian, 36, 54
Wallston, B. S., 238
Wallston, K. A., 238
Watson, J., 36, 66
Weaver, B. R., 82, 87
Wellness. *See* Health
Western Reserve University, 70
Wilson, Woodrow, 35
Winslow, C. A., 54
Women
  education and, 49, 52
  history and, 48
  status of, 48, 53, 191–192
Women's Movement, 36–37
Woodham-Smith, C., 49
Woolsey sisters, 31
World Health Organization, 226
World War I, 32–33
World War II, 33–34

Y

Yale University, 55, 70